Lecture Notes in Medical Informatics

Edited by D. A. B. Lindberg and P. L. Reichertz

21

Influence of Economic Instability on Health

Proceedings of a Symposium organized by the
Gesellschaft für Strahlen- und Umweltforschung,
Institut für Medizinische Informatik und Systemforschung,
with technical support from the World Health Organization,
Regional Office for Europe
München, Federal Republic of Germany
9–11 September 1981

Edited by J. John, D. Schwefel, and H. Zöllner

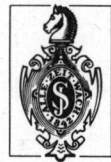

Springer-Verlag
Berlin Heidelberg New York Tokyo 1983

Editorial Board

J. Anderson J. H. van Bemmel M. F. Collen S. Kaihara A. Levy
D.A.B. Lindberg (Managing Editor) H. Peterson A. Pratt
P. L. Reichertz (Managing Editor) W. Spencer C. Vallbona

Editors

J. John, D. Schwefel
Gesellschaft für Strahlen- und Umweltforschung mbH München (GSF)
Institut für Medizinische Informatik und Systemforschung (MEDIS)
Ingolstädter Landstraße 1, 8042 Neuherberg, FRG

H. Zöllner
World Health Organization
Regional Office for Europe
8, Scherfigsvej, 2100 Copenhagen, Denmark

Programme Committee

W. van Eimeren, GSF, MEDIS, Neuherberg, FRG
H.M. Brenner, Johns Hopkins University, Baltimore, USA
D. Schwefel, GSF, MEDIS, Neuherberg, FRG
W. Wlodarczyk, Institute of Occupational Medicine, Lodz, Poland
H. Zöllner, WHO-EURO, Copenhagen, Denmark

ISBN 3-540-12274-5 Springer-Verlag Berlin Heidelberg New York Tokyo
ISBN 0-387-12274-5 Springer-Verlag New York Heidelberg Berlin Tokyo

This work is subject to copyright. All rights are reserved, whether the whole or part of the material is concerned, specifically those of translation, reprinting, re-use of illustrations, broadcasting, reproduction by photocopying machine or similar means, and storage in data banks. Under § 54 of the German Copyright Law where copies are made for other than private use, a fee is payable to "Verwertungsgesellschaft Wort", Munich.

© by Springer-Verlag Berlin Heidelberg 1983
Printed in Germany

Printing and binding: Beltz Offsetdruck, Hemsbach/Bergstr.
2145/3140-543210

PREFACE

The worldwide economic recession of the last years - sometimes described as an outright depression similar to the one of the early thirties - has led many health policy analysts and even policy makers to revive the old question of whether, and in what respect, there is a close relationship between economic development and health. In tackling this question, today's health services research looks rather helpless: even if a truth has the appearance of a truism, it will not necessarily be acknowledged in practice. While it is an established fact that social as well as (macro)economic conditions or events have an important influence on the health of people, this subject has been rarely pursued by medical or epidemiological research and rather has been treated - in industrial countries at least - as a quantité négligeable. Yet, this ahistoric and even parochial attitude must be questioned on methodological as well as political grounds.

- As to methodological aspects, further investigation into the relationship between health and the economy is essential in order to identify the real relevance, i.e. opportunity costs, of medical care; even more important, it might also direct attention to the interfaces - fairly neglected by our over-specialized system of sciences - between biometrics and econometrics, medicine and epidemiology, epidemiology and socio-economics. It is, hence, an area of research from which methodological development can receive major stimuli.

- As to political aspects, side-effects of (international) economic developments on health will become more frequent and noticeable in industrial countries as the worldwide recession continues to be a fact of life. Therefore, good social and economic policy is also good health policy and possibly vice versa; at least, social and economic policies have considerable health side-effects.

From its start in 1979, the working unit "Socio-Economic Methods" of MEDIS - Institut für Medizinische Informatik und Systemforschung of the Gesellschaft für Strahlen- und Umweltforschung (GSF) - has taken up the above-mentioned methodological as well as socioeconomic problems. At the same time, the European Regional Office of the World Health Organization (WHO-EURO) has formulated programmes in relation to health and socioeconomic policy. In 1980, WHO-EURO organized the planning meeting for the "Study on the influence of economic development on health", in which MEDIS researchers took part.

The Proceedings published in this volume stem from the GSF-MEDIS-Symposium on the "Influence of economic instability on health" held in Munich, 9 to 11 September 1981, which served as the second meeting within the WHO study on this topic. The main purpose of this publication is to illustrate the different points of view and procedures of the special branches of science analyzing the relationship between health and economic development. The volume includes contributions ranging from epidemiology, economics, psychology and psychiatry to history and sociology; with regard to the methods applied, the spectrum stretches from case (control) and cohort studies to macro-indicator models.

This volume cannot solve all the scientific differences and disagreements in this field; it will, however, offer more than a random selection of opinions. The contributions can only represent facets of a complex of problems: not one subsection could be covered wholly and in a fully scholarly manner. Mutual misunderstandings and perhaps even prejudices - e.g. between socio-economic research and epidemiology - had to be tolerated, since the methodological conflict has so far proved insoluble. Given that the state of the art in this field of research is still fragmentary, even highly diverse and isolated research projects might help to complement or correct each other. It should also be mentioned that the scientific activities dealt with are still in a state of flux; but even if papers of 1981 seem to be outdated in 1982 they will, nevertheless, decisively influence the terms of reference for many a long-term research project of today.

The Symposium also gave an opportunity to present and discuss papers that focussed on problems of future research. Particular emphasis was given to the scope, strengths and limitations of the various research designs presented and the research strategies aimed at producing useful information and guidelines for policy-makers in the near future. It is hoped that investigation into the relationship between the economy and health might eventually result in some practical advice for social and economic policies just as biological and medical research has guided the forms and methods of medical therapy, and epidemiological studies have triggered and directed broad intervention programmes.

Conclusive answers on the relationship between economic instability and
health cannot be offered by this book. It would therefore be premature to
state consequences for health, social and economic policies. However, the
challenge which the papers of this volume represent for health services
research is not to be overlooked. In the years to come, WHO-EURO will continue to promote research activities in this field; by publishing these
Proceedings, the editors hope to stimulate further research into this
important issue.

This volume will be opened by a report on the Symposium which Mr. K.Barnard
(Nuffield Centre for Health Services Studies, Leeds/UK) has written.
This report summarizes the scope, purpose and results of the Symposium,
introduces the individual papers, and explains the importance of the
meeting within the WHO activities with regard to health and health
research policy. The Proceedings are supplemented by a WHO report -
rapporteurs: M.Harvey Brenner (John Hopkins University, Baltimore/USA)
and Detlef Schwefel (GSF-MEDIS, Neuherberg, FRG) - on the planning
meeting for the "Study on the influence of economic development".

February 1983

J. John   D. Schwefel   H. Zöllner

TABLE OF CONTENTS

K. Barnard: 1
Influence of economic instability on health.
Report on the Symposium

PART 1 26
Recent empirical research: Aggregate-level analysis

    M.H. Brenner: 27
    Mortality and economic instability:
    Detailed analyses for Britain

    J. Søgaard: 85
    Socio-economic change and mortality - a multi-
    variate coherency analysis of Danish time series

    J. John: 113
    Economic instability and mortality in the Federal
    Republic of Germany. Problems of macroanalytical
    approach with special reference to migration

    W. Włodarczyk, Z. Szubert, M. Bryła: 139
    An attempt to analyse some dependences between
    economic and health status in Poland in the
    years 1959-1979

    J.M. Winter: 169
    Unemployment, nutrition and infant mortality in
    Britain, 1920-1950

    M. Colledge, M. Kingham: 200
    Involuntary unemployment and health status:
    A regional case study utilising sociological
    and micro-epidemiological perspectives

PART 2 224
Recent empirical research: Individual-level analysis

    R. Catalano, D. Dooley: 225
    The health effects of economic instability:
    A test of the economic stress hypothesis

    C. Brinkmann: 263
    Health problems and psycho-social strains of
    unemployed. A summary of recent empirical
    research in the Federal Republic of Germany

    L. Fagin: 286
    Unemployment: A psychiatric problem as well?

D. Fröhlich: 293
Economic deprivation, work orientation and
health conceptual ideas and some empirical
findings

N. Beckmann, K.-D. Hahn: 321
Unemployment and life-style changes

S.V. Kasl: 338
Strategies of research on economic instability
and health

K. Preiser: 371
Methodological problems in the measurement of
health consequences of unemployment in sample
surveys

PART 3 386

Further research: Proposals and strategy

I.P. Spruit: 387
Unemployment, the unemployed, and health.
An analysis of the Dutch situation

C.A. Birt: 427
Prevalence of unemployment amongst those
becoming ill

G. Westcott: 433
Proposed research on the effects of unemployment on health in Scunthorpe

H. Salovaara: 449
Outline of a study on the immediate and long-
term ill-effects of a plant shutdown in a
rural community

A. Kagan: 451
Some suggestions for future research on
economic instability and health

S.J. Watkins: 461
Recession & health - a research strategy

K.-D. Thomann: 480
The effects of unemployment on health and public
awareness of this in the Federal Republic of
Germany

Study on the influence of economic development on 492
health. Report on the WHO Planning Meeting

List of participants/authors 523

Acknowledgements 528

INFLUENCE OF ECONOMIC INSTABILITY ON HEALTH
Report on the Symposium
Munich, 9-11 September 1981

Keith Barnard[1]

1. Introduction

The Symposium 'The Influence of Economic Instability on Health' was held in Munich, 9-11 September 1981, under the auspices of MEDIS (Institut für Medizinische Informatik und Systemforschung - Institute for Medical Informatics and Health Services Research), a division of GSF (Gesellschaft für Strahlen- und Umweltforschung), with technical support from the WHO Regional Office for Europe. The meeting, the second within the WHO Study on the Influence of Economic Development on Health, was attended by 30 participants from 8 countries (see list of participants).Prof.Dr.W.van Eimeren, Dr. D. Schwefel and Dr. C. Wlodarczyk chaired the Symposium on a rotating basis while Mr. K. Barnard acted as Rapporteur and Dr. H. Zöllner as Secretary. Professor W. van Eimeren, Director of MEDIS, opened the Symposium and welcomed participants on behalf of GSF/MEDIS. Both Professor van Eimeren and Dr. Zöllner in their opening remarks stressed the importance of the subject matter of the Symposium to their organizations. Dr. Zöllner offered a welcome on behalf of Dr. Leo A. Kaprio, Regional Director of the WHO Regional Office for Europe, and thanked MEDIS for organizing and sponsoring the Symposium.

1.1 The European Strategy for Health for All by the Year 2000

In October 1980 the Member States of the WHO European Region at the 30th session of the Regional Committee adopted a Regional Strategy for Health for All by the Year 2000 which consists of three main elements: the promotion of life styles conducive to health, the reduction of preventable conditions, and the reorientation of the health care system to cover the whole population. The interest of the Regional Office in the influence of economic development was to be seen in the context of that Strategy: the

---

[1] with the assistance of Professor M. Harvey Brenner (section 2) and Ms Gill Westcott (section 3).

evolution of technology will affect the quality of life and the environment, and structural changes can be expected in industry, agriculture and service sectors. If chronic unemployment continues to grow in some countries and if there are continual changes in the employment situation in others, it may be argued, this is likely to lead to the emergence of groups subject to deteriorating health and other risks, with consequent psychosocial disorders and social deprivation. As it was put to the planning meeting (Copenhagen, 11-13 November 1980) of the Study: "The Regional Office was seeking scientific evidence and expert advice on the influence of economic development on health" (Report, p. 494).

1.2 Planning Meeting (first meeting) of the Study, Copenhagen, November 1980

The meeting had taken as its starting point the macro-level analysis carried out by Prof. Harvey Brenner (1979) on US and UK demographic and economic data which could be taken to suggest that - while economic growth through improved living standards contributed to the long-term decline in mortality rates - economic instability, particularly as manifested in increased unemployment, led to increased mortality. The meeting noted the policy significance of establishing conclusively the cause-effect linkages that related economy and health, of developing reliable forecasting of the relevant trends, and of studies directly focussing on population groups suffering most from economic change, recession and unemployment.

The meeting concluded that studies carried out at different levels of analysis would give a better understanding of the situation in within 3 - 5 years. At the macro-level, studies would be welcome which adapted, replicated, and tested Brenner's approach to the estimation and prediction by multiple regression of a relation between steady economic growth and overall mortality and between short-term instability and mortality. At more disaggregate levels, using different methodologies, studies were also advocated which focussed on: the economic and social experience of different regions and communities within a country; on the experience of potential high risk social groups, and indeed on individuals who had experienced the effects of economic instability and unemployment. Lastly the meeting recognised the need to attempt to link studies at different levels and to draw internationally valid conclusions.

1.3 Objectives of the Symposium (second meeting), Munich, September 1981

The purpose of this meeting was to review recent research and experience as called for by the first meeting, and to make further progress if circumstances permitted in the drawing up of protocols for the study. MEDIS in their call for papers drew attention to the unsatisfactory know-how in research concerning the influence of economic instability on health. They indicated that the Symposium would seek to reduce the deficit of knowledge by:
- giving publicity to new research results and to present research activities, and
- offering scientists an opportunity to exchange ideas and experiences.

They wished the Symposium to examine particularly:
- studies using a macroanalytical ecological approach,
- studies examining the elements of the theoretical rationalisation of macroanalytical ecological models (clinical, epidemiological and social science studies of the impact and consequences of undesired and adverse economic events on groups and individuals).

The Symposium would conclude with a consideration of possibilities in the field of research strategies and programmes.

1.4 Organisation of the Symposium

The meeting began with a statement of the questions raised at the Copenhagen meeting: e.g. reservations about the validity and reliability of the indicators available and used; the lack of an articulated elaborated theory of the presumed relationship between the phenomena; the credibility problem of findings seeming to contradict common sense; the importance of reconciling the findings of different disciplines (with their different research foci and techniques); traditional social research hazards such as the Hawthorne effect; the crucial importance of predictive power if research findings were to be seen as policy relevant.

Against that background of research issues the Symposium was divided into 3 sessions each occupying one day:

SESSION 1 - Recent empirical research: Aggregate-level analysis (macro-level)

SESSION 2 - Recent empirical research: Individual-level analysis (micro-level)

SESSION 3 - Further research:
Proposals and strategy

Each of the three sessions started with brief presentations of selected formal papers and continued with an extensive open discussion, the main intention of which was:
- to identify the strong and weak points of the various research designs and approaches as well as the possibilities of interconnection,
- to suggest priorities for further research based on the present state of art in research regarding the connection between economic instability and health,
- to stimulate the evolution of study designs for an international comparative study and the co-ordination of research proposals presented at the Symposium as well as to foster co-operation between the study groups attending.

2. Summary of Recent Empirical Research

During the first two sessions the Symposium received a number of scientific papers presented by participants. An indication of the contents of these papers now follows:

2.1 The Papers

2.1.1 Macro Studies

2.1.1.1 M.H. BRENNER
Objectives
(1) To study the implications of economic growth and recession on several causes of death in post-war Britain, controlling for the effects of behavioural risk factors (alcohol and cigarette consumption) and use of health services.

(2) Presentation of the simple economic change model without controls for behavioural risks and use of health services for eight countries, i.e. US, Canada, UK (England and Wales), France, Federal Republic of Germany, Italy, Spain and Sweden.[2]

---

[2]) Because of lack of space not included in this volume.

Method
Multiple regression and time series analysis at the national level.

Results
As regards total mortality, infant mortality and mortality due to cardiovascular disease, suicide, homicide and cirrhosis of the liver in post-war Britain, the author found the basic beneficial influences of economic growth and the deleterious influence of recession (especially unemployment). While the simple model of economic change can be seen to affect mortality in the eight sample countries, it is important to control for other epidemiological risk factors especially during the post-war era.

2.1.1.2 J. SØGAARD

Objective
Elaboration of the Brenner-type model via:
(1) spectral, rather than regression analysis
(2) multiple equation systems, rather than single multiple risk factor equations
(3) application of this methodology to Denmark for 1921-1978

Method
By spectral analysis of cycles of 4-8, 8-15 and 15 and over years duration, economic, health-risk factors and mortality rate are examined for interdependence. Data are first detrended via first differences. Lagged effects of economic and health risk data are built into the spectral analytic procedure. Path analysis is also used in order to infer direct versus indirect causation.

Results
The author regards the findings as a first-stage product in an exploratory research effort. He felt that the preliminary findings may be biased by inability to adjust for changes in age structure and problems in the overall quality of the mortality data. The independent variables of economic growth, unemployment (with adjustments for lost wages), alcohol and cigarette consumption, and the divorce rate were examined with regard to mortality caused by heart disease (males), respiratory disease (males), infant causes, accidents (males), suicide (20-44 year old males).
This technique yielded a positive correlation of unemployment to mortality for suicide only. In several other cases of mortality, the alcohol

and cigarette consumption variables were found to play an important role.

2.1.1.3 J.M. WINTER

Objective

Analysis of economic changes and infant mortality rates in England and Wales, 1920-1950.

Method

In this partial attempt to replicate Brenner's analysis of US infant mortality over 1915-1967, the author uses a pre-regression analysis model, based on graphic techniques and the single variable of unemployment. This procedure followed an earlier (1973) method by Brenner used to discriminate very long-term trends in pathology from their cyclic fluctuations.

Findings

A positive relation between unemployment and infant mortality rates was found only in the case of the first seven days of life, and not thereafter. Winter asks whether this positive relation may be inaccurate since explanation is lacking of why economic deprivation should effect early rather than late infant mortality. He feels, further, that the appropriate explanation of trends in infant mortality are to be found in nutrition and that long-term trends are more appropriate for analysis than fluctuations.

2.1.1.4 J. JOHN

Objective

Re-estimation of Brenner's model for the Federal Republik of Germany, 1952-1979.

Method

Time series regression analysis of total mortality rates, by age and sex. Study was unable, as yet, to incorporate risk factors to post-war mortality such as alcohol, cigarette consumption and recessional factors as in Brenner's post-war model. The replication effort was based on economic growth trend, unemployment rates and rapid economic changes as the independent variable.

Results

The unemployment rate was positively associated with male and female in-

fant mortality, and with female mortality for the 20-24 age group. The
author argued strongly that it was necessary to take account of foreign
worker immigration before proper estimation of the significance of the
Brenner post-war model could be carried out. In addition, the paper made
clear that multi-collinearity among the lagged unemployment variables
(0-5 years) could have been responsible for the absence of a stronger
finding for the unemployment factor. Finally, the use of a linear,
rather than an exponential trend of economic growth (as in Brenner's
model) could have also minimized the strength of his findings.

2.1.1.5 W.C. WŁODARCZYK et al.

Objective

Analysis of dependencies between changes in population, and economic
and health status in Poland 1959-1979.

Method

Systems analysis of interrelations among indices of:
(1) Somatic Health (total mortality rate, malignant neoplasm mortality
    rate, infant mortality rate; incidence rates of malignant neoplasms
    and sexually transmitted diseases; natural abortion rate for women
    15-49 years of age; sickness absenteeism rate from: malignant neo-
    plasms, nervous and psychiatric diseases, cardiovascular diseases
    and viral hepatitis);
(2) Psycho-social Aspects of Health (suicide rate; induced abortion
    rate for women 15-49; migration; divorce rate; alcohol consumption
    rate; tobacco consumption rate);
(3) Economic Status of the Population (national income per capita;
    investment expenditure per capita; investment expenditure as a pro-
    portion of state budget; health and social welfare as a proportion
    of overall investment expenditure);
(4) Health Care Resources (health expenditure as a proportion of state
    budget; and physicians, nurses and hospital beds per capita).

Results

Among the large number of interesting findings in this multiple time-
series and bivariate intercorrelation study are the following: Intercorrelation within each of the four sets of indices tend to be positively correlated, for example, the mortality and sickness absenteeism
data are positively related. This indicates considerable stability and
validity of the data themselves. The psycho-social aspects of health
tend to be related to the somatic aspects, for instance, the suicide

rate is correlated with mortality rates from major causes and with absenteeism. Indicators of economic well-being appear to be strongly correlated to somatic (e.g. total mortality) and psycho-social (e.g. suicide) indices.

The authors are encouraged by their statistical results, but advocate caution in their interpretation.

2.1.2 <u>Micro Studies</u>

2.1.2.1   <u>L. FAGIN</u>
<u>Objective</u>
A clinical picture, in depth, of the effect of unemployment on unemployed male workers and their families.

<u>Method</u>
Longitudinal clinical interviews of a sample of 22 unemployed male workers and their families.

<u>Results</u>
Health deteriorated in a number of members of the families following the event of unemployment, and these subjective changes in health were not restricted to the breadwinner but were also experienced by the wives and children. Reactions included a moderate to severe depression, and use of antidepressants, tranquilizers or sleeping pills. A great variety of psychosomatic illnesses tended to recur among those who had had an earlier history of them. Disabled people who had managed to keep their disabilities under control during most of their working lives, suffered serious and rapid decline in their physical handicaps.

The study concluded that there was sufficient evidence to suggest possibility of a causal relationship between unemployment and ill-health. It is the responsibility of government, social planners and economists to bear this in mind when making decisions. Also suggests the health care profession be alerted to methods of dealing with the implications of unemployment for ill-health.

2.1.2.2 <u>C. BRINKMANN</u>
<u>Objective</u>
Review of recent studies in the Federal Republic of Germany of factors associated with unemployment as it affects the unemployed - including subjective state of health and psycho-social strains.

Method
The studies reviewed (both published and forthcoming) were based on relatively large samples.

Results
Subjective state of health appears to be adversely influenced by the experience of unemployment - a situation that is compounded by health hazards in adjusting to a new job (i.e. the problem of re-employment and re-integration). Psycho-social strains were felt to be a greater burden by the unemployed than financial burdens. A smaller study (N = 147) found increased 'depressive signs'. The researchers emphasise the heterogeneity of their findings; and that the long-term consequences of unemployment (over 2 years) were beyond the scope of these studies.

2.1.2.3 D. FRÖHLICH
Objective
Development of and testing of analytic frame of reference to answer such questions as: Why does unemployment affect the unemployed deleteriously - especially in terms of health status? Which aspects of unemployment cause deleterious effects?

Method
Interview of 950 unemployed males in 1976 probing the areas of physical, mental and social well-being. Self-reports provide the basic data.

Results
The effects of unemployment are strongly modified according to whether the subjects were instrumentally work-orientated (i.e. concentrated on economic gain) or expressively work-oriented (i.e. focus on work as important in itself). In general, the unemployed who had an expressive work orientation showed considerably more damage to health and social well-being. Economic deprivation per se was more important in leading to social withdrawal.

2.1.2.4 S.V. KASL
Objective
Study of 100 low-skill blue collar workers undergoing unemployment due to a permanent plant shutdown to ascertain changes in physical and mental health.

Method
Longitudinal surveys from prior to until 2 years after the plant shutdown.

Results
Short-term acute 'stress' effects of the job loss were shown even though the great majority were relatively rapidly re-employed. Longer-term deleterious effects could not be demonstrated. Author questions the generalizability of his findings.

2.1.2.5 P. CATALANO and D. DOOLEY
Objective
To study the effects of economic change on life stresses and subjective indications of ill-health.

Methods and Results
Longitudinal survey of a cumulative total of 6190 subjects analysed over time (quarterly samples drawn from the same population). The first hypothesis is that controlling for socio-economic and demographic characteristics as well as for non-economic, non-illness events, respondents who experience economic life events will be at greater risk of illness or injury than those who do not. The second hypothesis is that respondents interviewed during periods of economic instability will be at greater risk of illness/injury than those interviewed during periods of less economic change. Both hypotheses are supported.

This and similar research challenges the political systems to devise decision processes that allow a full accounting of the health costs as well as of the economic benefits likely to accrue to groups and regions affected by policy options.

2.1.2.6 N. BECKMANN and K.-D. HAHN
Objective
To present a dynamic life-style model, emphasising society and the individual as systems and parts of each other's system. Systems have the ability to adapt in different ways more or less adequate.
Illness related to unemployment is one way to cope. The systems view should help to generate hypotheses and develop instruments in order to recognise the mechanisms by which the system works.

Methods and Results
Development of an inquiry instrument administered to unemployed workers attending courses provided for them. Responses fed back with interpretation to the respondents. In an action-research framework this provides means of discussing with the respondents possible means of coping.

2.2 Discussion of Research Methods and Results

2.2.1 Macro Studies

The meeting noted that the findings of the studies as presented to them were not prima facie compatible. At this stage it was necessarily a matter of speculation whether the differences would be accounted for by differences in analytical technique, in variables used or excluded, in time frame, or whether the units of measurement were in fact measuring different phenomena under a common label. Thus it might be that the different studies were addressing different aspects of very complex phenomena or measuring the same aspects in different ways or recording different realities.

There were certainly strong reservations entered by some participants regarding the concept of unemployment and its usual measurement in published statistics. Thus there were dangers of regarding unemployment, income loss, job loss and premature retirement as comparable phenomena, a view likely to be strongly contested by sociologists and anthropologists among others; and the experience of unemployment was likely to be qualitatively different in a period of recession when the prospect of an early return to employment is remote and unemployment in a buoyant economy when the prospect of re-employment was good.

At the same time there were reservations expressed about the validity of using aggregated data in the form of national annual statistics, i.e. what were the intrinsic merits of accepting a year basis rather than some longer period such as the life of a parliament which might be more meaningful in terms of observing government policy and its effects. Likewise statistics relating to the nation state might conceal significant variations in economic circumstances, culture and health status of its population. In which case could it ever be a worthwhile attempt to predict changes in mortality in one country on the evidence of an association between economic change and mortality in another country? In short, were the quantitative foundations of macro studies right or not?

Perhaps a more fundamental challenge to the proponents of macro studies lay in the assertion that aggregate data and ecological associations have over the years offered both false and useful leads and that it was difficult to determine which leads were likely to prove useful. Indeed it was all too easy to fall into the trap of the ecological fallacy of generalising from statistical associations at the macro level to the impact and consequences for the individual. Macro studies were not yet able to compute attributable risks arising from unemployment, or to establish whether it was the unemployed themselves who were at greater risk. Opponents characterised the work of macro studies as lacking in testable hypotheses and failing to make explicit the assumed intervening variable in each case.

These criticisms suggested the need to distinguish between what so-called macro studies have, cannot, and might achieve. They have through correlation and regression analysis suggested hypotheses. They cannot test hypotheses through association alone; they might predict and, in turn, be useful for planning purposes. However, it was suggested that prediction would need to be backed by more powerful and persuasive corroborating evidence from studies designed to permit causal inference to be drawn. In practice there were too many actual or potential intervening variables to make 'proof' by prediction acceptable for policy makers' purposes, and it was therefore unlikely to be enough merely to describe a relationship and establish its regularity.

In this discussion it was initially implicit and later made explicit that macro level studies were more likely to be carried out by econometricians and micro level studies by epidemiologists testing hypotheses as to what impact a given agent has on people. In mitigation it was pointed out on behalf of the econometricians that they normally worked within a framework of well established theory of causal connections and this condition very often did not exist in respect of epidemiological explanations: macro level relationships were ultimately dependent on theory postulated at the micro level.

If, as was said, it is the level of analysis that dictates the level of discussion of causal explanation, then one might reflect on the gains and losses of moving from the micro to the macro level, as suggested by one participant, at the micro level there is likely to be greater confidence in the results based on an awareness of the full context of the study, but great hesitancy about generalising from those findings: moving to the macro level one loses that detail but becomes more confident in generalising which is clearly a necessary if not sufficient condition for public policy making.

2.2.2 Micro Studies

It will be noted that the range of studies presented at this session was much broader than for the macro session: from indepth clinical studies of small samples (albeit using a variety of research instruments) to epidemiological studies of limited samples with control groups to a 'sub-macro' study that used both published statistics and commissioned survey data relating to a locality representing an identifiable political and economic entity. It was pointed out early in the discussion that the level of analysis selected should depend on the theory brought to bear on the issue to be studied. It was further suggested that some studies had been marked by an absence of theoretical structure and that the use of different research methods by different researchers had as a necessary consequence the loss of replicability and of consistency of findings. Conversely the application of the same method and the subsequent discovery of the same type of findings would generate confidence in that form of research.

The image of a collection of micro studies was evoked as a 'book of short stories', contrasted with macro studies as the 'picture on the front cover'. While macro studies might be indected for being solely concerned with that picture and not with the variety of the contents inside, micro studies generally suffered from not being related one to another. The reality was that one small study could never be authoritative; in small scale studies measures of serious health events are not possible. Since mortality and severe morbidity are rare, large samples are imperative and studies under the critical sample size can only pick up minor events. If the book of 'short stories' were to have credibility it needed a common theme and a coherence which was convincing not only to the scientist but to the policy analyst and the practical decision maker.

An alternative approach was the large long-run (10 years at least) cohort study focussing on economic dislocation, conducted in an exacting fashion credible to all disciplines and using a model in which all

selected variables fitted. In this way use could be made of previous
micro studies which had identified pathways and possible means of
measuring the phenomena experienced by individuals and communities as
a consequence of economic dislocation. In any event it was now vital
to recognise the interdependence of all disciplines in the acquisition
of new knowledge at every level of analysis.

While there was substantial support for emphasizing large-scale prospective studies, there was also dissent. It was suggested that in
some circumstances it might be cheaper and more practical to attempt
retrospective studies of those who had become ill. It was also disputed
whether prospective studies were necessarily the ideal; the experience
of being unemployed was unlikely to be the same over time since economic
and social circumstances were changing. Counter arguments advanced for
long-run studies were the opportunity to monitor 'trigger events' which
caused changes in the phenomena being studied; and the desirability of
following over time the adaptive behaviour of the human organism (bear-
ing in mind that the studies on responses to unemployment had been a
relatively short duration - often under 2 years). It was also argued
that it was not right in the studies being contemplated only to concentrate on dramatic events; it was no less legitimate to focus on short
run events/effects.

<u>The fundamental questions are:</u> What aspects (or correlates) of economic
change pre-disposes what kind of people through what kinds of mechanisms
to what kind of diseases? What kind of interventions will protect against
such ill-effects?

To take an example: On the assumption that one accepted that life events
led to stress which led in turn to ill health, how was one to define
stress in such a way as to permit the formulation of testable hypotheses?
The need was to bring the disciplines together to harness different expertise, to identify what issues of social importance should be adressed
within what time frame, and to formulate hypotheses that are likely to
be helpful. In deciding on a study it was necessary to identify first
the problem and study focus and not the techniques to be used. At one
level the challenge was to transfer existing knowledge into public information. At another there was a more fundamental challenge to researchers before they could confidently advise decision makers.

2.3 The Tentative Picture Emerging

The evidence from the various studies presented needs more systematic review than has so far been possible. The accumulated multi-country evidence of Brenner is persuasive in suggesting links between economic change and health if one accepts his assumptions and methodology. Catalano and Dooley report that the effect of economic life events on the odds of ill-health and injury was significant, controlling for individual characteristics <u>and</u> non-economic non-health life events. But at the same time they say that the unemployment and employment change macro variables were <u>not</u> related at all to life events or health. At the same time the discrepancies between Brenner's findings and those of John and Søgaard need further scrutinizing before it can be deduced whether they dispute Brenner's findings.

Reviewing the micro studies, there is as yet no clear simple picture of a relationship between economic change and ill-health, but some recurring themes may be noted. There may be variations in response to adverse economic events dependent on their attitude to work as instrumental or expressive (Fröhlich), the level of income maintenance in unemployment, the level of social support, the availability of an alternative social role after job loss, and the strength of the work ethic in the subject. Those affected adversely are more likely to exhibit depression and/or psychosomatic symptoms but for those for whom work had been an unpleasant experience, it was conceivable that health status would improve during a period of unemployment. The variety of phenomena observed make it important to develop a more integrated research strategy that is geared to establishing the link between all economic experiences and health.

3. Outline of Future Research Strategies and Projects

The first two sessions of the Symposium revealed the variety of phenomena to be studied within the framework of economic change or instability and health. In particular participants noted similarities and differences in the findings of studies using a variety of techniques at different levels of analysis, different types of data, locations, time spans, and not least implicit or explicit hypotheses. It became apparent that all approaches could make some contribution to our understanding, by contributing an addition to knowledge, by corroborating or challenging existing conventional wisdom or by suggesting new more closely focussed hypotheses. The purpose of the third session was to stimulate thought on the future direction of the study through presentations on potential research strategies, which were argued for in terms of strategic direction, research methodology, and what might be described as the appropriate 'conceptual arena'. The meeting also noted the suggestive evidence available that there was little awareness yet among many health professionals, political and administrative decision makers and the general public of existing research findings and their potential policy significance (Thomann). The meeting therefore expressed the view that it was now timely to move towards a manifestly purposeful research strategy with a clearly expressed rationale; and to make yet more conscious efforts to heighten professional, political, and public awareness of the inter-connectedness of economic activity and health. The meeting was further stimulated in moving towards its conclusions and recommendations by having the opportunity of commenting on certain specific research projects which had been consciously prepared within the framework of the study.

An indication of the contents of the relevant presentations on strategy and project proposals referred to above now follows:

3.1 Outline of New Research Proposals

3.1.1 C.A. BIRT proposed a study in an industrial urban area in North-West England to test the hypothesis that the incidence of certain conditions does not differ significantly between people who are employed and those who are unemployed, in each age and sex group. A retrospective study covering a 36 month period would be made of those admitted to the district hospital or dying elsewhere within the study area from any of the following:
- acute myocardial infarction (ICD 410)
- cerebrovascular disease (ICD 430-438)
- poisoning (ICD 965-967, 968 and 980)
- malignant tumours (ICD 140-206)

Information on personal details, diagnostic information, admission details, social information and employment information will be collected. The incidence of the conditions being studied can be calculated using quarterly employment data for the area, for those in employment and those who have been out of work for varying periods.

3.1.2 H. SALOVAARA proposed a study of 250 workers served by an Occupational Health Centre and currently employed in a telecommunications plant which will close in 1982. The plant is in a town in southern Sweden offering scarce alternate employment opportunities to those becoming unemployed. Certain data exist to facilitate: a retrospective study of the workers (mainly women) during an earlier prosperous period and the subsequent (recent) period of uncertainty about the future of the plant; a short-term follow-up during the transition phase from employment to unemployment; and a long-term follow-up during the ensuing unemployment period (say up to 10 years).

Various sorts of intervention will be tried with this group. There will be two control groups available: an employed group from the same town, and a comparable unemployed group in the same neighbourhood but not served by the Occupational Health Centre. The 300 employees who left voluntarily during the period of uncertainty will also be followed up. The spouses and children of the employees would also be examined, and conclusions sought about the total costs of a shutdown. It was hoped that recommendations may follow on how to minimize the damage to workers and their families in similar situations in future.

3.1.3 G. WESTCOTT outlined a research design to study the health impact of unemployment on steel and other workers made redundant between January 1980 and December 1981 in an urban industrial area in North-East England. In addition to identifying any such effects on the unemployed, as compared with their own employed past and with a matched control group still in employment, it is proposed to study reasons for different health responses among the unemployed. The sample of 500 will come from two firms declaring large scale redundancies, and will be interviewed at home at 4-monthly intervals for up to two years. Particular attention will be given to the following factors in determining the impact of unemployment: age, previous employment history, spouse's employment, social support, financial status, the nature of job loss and whether meaningful life activities are found. Information will be fed back to local voluntary and statutory organisations.

The results of a pilot study were reported, suggesting that the proposed questionnaires for measuring health and collecting socio-economic data were sensitive to the required degree, and capable of testing the hypotheses considered.

3.2 Further Research Needs

3.2.1 A. KAGAN took as his starting point that it was probable (but not proven) that economic change causes health risks through psycho-social stress, in that it fitted the general theory of social change and stress. The purpose of research therefore could be to establish whether harm can come from economic change; and if so whether that harm could be minimised. Research must be conceived to show causal relationships through the testing of hypotheses and to evaluate interventions designed to mitigate the effects of ill-health or lower levels of well-being resulting from economic change.

He took as a fundamental working assumption that economic change causes inappropriate stress responses/precursors of disease if it causes psycho-social stresses such as threats to survival, security, or being in control of one's circumstances.

The above could be fashioned into what he termed 'key hypotheses' to be tested. This would lead to a better understanding of how the social change-stress system works, how intervention should be conducted; if key hypotheses were sustained or corroborated then it would be possible to detect the effects of socio-economic change early. These were 'key' hypotheses in that if they were confirmed the true nature of the phenomena would be revealed; and if refuted it would change fundamentally current thinking about the most relevant and fruitful future research.

Equally central to his strategy was the conduct of evaluation studies which would show the benefits (and harm) arising from various interventions: _who_ benefited, what costs were incurred and by whom? Evaluation studies would be a conscious and systematic programme of 'learning from mistakes'.

Lastly it was necessary to collect quantitative data on factors thought to be important in the economic change-stress-health service system. If it was possible to quantify relationships between factors thought to be important, it would then be possible to develop simulation models, i.e. to model different situations and interventions and to predict consequences.

It was, he felt, possible to find, say, 12 locations where it would be possible with the co-operation of all concerned (e.g. redundant workers, their families, managers of enterprises, and the medical services) to mount studies over a period of one to three years. If such a programme was carried out in a co-ordinated way, comparable data could be collected and pooled, the same key hypotheses tested and a simulation developed of the society-stress-health service system.

3.2.2 <u>I.P. SPRUIT</u> reviewed and summarized the Dutch studies so far available in this area. She drew out a hypothetical formulation of the process from unemployment to disease and a holistic representation of the hypothesized experience of unemployment and disease. Of particular interest was the existence of a high work ethic found to be a prevalent feature of Dutch society, which should be included with unemployment among the possible causes of resultant ill-health.

Aggravating factors found include certain 'negative' conditions existing at the time of termination of employment, such as being of higher age, engaged in specialized work, being a married woman of ex-self-employed; being dismissed or experiencing other types of involuntary termination which might be associated with personal failure; previous unemployment; and the current high unemployment rate. All these factors lead to a reduction in the estimated chance of re-employment and contribute (perhaps with other personal and family problems) to a strongly negative experience of unemployment and a sense of failure. This state which may be characterized by guilt, stress (with accompanying physiological changes), and a less healthy lifestyle, may lead to a loss of desire to work, and to health complaints and social problems. On the other hand it could in some cases lead to a willingness to accept less attractive work. Further research might be directed to testing the hypotheses about the links between the subjective experience of unemployment and the health consequences.

3.2.3 <u>S.J. WATKINS</u> considered alternate hypotheses which might account for an association at the national level between unemployment and health indicators. These were:
- Unemployment leading to stress
- Economic failure and lower income
- Deterioration of working conditions in adverse labour market conditions
- Deteriorating social services
- Changed personal lives

Research was needed to study the effects of recession on lifestyle and stress across income groups, not merely among the unemployed.

Suggestions were made for research also in situations where fear of redundancy can be separated from pressure on work conditions, social effects of unemployment from loss of income etc. The health of those receiving state benefits should also be documented. Conditions for an ideal study of the effects of unemployment per se in a situation of plant closure were outlined, and it was suggested that the opportunity be taken when this relatively rare natural experiment presented itself.

3.3 Guiding Principles for Future Research

Kasl introduced a set of general methodological issues as regards macro studies and Brenner gave a similar presentation on micro studies. From these presentations and their discussion there emerged the following checklist of methodological guiding principles for future research.

(a) Since "micro" vs. "macro" approaches is an oversimplification specify what units of observation are actually available to the scientist: individual, family, social network, organization, community region, nation, etc. Determine to which degree they have been or should be studied equally diligently.

(b) Try to understand the consequences or advantages (benefits) and disadvantages (costs), in terms of likely differences in research effort as well as in knowledge and policy relevance, of changing the units of aggregation (temporal, geographical, sociopolitical); check whether certain levels of aggregation require a unique research approach and information basis and/or are capable to make unique contributions to scientific knowledge or policy-making.

(c) Choose the proper research hypothesis and units of observation, and thus the appropriate level of analysis. Keep in mind that certain research questions require research across different levels of analysis.

(d) Review the major types of research designs, i.e.: (a) fully prospective subjects identified prior to start of unemployment; (b) longitudinal but not prospective subjects are followed but start of study is after the event; (c) prospective study done in retrospect - start of study is after the unemployment has begun, but subjects are part of a cohort assembled earlier (e.g. all factory workers at a plant from 5 years ago) and data from earlier are available; (d) cross-sectional community surveys; (e) case/control designs with specific dimensions of matching; and

(f) multivariate retrospective time series analysis at the national or regional level.

Determine to which degrees these designs have à priori strengths and weaknesses, and which degrees it depends on the actual execution of study and the types of questions being asked. Can any research design be labelled, à priori, as "useless", as "essential", as "unrealistic", as "too expensive", etc.?

(e) Review alternative methods for specifying behaviourally and/or biologically valid dependent variables or impact criteria. Can any be labelled as "important", as "trivial", as "immeasurable at present" and so on? Should any priorities be set? What proxy indicators (e.g. risk factors instead of disease outcomes) are useful, or useless? Also determine which special features are required for cross-level analysis, if relevant.

(f) Since the two directions of causality are not mutually exclusive (e.g., those in prior poor health are at greater risk for experiencing some form of economic instability, which, in turn, may accelerate the downward course of their health), an effort should be made to address both. In how far will retrospective accounts be useful?

How good must be the initial assessment of physical and mental health status if subjects are studied where the self-selection process has already taken place and cannot be reconstructed?

Determine which research designs minimize self-selection and provide us with some baseline information on subjects from the past, etc.

(g) Determine the relative merits of naturalistic research of adverse impact versus controlled studies of benefits of various policies/programmes/interventions. Note that hypothesis testing per se does not lead to concrete policy conclusions and recommendations, except where relevant operational policy variables are explicitly included.

(h) If working at a low level of aggregation ("micro") attempt to use research designs and subject populations which offer the greatest promise of generalizable findings, lest results are highly specific to occupational subgroups, to types of experiences, to stages of adaptation, to social settings and social support systems etc. Include a number of "context variables", such as information about (a) the economic climate; (b) social insurance policies applicable to subjects being studied; (c) the type of experience being studied and its exact nature (financial aspects, career, job change, reduced hours, layoff, etc.).

(i) If working at a high level of aggregation ("macro"), attempt to use units of observation which are, or can relatively easily, be disaggregated in terms of those regions, sociodemographic subgroups and outcomes which are typically used at lower levels of research focus. The research methodolgy should also be structured in such a way as to provide useful leads, suggestions or hypotheses for more detailed studies.

(j) When using archieval or institutional data, i.e. information collected for the purpose of routine adminstration and management, check the quality of data and decide when to accept or reject a new data source. Choose a research design which, beyond describing the past, can tell something meaningful about the present and the near future, i.e. has a forecasting usefulness.

(k) When using a prospective research design, determine the length of observation period needed before the full impact of a particular experience can be described. Note that different experiences may call for different lengths of observation.

(l) When using a multivariate analysis be sure not to confuse association with explanation. Note that the value of statistical regression coefficients is not sufficient to justify that one "model" is better than another. Be sure to carry out internal checks on the way that data analysis is being carried out so that technical problems (e.g. excessive error variances when working with associations among strongly intercorrelated variables) are avoided. Attempt to differentiate "spurious" and "real" associations.

4. Conclusions and Recommendations of the Symposium

4.1 Conclusions

(1) There are several levels (country, community, industry, group, family, individual) at which studies need to be conducted. There is an impression, however, that investigators sometimes choose a particular level of study merely because it conveniently fits their analytical skills.

(2) No discipline working in isolation (economics, sociology, epidemiology, psychology etc.) can reveal the complex relationships that link economic activity and health. For further progress to be made it is necessary to move forward to more interdisciplinary research based on a common understanding of the phenomena to be studied, as well as a clear understanding of each other's disciplines and of the strengths and weaknesses of their methods.

(3) There is an urgent need to synthesize the work done so far, as regards the economic and health behaviour of regions and communities experiencing periods of instability and the behaviour of members of groups suffering adverse economic experience (firms, families and categories of workers). Only then shall we know whether the orders of magnitude found in research are similar or whether differences in findings are due to different methodologies or different experience of economic development and health.

(4) Short-term and long-term studies are not merely alternatives. If research is to have any impact on policy and decision-making, it is necessary to commission studies of relevance to short-term policy. At the same time it is legitimate to argue for longer-term cohort studies serving the purpose of basic research, since the economic structures of industrialized countries are undergoing fundamental technological and institutional change.

(5) Given the potential social, economic and health significance of the research findings, presented at the Symposium, it is a matter of regret that (notwithstanding some execptions) there is still a marked lack of awareness of the issues by both the health professions and the general public.

4.2 Recommendations

(1) The study should focus its research effort on:

(a) the health effects of major structural changes in the economy of a local or regional community, e.g. the loss of a major employment source or, inversely, a rapid upturn in the economy; and

(b) the health consequences for groups of the population most obviously affected directly by an economic change, especially the older workers.

This effort at the disaggregate ("micro") level should embrace prospective, retrospective and case-control studies using epidemiological and other methods. It should include in the near future multinational research on long-term health effects.

(2) A further meeting should be convened in 1982 or 1983 in order to:

(a) consolidate the knowledge gained from completed research in the above-mentioned communities and population groups, and draw the attention of policy-makers to implications for health and social policies; and
(b) review research in progress and proposed research regarding their potential contribution to policy information.

(3) The Regional Office should promote public and professional awareness of the interconnections between health and economic change, and should promote intersectoral concern. This should include:

(a) setting up an international clearing-house for the exchange of information on current research, research findings and methodologies; the offer by MEDIS - Institut für Medizinische Informatik und Systemforschung - of GSF to act as clearing-house in 1982/1983 is welcomed;
(b) promoting the exchange of models and data sets among the scientists conducting multivariate analyses at the highly aggregate ("macro") level, and monitoring the progress of these exchanges; the offer by the Department of Community Medicine of the Johns Hopkins University, Baltimore, to act as clearing-house in 1982/83 is welcomed; and
(c) circulating widely the reports on the two meetings within the study; the offer by GSF/MEDIS to publish the papers of the Symposium is welcomed.

Addendum of the Editors to K. Barnard's Report
───

Special reference is made to the papers of K. Preiser (Forschungsgruppe Arbeit und Gesundheit, Dortmund/FRG) and of M. Colledge and
M. Kingham (School of Behavioural Science, Newcastle upon Tyne/UK).
Colledge and Kingham illustrate the possibilities of an interpretative
link between macro-sociological and micro-epidemiological perspectives
of observation by means of a regional case study on the relationship
between unemployment and health. Preiser discusses some methodological
problems of sample surveys in the measurement of health effects of
unemployment. These papers had been prepared for the symposium but
were not personally presented by the authors. They are, therefore,
not dealt with in K. Barnard's report. Since the editors regard both
papers as a real gain for the discussion, they are both included in
this volume.

Part 1

RECENT EMPIRICAL RESEARCH:

AGGREGATE-LEVEL ANALYSIS

MORTALITY AND ECONOMIC INSTABILITY: DETAILED ANALYSES FOR BRITAIN

M. Harvey Brenner

School of Hygiene and Public Health &
Department of Social Relations
The Johns Hopkins University
Baltimore, Maryland, U.S.A.

During the past decade, disturbances to the economies of industralized nations, and to that of the United Kingdom in particular, have again raised the question of the relative importance of a growing and stable economy to the health of a population. The question is whether, in a modern society, national health levels could be seriously damaged, or at least fail to improve, in the context of extraordinarily high unemployment rates, periods of violent inflation, general decline in manufacturing employment, and increased regional disparities in wealth and economic development.

The importance of this question is underlined by consistent observations that mortality and morbidity rates are, to a large extent, predictable on 1) a micro basis by individual socioeconomic status (1) and on 2) a macro basis by level of national real income per capita (2), (3) and in county and metropolitan areas by prevalence rates of unemployment and low income earners (4), (5). That there is also a dynamic inverse relation between the national economic level and mortality rates, with mortality rate increases following economic adversity and mortality rate declines following long-term economic growth, has been documented for various periods in the United States (6), and for 1936-1976 for England and Wales (4).

The analysis of the mortality trends of England and Wales, however, included effects of two periods (the last part of the Great Depression and the Second World War) of limited generalizability to the economic conditions of the recent past. It did not separately analyze the post-War period, which involved two important changes: 1) a major transformation of the mortality structure toward chronic diseases, which are influenced by man-made risk factors associated with affluent societies; and 2) the rise of "welfare state" policies specifically designed to minimize the relation between low socioeconomic status and ill health.

Hypothesizing on the basis of currently available evidence, that the dynamic inverse relation between the state of the national economy and mortality rates continues, one may ask: what variables related to the economy have recently had the most powerful influence on changes in mortality? Specifically, has the long term trend of economic growth maintained its traditional predominant role in reducing the mortality rate? Or have the presumably countervailing deleterious health risks, either intrinsically associated with economic growth (e.g., environmental contamination, hypernutrition, and sedentariness) or with behavioral risks made possible by economic growth (e.g., excessive alcohol use, cigarette smoking), significantly reduced its essentially beneficial effect?

Has economic recession, as measured by the rate of unemployment, continued to produce its traditionally harsh effects on health despite the offsetting factors of lower durations of unemployment, substantial unemployment compensation and easier, more financially secure retirement?

---

* A negative answer to this question has been given by Gravelle et al. (14). Several methodological and substantive errors invalidate their Conclusions (15).

More generally, nave there been important ameliorative effects on the socioeconomic status - mortality relationship based on the welfare state legislation in general and the national health service in particular?

In extending this analysis of England and Wales mortality patterns, it is important to test the generalizability of the England and Wales results to another region of the country. A comparative analysis of Scotland provides data on a region that is both similar to and different from England and Wales in some significant respects. It is similar in some aspects of its total economy, trade, foreign relations and welfare policies. It differs from England and Wales in being less economically developed and industrial, less wealthy, and more subject to high unemployment. It also differs in having a somewhat different culture (e.g., spirits, rather than beer, is the traditional alcoholic beverage), history and climate.

The test is of the applicability of the overall economic change model--which is expected to apply--and of the specific measurements-- which are expected to be different to the extent that the England and Wales/Scotland differences mentioned above are important. In particular, it would be anticipated that recessional variables might have a more damaging impact on mortality in a less wealthy region with fewer resources to fall back upon in adversity.

Extension of the Economic Change Model of Mortality

In principle, the "economic change model of mortality," which assumes that the principal factors in mortality trends arise from major changes in the structure of the national economy, can be elaborated for the purpose of examining these issues. It is essential, however, that each of the key concepts in this model be retained and be appropriately measured.

The present study explicitly takes into account, and separately examines both beneficial and adverse factors associated with, and made possible by, economic growth, but which are only loosely correlated with it. The major beneficial factors in this category that are investigated in this paper involve the provision and utilization of health services. The adverse factors are cigarette consumption and the overuse of alcoholic beverages. Theoretical and measurement problems at present preclude the separate study of beneficial and adverse factors to health that are intrinsic to economic growth and are reasonably well accounted for by its general trend. The beneficial factors include those that would be subsumed in the standard of living (nutrition; climate control via housing, clothing and use of fuel; parasite control; education; comfortable working conditions; and adequate monetary and social remuneration for work) and the potential for societal investment in the development of new knowledge and its application. Factors which may damage health and are intrinsic to economic growth include industrially produced toxins, and adverse implications of increasing reliance on non-human energy sources such as the decline in cardiovascular fitness and over-consumption of calories.

Recession-Related Factors

It is also important to know the full range of adverse economic implications of recession as they relate to health. In previous work, the totality of recessionary effects were measured by the overall unemployment rate alone. In this study, the effects of general recession are separated from those of income loss and from employment loss specifically--especially as it becomes an unusually great burden, proportionately, on a particular age-sex subgroup of the population. It is assumed that the effects of recession, and a high national unemployment rate, will adversely affect those who work as well as those who lose their jobs. The reason for this is that the realistic threat of loss of career, livlihood and relations with work-associates, sustained over a considerable period, may generate for much of the population a series of stresses nearly equivalent to employment loss. Part of this threat to the employed worker or small business owner will be reflected in the sharp reduction of working hours during economic slowdowns.

The Problem of Rapid Economic Growth

Apart from long term economic growth and recessional loss, some of the impact of rapid economic growth, which coincides with the economic upturn in its positive relation to longer-term growth, is adverse. The "recovery" or early phase of upturn following recession, can be especially stressful for the unemployed who are at this time trying to reintegrated into the economy. After a severe recession, the actual recovery of industry and reintegration of those who experienced economic loss may not take place until relatively late in the upturn, or at a time near to the "crisis" point in the business cycle. This point, at which reintegration possibilities temporarily decline, occurs on the average of two years after the lowest level of recession.

The early and major part of the reintegration problem is measurable by the same variables which indicate severe recession (i.e., the unusually heavy burden of unemployment on a particular age-sex subgroup). An implication is that "annual changes in real per capita income" unlagged, which are positively associated with rapid economic growth and can therefore be taken as a measure of the reintegration problem, can be shorn of their correlation to this problem through statistical control. In that case, the meaning of annual changes in real per capita income will be literal. The effect of longer-term recession on reintegration that is slowed down by the "crisis" period can be measured by annual changes in real per capita income at a lag of two or three years.

Random Shocks

An additional set of factors--"random shocks" to the population--need to be taken into account if one is to be able to use this elaborated economic change model for detailed explanation or prediction. These types of factors include extremely disruptive phenomena which have a deleterious effect without necessarily disturbing the economy (e.g., climate irregularities such as unusually severe winters or minor epidemics), or those which damage the economy and the population in ways that go beyond the usual economic prediction, (e.g., natural disasters, political or international economic crises).

One such shock, namely the oil price crisis, occurred in Europe during late 1973 and 1974. While this crisis ushered in the subsequent international recession, its effect in the United Kingdom in 1974 did not bring about immediate loss of per capita income or employment loss (7) both of which could be measured in our analytic model. Rather its very short-term impact, which was heightened by a miners' strike, was to immediately reduce the supply and sharply increase the price of energy, and with it the overall inflation rate. This radical effect during the single year of 1974 cannot be measured adequately by our economic or health risk indicators, yet this acute disturbance is said to have brought about stunning economic hardship to small business persons and to the economically weaker and non-active groups in the population "such as the unemployed, handicapped, sick, those suffering from employment injuries and occupational diseases, the retired, and workers with lower wages and salaries" (8). To the extent that this crisis did cause economic loss, one would hypothesize that it should have had deleterious effects on health.

DATA

1. Data are nearly all from standard published sources and are listed in Table 9.

2. In order to assure maximum comparability for cause-specific mortality between England and Wales, and Scotland, the data were obtained from the ICD-classified, World Health Organization, <u>Epidemiological and Vital Statistics</u> from 1950-1961, which was superceded in 1962 by WHO <u>World Health Statistics Annual</u>. The ICD listings in these publications have changed in 1965 and 1968. Table 10 below shows the numerical classification used for data collection in this study. It has been suggested by at least one authoratative source that, on the grounds of etiological similarity, major cardiovascular diseases should be grouped under a single heading (9). More traditional sources, however, prefer a separation of the major causes on diagnostic grounds. In this study, both methods are adopted and the cause groupings are separately examined.

3. Annual data on the age-sex composition, and size of the labor force were unavailable for England and Wales, and Scotland, separately. Therefore, for the two regions, 1952-76, the denominator for the total and age-sex specified unemployment rates is the total population over age 15 and the sex-specific population respectively. The age-sex specific unemployment ratio is calculated as the age-sex specific unemployment rate divided by the total unemployment rate. For 1977-79, annual data on the age and sex composition or total size of the unemployed population, for England and Wales, and Scotland separately, are as yet unavailable, or are not continuous with the available time series on unemployment during 1952-76. Analyses for the period 1950-79, therefore, for each of the two regions, utilize the unemployment ratio for the United Kingdom as a whole, measured in the conventional manner with the civilian labor force over fifteen years of age as the denominator.

4. The overall time-span of the analyses was shortened by constraints on the availability of annual data for some of the independent variables. In addition, time-lagged relations for several of the independent variables necessitated minor variations in the starting dates of some of the analyses.

Development of Post-War Equations

The equation for total mortality is an extension of that used for the analysis of England and Wales mortality for 1936-76. As in that earlier analysis, the exponential trend of real per capita income and the unemployment rate are the main indices of long-term economic growth and recession, respectively. Controls for adverse and beneficial factors to health, made possible by but only loosely correlated with economic growth, were added--namely, per capita cigarette and alcohol consumption (also, the ratio of spirits to total alcohol consumption), the ratio of health care to total government expenditures and hospital bed utilization per capita.

The recessional indicator of unemployment is supplemented by age- and sex-specific unemployment ratios, average weekly hours worked in manufacturing industries (unlagged), and annual changes in real per capita income (at zero or one year's lag). Random shocks to the population are indicated by instances of unusually cold winters and the immediate (1974) effects of the oil crisis.

These variables were tested in an equation to account for total (see Table 1) and age/sex-specific mortality rates for England and Wales over 1954-76. The applicability of this extended general model to different causes of death was then tested. The mortality categories chosen included: those that are numerically important (the cardiovascular diseases), especially sensitive to the economic environment (infant mortality), and reactive to mental stress (suicide, homicide, motor vehicle accidents). All of the variables that proved statistically significant for total mortality in England and Wales (Table 1) were tested for significance for each of the causes and infant mortality.

Additional variables were used to supplement the equations for individual causes of death. Specifically: for cirrhosis of the liver, the three major alcoholic beverages were represented (in ratio to total alcohol consumption); for suicide, bankruptcy rates were added to identify recessional losses of higher socioeconomic groups; for homicide and motor vehicle accidents, the proportion of the population aged 15-24 was added to more clearly specify the population at risk of responsibility for these behaviors; and for motor vehicle accidents, the per capita miles travelled by automobile were added.

On account of the relatively short series available for analysis, resulting largely from the small unemployment data sample, an additional test was performed in order to determine whether having substantially increased degrees of freedom would be likely to alter the overall results. This test involved "pooling" the regional samples for England and Wales and Scotland into a single sample of years (n=44), but keeping the sexes separate. While the tests demonstrate the overall generalizability of the model to samples of larger size and greater degrees of freedom, the coefficients of each of the independent variables are not interpretable in precisely the same manner as if the regional samples had not been pooled.

The Chow test was performed on all predictive equations for the years 1955-1976. This test examines whether relations are stable, robust and consistent when years sampled are split in half (i.e. 1955-1965, 1966-1976). In order to perform this test on equations for total and infant mortality, and mortality for seven causes of death, occasionally variables had to be deleted to accomodate degrees of freedom requirements for split samples of eleven years. Nevertheless, of the eighteen equations tested, only one (for suicide in Scotland) did not pass the Chow test -- i.e., in one case there is statistical evidence of unstable relations (see Table 12).

Finally, in a few cases, specific variables were not found statistically significant. Of these, several were omitted in the final equations because (1) their t values were near zero, (b) their presence as statistical controls was not required, and (c) their presence tended to damage the statistical significance of the overall equations (F or DW values). Several other variables whose t values were greater than zero, but not technically significant, were retained in the final equations if (a) they were needed for statistical control, and (b) their presence did not damage the statistical significance of the overall equations.

Analysis of Lag Relations

Analysis of the lag structures of each of the time-series relations was accomplished in the following four stages: (a) theoretical specification of the relevant time span over which the relation may lag; (b) estimation of the actual range of statistically significant lagged relations; (c) narrowing of the range of significant lagged relations under conditions of multi-variate statistical controls; and (d) selection of optimum lag, within previously determined range, under multivariate controls.

The last stage, of selection of the optimum lag, is the most difficult since, in fact, the relations usually take place over several years and the "optimum" lag is either the strongest or the average. The ideal procedure, when degrees of freedom permit, is to express the relations in distributed lag form (typically polynomial). This method was used in the analysis of England and Wales mortality rates for 1936-1976 (4), which involved a longer time span and fewer independent variables. While the equations presented here are, on the whole, statistically robust, they express less than the entire impact of the independent variables on mortality.

Hypothetical lag relations

Specific hypotheses were developed to identify the years of lag within which, theoretically, the empirical relations should occur. First, with respect to the impact of economic trends and fluctuations on mortality rates (see Tables 13-15):

a. The exponential trend in real per capita income, as well as annual changes in real per capita income, were hypothesized to show inverse relations to mortality rates for all causes examined within a lag of one year.

b. Similarly, representing "cyclic" changes in economic activity, the average weekly hours worked in manufacturing industries were hypothesized to show an inverse relation to mortality for all causes examined within a lag of one year.

c. The overall unemployment rate was hypothesized to show two different temporal relations to total mortality and to that for the chronic diseases: one at under 5 years lag, the other at between 6 and 10 years lag. Infant mortality and mortality due to suicide, homicide and motor vehicle accidents were hypothesized to be related to unemployment at within 2 years lag.

d. The unemployment ratios for males at the ages 20-40 and over 40 were hypothesized to show relations to each of the mortality causes that were identical to those shown for the overall unemployment rate, except that relations at lags of 6-10 years were not expected for the male ratios 20-40 and over 40.

e. The unemployment ratio for males under 20 years of age was hypothesized to show relations only to homicide and motor vehicle accidents within two years.

f. The unemployment ratio for femals aged 20-40 years was hypothesized to show a relationship to infant mortality within two years.

Second, with respect to the impact of health risk and health service factors on mortality rates (see Tables 16-18).

a. For heavy alcohol consumption, a relatively short lag period of within 5 years was hypothesized for total mortality and all causes studied except for infant mortality where the hypothesized lag was for under 2 years. Relatively long lags of between 10 and 20 years were hypothesized for total mortality and the chronic diseases examined (incorporating the problem of long-term alcohol damage).

b. For cigarette consumption, relatively short lags of within 5 years were hypotthesized for total mortality and the chronic diseases studied, while in the case of infant mortality within 2 years was thought appropriate. As in the case of heavy alcohol consumption, cigarette consumption lags of between 10 and twenty years were hypothesized for total mortality and for the chronic diseases studied.

c. In the case of health services, beneficial influences on mortality were expected for total mortality and all causes examined except for suicide and homicide; for infant mortality the inverse relations were expected within two years.

d. Cold winter temperatures were hypothesized to exert a deleterious influence on total mortality and on the chronic disease causes of death examined.

Findings

1. The exponential trend in real per capita disposable income is the single most prominent explanatory factor in these analyses, and shows an inverse relationship to mortality rates for each cause, except for homicide where it is not significant.

   Other measures of long term economic growth were also tested, particularly the real Gross National Product, but were found to be inferior predictors, probably because the equations also contain indicators of government transfer payments in the form of health care benefits.

2. Annual changes in real per capita income, unlagged or with a one-year lag indicate, literally, short-term changes in income. (The usual association of this variable with the rapid economic growth problem of reintegration is obviated via statistical control achieved by the presence of age-sex-specific unemployment ratios.) This factor is inversely related to heart disease mortality and homicide, to total cardiovascular mortality for Scotland and to cerebrovascular mortality for England and Wales.

3. The unemployment rate was examined for lagged relations to mortality within the 0-5 year range. A positive relation at zero or one year lag was found for nearly all causes of death except for infant mortality where no relation is found for Scotland, and suicide where the relation is found only for Scotland and at a two-year lag.

The question of whether the rates of long duration of unemployment (over 28 weeks) was a better predictor of the mortality rate than the total unemployment rate without regard to duration was extensively examined. Superior age-specific mortality predictions were obtained for the 20-49 year old groups when the unemployment rate was specific to long duration. When age is not considered, however, mortality for the great majority of causes is more closely correlated with the total unemployment rate, probably because this recessional indicator is not limited to populations that are unusually vulnerable to long-lasting unemployment.

4. The total unemployment rate for the United Kingdom was used to analyze the effect of longer recessional lags of from 6 to 15 years on mortality, since the region-specific unemployment rates are only available from 1952 onwards. A 10-year optimum lag of the unemployment rate was found significant for England and Wales total mortality, while a six-year lag was found in relation to Scottish total mortality.

5. The 20-40 year old male unemployment ratio tends to indicate severe recession as well as a particularly heavy burden of unemployment on 20-40 year olds. It was examined for lagged relations of from zero to five years and shows a range of relations of 0-3 years. It is nearly as important a factor as the total unemployment rate but is not significant in cerebrovascular disease, homicide and infant mortality, or in motor vehicle accidents in Scotland.

6. The over-40 year old male unemployment ratio was significantly related to total, cirrhosis and cerebrovascular mortality in England and Wales.

It also showed significant relations to homicide, which may reflect a deleterious economic situation for the parents of youths involved in violence. The range of impact of this variable covers 0-3 years.

7. The under-20 year old male unemployment ratio is a significant factor in the homicide mortality rate in England and Wales at a three-year lag and in Scotland without lag.

8. The 20-40 year old female unemployment ratio is significantly related to infant mortality in both regions without lag.

9. Average weekly hours worked in manufacturing industries, unlagged, show an important inverse relationship to total mortality and all causes except suicide and homicide, especially in England and Wales. For Scotland, this relationship is found for total mortality, heart disease, cirrhosis and suicide.

10. Annual changes in real per capita income at a two-year lag is meant to reflect the late stages of rapid economic growth, which creates reintegration problems at a time when the economy is near its "crisis" point. This indicator of slow economic recovery is significantly and positively related to total mortality in Scotland.

11. Cigarette consumption per capita is positively related to the total and all categories of cardiovascular mortality at an optimum five-year lag for both England and Wales and Scotland. It would also have been desirable to examine these data for longer-term relations, but this was precluded by the limitations of degrees of freedom. In infant mortality, the relation to cigarette consumption is at a two-year lag, perhaps

reflecting an effect on late infant death associated with developmental abnormalities. Cigarette consumption in relation to total mortality is at a five-year lag in England and Wales and a two-year lag in Scotland.

12. For alcohol consumption per capita, as in the case of cigarette consumption, degrees of freedom limitations prevented an analysis of the important long-term relations. Nevertheless, the alcohol consumption variables are important in several causes of death. Total alcohol consumption per capita shows a two-year lagged relation to infant mortality in both regions, and a one-year lagged relation to suicide in England and Wales.

Alcohol consumption was also investigated according to beverage type by using ratios of each beverage type consumed to total alcohol consumption. This method of calculation avoided multicollinearity among the beverages. All three beverages were found to influence cirrhosis of the liver mortality in both regions over a range of 0-3 years. In both England and Wales and Scotland, spirits exert the greatest influence on cirrhosis, followed by wine and then beer -- perhaps a direct reflection of the absolute alcohol content of each beverage.

The specific ratio of spirits to total alcohol consumed per capita is related to cardiovascular and heart disease mortality, and to suicide, homicide and motor vehicle accident mortality in both regions, at lags ranging from 0-3 years. In Scotland, total mortality is also influenced by this variable unlagged. It is difficult to know to what extent the spirits consumption ratio actually represents a pure ethanol effect or is instead a measure of the extent to which spirits are the favored beverage under stressful conditions.

13. Health service availability, as measured by the proportion of total government expenditure spent on the National Health Service (separately measured for the Health Services in England and Wales and Scotland) exerts a substantial beneficial effect on mortality rates in Britain unlagged and lagged by one year. For both regions total, cerebrovascular and infant mortality show the beneficial effect as does total cardiovascular and heart diseae mortality in England and Wales, and cirrhosis mortality in Scotland.

14. Hospital bed utilization per capita might ordinarily be taken as an indicator of morbidity, except for the presence of general health risk factors in the equations predicting mortality. These health risk factors act as statistical controls on morbidity, in which case the hospital bed utilization variable is more likely to measure the ability of the population to obtain hospital treatment. Beneficial effects of this variable, measured separately in each of the two regions, are found unlagged in England and Wales and Scotland, for total mortality and specifically for cerebrovascular disease in England and Wales.

15. February temperatures as an indicator of "random" (i.e., unpredictable) climatic changes implicating especially severe winters, show significant unlagged relations to total, cardiovascular and heart disease mortality rates. Although January is usually a colder month than February, the latter shows higher variability in its temperatures, and is the superior empirical predictor of mortality rates in Britain. An interesting additional finding is that suicide in England and Wales shows a marginal tendency to increase during the colder, and perhaps darker, winters.

16. The effect of "random shock" represented by the oil crisis is measured to some extent in England and Wales by a binary variable (i.e., value of 1 for 1974, and zero for other years) in relation to total mortality, where the data end in 1976. The binary variable is a traditional but crude measure of discontinuity; it indicates that some disturbance occurred, but nothing of the disruptive nature of the event.

17. The 1974 shock to mortality is more easily observed when the predictive power of the equations for total mortality are tested over the period 1972-1976 (Table 11). Of the sixteen predictions for England and Wales and Scotland which do not include those for the year 1974, the error rate is less than 1.5 percent and usually less than one percent. For 1974, however, the predictive errors for Scotland are 3.5 percent from 1973 and 1972. For England and Wales, those errors are 6.5 (from 1973) and 6.4 (from 1972) percent respectively. The short-term impact of the oil shock on mortality appears to have been greater in England and Wales than in Scotland as judged by the binary variable relationship and the predictions.

18. It is clear that the region-specific totals and age-sex specific unemployment rates are important to the explanation of the British mortality trends. Since these data were not as yet available for the years after 1976, no precise predictions were attempted for subsequent years. Nevertheless, it was thought desirable to estimate general explanatory equations for at least total mortality up to 1979 (the last year for which mortality data are available) based on cruder estimates (Table 8). These equations are statistically satisfactory and are generally similar to those in which the data end in 1976 (Table 1 and Figure 2).

19. More recently (i.e., since the first edition of this paper was produced), new data became available for mortality rates and for age and sex-specific unemployment rates for England and Wales, and Scotland, permitting analyses through the year 1979. Analyses have therefore been constructed for pooled regional data (England and Wales, and Scotland treated as a single time series) in the case of total and cardiovascular mortality. The purpose of these analyses was to observe whether the basic relations could be reconstructed with larger samples, given the relatively large number of independent variables. Tables 19-20 demonstrate a satisfactory replication with pooled data through 1979.

20. Similarly, the data for the two regions extended to 1979 were combined to create total and cardiovascular mortality rates for Great Britain. Since several of the independent variables can be obtained only at the U.K. level, it is useful to observe whether more refined analyses can be performed with mortality rates that more closely approximate the U.K. The results (Tables 21-22) show improved tests of significance for some of the independent variables, and improved Durbin-Watson statistics.

DISCUSSION

The principal factors which have influenced post-war British mortality trends involve (1) economic growth and stability, (2) behavioral risks which tend to be loosely correlated with economic growth and (3) the availability and utilization of health care services. Unpredictable climate changes--especially severe winters--and other "random shocks" to the society such as the oil crisis also appear to have influenced the mortality rate.

The long-term trend in growth of real per capita income has maintained its major traditional role in continuously lowering mortality rates. These findings remain even with statistical controls for the effects of beneficial (health services) and deleterious (cigarette consumption and overuse of alcohol) factors made possible by economic growth, but not intrinsic to it.

Health services provision and utilization are themselves found to be highly beneficial to health, and tend to lower the mortality rate, especially for the youngest and older populations. These findings are precisely consistent with observations by Cochrane, et. al. (2) that, among eighteen industrialized countries analyzed cross-sectionally, the proportion of government expenditures allocated to health services is inversely related to age-specific mortality rates. A second observation by Cochrane, et. al. (2), that the ratio of physicians to the population is either unrelated or slightly positively associated with mortality rates cross-sectionally ("the anomaly that wouldn't go away") (10-11) may in fact disappear with more stringent statistical controls. A second possibility is that the anomalous finding may reflect true maldistributions of health services (12), especially in societies where provision and utilization of health care is subject to substantial market influences.

The effects of behavioral risks made possible by societal affluence have a pronounced impact on many causes of mortality. The effects of cigarette consumption on mortality trends are especially obvious in total, cardiovascular and infant mortality. The deleterious impact of overuse of alcoholic beverages is measurable in mortality trends for the external causes of death, infant mortality and perhaps for cardiovascular mortality, though the mechanism in the last group may be indirect.

The deleterious impact of economic recession is made plain by findings which indicate that several different indicators of economic loss simultaneously have a powerful positive relation to total mortality and all causes of mortality studied. The total unemployment rate <u>as well as</u> proportionally high unemployment rates among the populations aged 20-40, over 40, and under 20 correlate significantly with increased mortality rates for different causes. <u>Recessional</u> declines in average weekly hours worked (in manufacturing industries) show strong relations to increased mortality as do short-term losses in income (except in the case of motor vehicle accident mortality). These findings demonstrate that the implications of recession for health go far beyond unemployment alone. It is clear that the chronic realistic <u>threat</u> of economic loss and the breakdown of social networks increase the risk of mortality to workers who do not lose employment, and to small business persons, during recessions.

Overall, the general "economic change-model" of mortality is seen to be applicable for the analysis of post-War and relatively recent health problems. This approach is found to be quite sensitive to the epidemiological characteristics of different causes of illness and mortality. Prediction possibilities are generally quite reasonable with the equations, aside from the problem of major exogenous shocks, and provided that all concepts in the model are accurately measured.

Excellent replications of total and cause-specific sub models of mortality were achieved in the comparison of England and Wales and Scotland. The dynamics of mortality in these two regions are very similar as is indicated by frequent mortality responses to the same factors. Some exceptions to the comparable findings between these regions are that Scotland shows greater sensitivity to cold winters and to high ratios of spirits-to-total alcohol consumption. Also, it appears that the 1974 effects of the oil shock were less damaging to Scotland, perhaps because it was less dependent on oil, considering its lower level of industrialization and greater reliance on hydroelectric power.

At the same time, Scotland tends to show more severe health responses to the effects of slow economic recovery after periods of recession. This may be due to the actuality of harsher and longer recessional periods in Scotland.

Coefficients

Writing some years ago on the subject of standardization of death rates, Hugh H. Wolfenden[13] emphasized that standardized rates are index numbers computed to facilitate comparisons between populations with differences in structure, that "no significance is to be attached to their absolute magnitudes", and that there is always the possibility that they appear to support conclusions that are actually unwarranted. He continued: "However useful for rapid practical purposes they may be in summarizing comparative mortalities, it still remains true that mortality comparisons are effected most completely by detailed examinations of the rates of mortality for each sex at each age or age group--to which a careful analyst would certainly turn when he has been alerted by any unusual standardized rate or in any circumstances of notable importance." Assuming that the current conditions of unemployment and economic stagnation in Britain are "circumstances of notable importance", it is incumbent upon those interested in the problem to seek the resources to pursue it with data specified for age and sex. Then it will be possible to determine more precisely the extent of economic effects, and other effects, on mortality and to understand which subgroups are most harmed and in need of special consideration.

The mortality rates used in these analyses, except for infant mortality, were standardized for age and sex by the direct method. The standard population is the U.S. for 1950; the age/sex specific death rates are those of the respective regions of the U.K. for the years shown, usually 1955-1976. These rates are, therefore, a kind of index number which differs from the crude rate (number of deaths divided by population) that is often reported as a summary measure of mortality for a population.

The ideal choice in this situation, as Wolfenden advised, would have been to use rates <u>specified</u> by age and sex and to calculate separate equations for each series of rates. This procedure, though superior technically, would have greatly increased the cost of the project because, depending on the number of age groups used, there would have been between 20 and 30 equations for each one in the present report (10-15 age groups x 2 sexes = 20-30 total). The money to run that many equations through the computer for each of the causes of death (or even a few of them) was simply unavailable. Therefore, we took the practical step, from a financial standpoint, of standardizing the rates to provide a summary measure of mortality in each year for each region, a measure the would not be affected by the aging of the population nor changes in the sex ratio at any age.

In addition to providing a summary death rate for each year for each cause, the standardization procedure does allow us to estimate the effects of various economic and social changes on the mortality rates in any region. In particular, we can address the questions of what conditions are related to mortality change and in which direction the relationship goes. These equations have all been tested for stability over time, using the Chow test. They were subjected to other statistical tests for significance of individual variables, significance of the equation as a whole, autocorrelation of residuals, etc.

The coefficients, however, are being asked to express in summary fashion (that is, by some kind of weighted average) the effects of predictors on persons at different ages and of two sexes--effects that often will vary by sex and age. This means the estimates will usually be less precise than they could be if the dependent variables were specified. Then effects of each predictor on a given mortality rate could be estimated separately for each age/sex group. The sum over all ages could be used to estimate the total effect of specified changes in an independent variable. This would be a desirable step, but it cannot be done with the analyses in hand.

The work to date does show, however, which variables would be likely to be effective predictors for most age/sex groups. Knowing this allows the research to continue in a productive direction, without having to test as many different equations as would need to be tested in the absence of the completed preliminary work. As a result of this work, it is clear that recession and economic growth, as well as health-related behaviors and health services, have had important associations over the 22-year period ending in 1976 with mortality rates from many causes, and for total mortality through 1979. This is important information as a basis for proceeding with more detailed investigation of the still unanswered questions.

SUMMARY

This paper discusses a first-stage analysis of the link of unemployment rates, as well as other economic, social and environmental health risk factors, to mortality rates in post-War Scotland.

This analysis is done within the context of an international study of the impact of economic change on mortality patterns in industrialized countries. After an initial series of studies in the United States, the basic "economic change model of mortality" was further developed and tested for England and Wales. Replications and additional development are now being carried on for Scotland. The background and initial results of the Scotland versus England and Wales comparison are reviewed in the present paper.

The mortality patterns examined include total and infant mortality and, by cause: cardiovascular (total), cerebrovascular and heart disease, cirrhosis of the liver, suicide, homicide and motor vehicle accidents.

Among the most prominent factors which beneficially influence post-War mortality patterns in Scotland as well as in England and Wales, are economic growth and stability and health service availability. A principal detrimental factor to health is, conversely, a high rate of unemployment. Among the additional detrimental risk factors to mortality trends are such behavioral factors as cigarette consumption and heavy use of alcohol. Environmental factors, such as unusually cold winter temperatures, also influence mortality rates adversely, especially in Scotland.

The reason that the unemployment rate is an important influence on mortality rates is that it is a general and sensitive indicator of the extent of the recession phase of the business cycle. The stressful effects of recession, as measured by the unemployment rate, are on the employed as well as on the unemployed and their dependents.

The employed population experiences substantial stresses of work and economic insecurity as a result of: (a) the threat of loss or damage to livelihood, career and social standing; (b) greatly intensified competition among firms for economic survival resulting in increased anxiety, time pressure, and work overload; (c) a general decline in confidence and diminished ability to plan for the future—especially as regards family formation and residential mobility; and (d) a deterioration in working conditions.

TABLE 1

MULTIPLE REGRESSION OF TOTAL MORTALITY RATES** ON ECONOMIC AND HEALTH RISK FACTORS, ENGLAND AND WALES, AND SCOTLAND: 1954 - 1976

	Exp Trend Real PCI*	Annual Changes Real PCI*	Unemployment Rate	Unemployment Male 20-40 Ratio	Unemployment Male 40+ Ratio	Unemployment Rate U.K.
ENGLAND & WALES						
Coefficient	-0.0132	-0.00338	0.355	5.099	7.250	φ
T Value	(10.206)c	(-1.899)a	(3.197)b	(7.675)c	(7.865)c	
Optimum Lag	0	0	1	2	2	
SCOTLAND						
Coefficient	-0.0248	φ	φ	0.704	.840	31.623
T Value	(-7.067)c			(2.351)a	(2.340)a	(3.160)b
Optimum Lag	0			1	0	6

TABLE 1 - continued

	Average Weekly Hours Mfg.*	Cigarette Consumption per Capita*	Spirits Consumption Ratio*	National Health Service Exp % Govt Expenditures	Constant	R^2	D.W.†	F
ENGLAND & WALES								
Coefficient	φ	0.00272	φ	-20.558	-3.534	.974	1.903	77.8 c
T Value		(8.730)c		(-8.604)c	(-1.552)			
Optimum Lag		5		0				
SCOTLAND								
Coefficient	-0.3444	0.00295	10.095	-14.016	32.759	.952	2.677	32.6 c
T Value	(-2.903)b	(4.676)c	(4.762)c	(-2.911)b	(4.581)c			
Optimum Lag	0	2	0	0	0			

*United Kingdom (Other data are specific to England and Wales, and Scotland, respectively.)

**Age and sex adjusted

φ T value near 0; variable subsequently omitted from the equation

† Cochrane-Orcutt technique used to minimize residual autocorrelation

a - $p < .05$
b - $p < .01$
c - $p < .001$

TABLE 2A

MULTIPLE REGRESSION OF TOTAL CARDIOVASCULAR DISEASE MORTALITY RATES**
ON ECONOMIC AND HEALTH RISK FACTORS, ENGLAND AND
WALES, AND SCOTLAND: 1955 - 1976

	Exp Trend Real PCI*	Annual Changes Real PCI*	Unemployment Rate	Unemployment Males 20-40 Ratio	Average Weekly Hours Mfg.*	Cigarette Consumption Per Capita*	Spirits Consumption Ratio*
ENGLAND & WALES							
Coefficient	-0.0084	ϕ	.0329	0.201	-0.217	0.0006	1.706
T Value	(-11.294)c		(6.189)c	(2.995)c	(-5.826)c	(4.292)b	(4.498)c
Optimum Lag	0		1	3	0	5	1
SCOTLAND							
Coefficient	-0.0092	-0.0040	0.0096	0.560	ϕ	0.0013	0.665
T Value	(-21.843)c	(-7.265)c	(5.482)c	(14.215)c		(13.716)q	(2.245)a
Optimum Lag	0	0	0	2		5	0

TABLE 2A - continued

	National Health Service Exp & Govt Expenditures	Feb Temp	Constant	R^2	D.W.†	F
ENGLAND & WALES						
Coefficient	-4.611	-0.0082	18.302	.979	2.083	55.755c
T Value	(-5.632)c	(-3.461)b	(8.418)c			
Optimum Lag	1	0				
SCOTLAND						
Coefficient	ϕ	-0.0159	7.835	.987	2.246	139.333c
T Value		(-6.143)c	(57.195)c			
Optimum Lag		0				

TABLE 2B

MULTIPLE REGRESSION OF HEART DISEASE MORTALITY RATES**
ON ECONOMIC AND HEALTH RISK FACTORS, ENGLAND AND
WALES, AND SCOTLAND: 1955 - 1976

	Exp Trend Real PCI*	Annual Changes Real PCI*	Unemployment Rate	Unemployment Male 20-40 Ratio	Average Weekly Hours Mfg.*	Cigarette Consumption Per Capita*	Spirits Consumption Ratio*
ENGLAND & WALES							
Coefficient	-0.0058	-0.0011	0.0240	0.169	-0.160	0.0004	1.618
T Value	(-11.126)c	(-2.060)a	(6.467)c	(3.602)b	(-6.147)c	(3.924)b	(6.097)c
Optimum Lag	0	0	1	3	0	5	1
SCOTLAND							
Coefficient	-0.0071	-0.0033	0.0085	0.511	-0.308	0.747	1.616
T Value	(-22.154)c	(-8.010)c	(7.250)c	(19.293)c	(-1.878)a	(8.850)c	(4.778)c
Optimum Lag	0	0	0	2	0	5	0

TABLE 2B - continued

	National Health Service Exp & Govt Expenditures	Feb Temp	Constant	R^2	D.W.†	F
ENGLAND & WALES						
Coefficient	-3.033	-0.0082	13.119	.966	2.167	34.365c
T Value	(-5.290)c	(-3.461)b	(8.615)c			
Optimum Lag	1	0				
SCOTLAND						
Coefficient	ϕ	-0.155	7.157	.986	2.45	106.669c
T Value		(-8.6)c	(7.440)c			
Optimum Lag		0				

a – $p < .05$
b – $p < .01$
c – $p < .001$

ϕ T value near 0; variable subsequently omitted from the equation
† Cochrane-Orcutt technique used to minimize residual autocorrelation

*United Kingdom (Other data are specific to England and Wales, and Scotland, respectively.)
**Age and sex adjusted

TABLE 2 C

MULTIPLE REGRESSION OF CEREBROVASCULAR DISEASE MORTALITY RATES**
ON ECONOMIC AND HEALTH RISK FACTORS, ENGLAND AND
WALES, AND SCOTLAND

	Exp Trend Real PCI*	Annual Change Real PCI*	Unemployment Rate	Unemployment Male 40+ Ratio	Unemployment Rate U.K.	Average Weekly Hours Mfg.*	Cigarette Consumption per Capita*
ENGLAND & WALES (1954-1976)							
Coefficient	-0.0048	-0.0054	0.0116	0.0624	1.202	0.0847	0.00018
T Value	(-7.348)c	(-1.914)a	(6.880)c	(2.861)b	(2.743)b	(-9.421)c	(4.414)b
Optimum Lag	0	1	1	0	11	0	5
SCOTLAND (1955-1976)							
Coefficient	-.288	∅	0.0035	∅	∅	∅	.00039
T Value	(-12.952)c		(2.688)a				(6.667)c
Optimum Lag	0		1				5

TABLE 2 C - continued

	National Health Service Exp & Govt Expenditures	Hosp. Bed Utilization Per Capita	Constant	R^2	D.W.†	F
ENGLAND & WALES						
Coefficient	-2.390	-167.371	9.397	.9914	2.524	153.409c
T Value	(-5.60)c	(-3.132)b	(7.806)c			
Optimum Lag	0	0				
SCOTLAND						
Coefficient	-15.890	∅	2.615	.971	2.033	132.762c
T Value	(-2.347)a		(33.719)c			
Optimum Lag	0					

*United Kingdom (Other data are specific to England and Wales, and Scotland, respectively.)

**Age and sex adjusted

∅ T value near 0; variable subsequently omitted from the equation

† Cochrane-Orcutt technique used to minimize residual autocorrelation

a - p < .05
b - p < .01
c - p < .001

TABLE 3

MULTIPLE REGRESSION OF CIRRHOSIS OF THE LIVER MORTALITY RATES**
ON ECONOMIC AND HEALTH RISK FACTORS, ENGLAND AND
WALES, AND SCOTLAND

	Exp Trend Real PCI*	Unemployment Rate	Unemployment Male 20-40 Ratio	Unemployment Male 40+ Ratio	Average Weekly Hours Mfg.*	Spirits Consumption Ratio*	Beer Consumption Ratio*
ENGLAND & WALES (1954-1976)							
Coefficient	-0.006	0.241	4.103	7.498	-0.657	22.849	0.833
T Value	(-2.208)a	(6.822)c	(5.252)c	(6.400)c	(-5.366)c	(11.176)c	(4.026)c
Optimum Lag	0	1	1	1	0	1	3
SCOTLAND (1955-1976)							
Coefficient	-0.0008	.003	ø	ø	-0.02	0.806	0.041
T Value	(-2.321)a	(3.657)b			(-2.48)a	(4.470)c	(4.421)c
Optimum Lag	0	1			0	1	1

TABLE 3 - continued

	Wine Consumption Ratio*	National Health Service Exp % Govt Expenditures	Constant	R^2	D.W.†	F
ENGLAND & WALES						
Coefficient	ø	ø	6.592	.981	2.358	96.087c
T Value			(1.155)	.984		
Optimum Lag			0			
SCOTLAND						
Coefficient	.252	-1.333	0.742	.873	2.049	10.365b
T Value	(2.520)a	(-3.044)b	(1.277)			
Optimum Lag	2	0	0			

*United Kingdom (Other data are specific to England and Wales, and Scotland, respectively.)

**Age and sex adjusted

ø T value near 0; variable subsequently omitted from the equation

† Cochrane-Orcutt technique used to minimize residual autocorrelation

a - $p < .05$
b - $p < .01$
c - $p < .001$

TABLE 4

MULTIPLE REGRESSION OF SUICIDE MORTALITY RATES**
ON ECONOMIC AND HEALTH RISK FACTORS, ENGLAND AND
WALES, AND SCOTLAND

	Exp Trend Real PCI*	Unemployment Rate	Unemployment 20-40 Ratio (Male)	Unemployment Male 40+ Ratio	Average Weekly Hours Mfg*	Bankruptcy	Alcohol Cons. Per Capita*
ENGLAND & WALES (1954-1976)							
Coefficient	-0.006	ø	0.014	ø	ø	0.165	0.013
T Value	(-6.259)c		(3.615)b			(3.302)b	(2.897)b
Optimum Lag	0		0			2	1
SCOTLAND (1955-1976)							
Coefficient	-0.00030	0.00068	ø	0.291	-0.00717	ø	ø
T Value	(-5.602)c	(2.839)b		(4.839)c	(-3.777)b		
Optimum Lag	0	2		0	0		

TABLE 4 — continued

	Spirits Consumption Ratio*	Feb Temp	Constant	R^2	D.W.†	F
ENGLAND AND WALES						
Coefficient	0.187	ø	0.424	.983	1.600	173.292 c
T Value	(3.788) b		(8.363)c			
Optimum Lag	0		0			
SCOTLAND						
Coefficient	0.240	-0.000505	0.629	.765	2.123	7.596 c
T Value	(5.327) c	(-1.776)	(4.955) c			
Optimum Lag	0	0	0			

*United Kingdom (Other data are specific to England and Wales, and Scotland, respectively.)

**Age and sex adjusted

ø T value near 0; variable subsequently omitted from the equation

† Cochrane-Orcutt technique used to minimize residual autocorrelation

a - p < .05
b - p < .01
c - p < .001

TABLE 5

MULTIPLE REGRESSION OF HOMICIDE MORTALITY RATES**
ON ECONOMIC AND HEALTH RISK FACTORS, ENGLAND AND
WALES, AND SCOTLAND: 1955 - 1976

	Annual Changes Real PCI*	Unemployment Rate	Unemployment Male <20 Ratio	Unemployment Male 40+ Ratio	Spirits Consumption Ratio*	% Pop. 15-24	Average Weekly Hours Mfg.
ENGLAND & WALES							
Coefficient	-0.00002	0.001	0.0001	0.005	0.033	∅	∅
T Value	(-4.520)c	(4.661)c	(3.255)b	(5.814)c	(9.774)c		
Optimum Lag	1	0	1	1	0		
SCOTLAND							
Coefficient	-0.0001	0.0001	0.004	0.010	0.031	0.168	-0.0009
T Value	(-6.795)c	(3.772)c	(2.556)b	(4.504)c	(2.329)a	(2.06)a	(-1.367)
Optimum Lag	0	1	1	3	1	0	0

TABLE 5 - continued

	Constant	R^2	D.W.†	F
ENGLAND & WALES				
Coefficient	-0.006	.957	1.950	67.044 c
T Value	(-4.416)c			
SCOTLAND				
Coefficient	0.003	.956	2.562	40.621 c
T Value	(0.093)			

*United Kingdom (Other data are specific to England and Wales, and Scotland, respectively.)

**Age and sex adjusted

∅ T value near 0; variable subsequently omitted from the equation

† Cochrane-Orcutt technique used to minimize residual autocorrelation

a - p < .05
b - p < .01
c - p < .001

TABLE 6

MULTIPLE REGRESSION OF MOTOR VEHICLE ACCIDENT MORTALITY RATES** ON ECONOMIC AND HEALTH RISK FACTORS, ENGLAND AND WALES, AND SCOTLAND: 1955 - 1976

	Exp Trend Real PCI*	Unemployment Rate	Unemployment Male 20-40 Ratio	Spirits Consumption Ratio*	Miles Traveled Per Capita*
ENGLAND & WALES					
Coefficient	-0.0011	0.0035	ø	0.362	49.361
T Value	(-4.946)c	(4.285)c		(2.478)a	(3.876)c
Optimum Lag	0	2		2	0
SCOTLAND					
Coefficient	-0.0005	ø	0.033	0.197	33.889
T Value	(-4.700)c		(3.667)b	(2.125)a	(4.416)c
Optimum Lag	0		2	3	0

TABLE 6 - continued

	% Population Age 15-24	Constant	R^2	D.W.†	F
ENGLAND & WALES					
Coefficient	0.871	0.651	.883	1.853	22.8 c
T Value	(2.212)a	(4.521)c			
Optimum Lag					
SCOTLAND					
Coefficient	1.277	0.170	.955	1.958	63.816c
T Value	(2.514)a	(1.540)			
Optimum Lag	1				

*United Kingdom (Other data are specific to England and Wales, and Scotland, respectively.)

**Age and sex adjusted

ø T value near 0; variable subsequently omitted from the equation

† Cochrane-Orcutt technique used to minimize residual autocorrelation

a - p < .05
b - p < .01
c - p < .001

TABLE 7

MULTIPLE REGRESSION OF INFANT MORTALITY RATES
ON ECONOMIC AND HEALTH RISK FACTORS, ENGLAND AND
WALES, AND SCOTLAND, 1955 - 1967

	Exp. Trend Real PCI*	Unemployment Rate	Unemployment Females 20-40 Ratio	Average Weekly Hours Mfg.*	Alcohol Consumption Per Capita*	Cigarette Consumption Per Capita*	National Health Service Exp & Govt Expenditures
ENGLAND & WALES							
Coefficient	-0.0652	0.0810	1.647	-0.521	0.676	0.00288	71.663
T Value	(-10.210)c	(4.239)c	(2.561)b	(-2.825)b	(2.648)b	(4.239)c	(-10.551)c
Optimum Lag	0	1	0		2	2	1
SCOTLAND							
Coefficient	-0.117	ø	3.781	ø	2.781	0.0104	-1267.16
T Value	(-12.201)c		(2.939)b		(4.550)c	(5.448)c	(-4.912)c
Optimum Lag	0		0		2	2	0

TABLE 7 - continued

	Constant	R^2	D.W.†	F
ENGLAND & WALES				
Coefficient	82.586	.994	2.384	309.8c
T Value	(7.209)c			
SCOTLAND				
Coefficient	70.030	.986	2.207	216.4c
T Value	(16.183)c			

*United Kingdom (Other data are specific to England and Wales, and Scotland, respectively.)

**Age and sex adjusted

ø T value near 0; variable subsequently omitted from the equation

† Cochrane-Orcutt technique used to minimize residual autocorrelation

a - p <.05
b - p <.01
c - p <.001

TABLE 8

MULTIPLE REGRESSION OF TOTAL MORTALITY RATES ** ON ECONOMIC AND HEALTH RISK FACTORS, ENGLAND AND WALES, AND SCOTLAND: 1954-1979

	Exp Trend Real PCI*	Unemployment Rate	Unemployment Rate U.K.	Average Weekly Hours Mfg. *	Annual Changes Real PCI* (Uncontrolled)
ENGLAND & WALES					
Coefficient	-.436	24.396	10.361	-.358	∅
T Value	(-5.284)c	(3.613)c	(2.182)b	(-4.033)c	
Optimum Lag	0	1	10	0	
SCOTLAND					
Coefficient	-.171E-01	.123	19.835	.914E-03	.806E-02
T Value	(-6.882)c	(3.315)c	(2.916)c	(-.822)a	(4.182)c
Optimum Lag	0	2	6	0	2

TABLE 8 - continued

	Cigarette Consumption Per Capita*	Spirits Consumption Ratio	National Health Service Exp % Govt Expenditures	Hospital Bed Utilization Per Capita *	Feb Temp
ENGLAND & WALES					
Coefficient	.136E-02	∅	-13.176	-1880.28	-.160E-01
T Value	(3.439)c		(-3.219)c	(-3.470)	(-2.030)b
Optimum Lag	5		1	0	0
SCOTLAND					
Coefficient	.914E-03	5.003	-104.711	-740.457	-.597E-01
T Value	(2.754)c	(2.807)c	(-3.593)	(-3.798)	(-5.135)
Optimum Lag	2	0	1	0	0

TABLE 8 - continued

	Constant	RHO†	R^2	R^2 in Chgs	D.W.†	F
ENGLAND & WALES						
Coefficient	69.872	-.509	.954	.815	2.105	41.539c
T Value	(5.278)c	(-2.955)c				
Optimum Lag	0					
SCOTLAND						
Coefficient	38.378	-.757	.981	.938	2.503	71.416c
T Value	(4.305)c	(-5.796)c				
Optimum Lag	0					

*United Kingdom (Other data are specific to England and Wales, and Scotland, respectively.)

**Age and sex adjusted

∅ T value near 0; variable subsequently omitted from the equation

† Cochrane-Orcutt technique used to minimize residual autocorrelation

a - $p < .05$
b - $p < .01$
c - $p < .001$

TABLE 9

BIBLIOGRAPHY

VITAL STATISTICS

Population:

1952 - 77   Annual Epidemiological and Vital Statistics. WHO, Geneva. Superceded in 1962 by WHO World Health Statistics Annual.

Mortality:

1952 - 77   Annual Epidemiological and Vital Statistics.

ECONOMICS

Unemployment:

United Kingdom - "Numbers Unemployed." Annual Abstract of Statistics. Central Statistical Office, HMSO, London.

England & Wales, Scotland - "Numbers Umemployed: Industrial Analysis"
- 1948 - 1965 - Ministry of Labour Gazette - "Unemployment by Industry"
- 1966 - 1968 - Ministry of Labour Gazette - "Unemployment by Occupation"
- 1969 - 1976 - Labour Statistics Yearbook - "Unemployed by Standard Industrial Classification"

Per Capita Income:

United Kingdom - "Personal Disposable Income." Annual Abstract of Statistics.

Average Weekly Hours:

Great Britain - "Average Weekly and Hourly Earnings and Hours," Annual Abstract of Statistics.

England & Wales - British Economy Key Statistics, 1900 - 70.

G.N.P.:

United Kingdom - Annual Abstract of Statistics.

Balance of Payments:

United Kingdom
- 1949 - 69 - "Balance of Payments, visible balance." B.R. Mitchell. European Historical Statistics, 2nd edition. Facts on File, New York, 1981.
- 1970 - 79 - "Balance of Payments, net trade." Main Economic Indicators, Historical Statistics 1960 - 79. OECD, Paris, 1980.

TABLE 9   A

ECONOMICS - (Continued)

Bankruptcies:

England & Wales, Scotland - "Bankruptcies" ("Sequestrations" in Scotland). Annual Abstract of Statistics.

Government Expenditure:

United Kingdom - "Summary of Government Expenditure on Social Services and Housing." Annual Abstract of Statistics.

HEALTH

National Health Service as % Government Expenditure:

"Government expenditure on the national health service." Annual Abstract of Statistics.

Hospital Bed Utilization:

England & Wales - Hospital and Family Practitioner Services." Annual Abstract of Statistics.

Scotland - "Hospital and Primary Care Services." Annual Abstract of Statistics.

MOTOR VEHICLES

Licenced Motor Vehicles - Annual Abstract of Statistics.

Miles Travelled "Passenger Transport in Britain: estimated passenger kilometers." Annual Abstract of Statistics.

ALCOHOL AND TOBACCO

Alcohol Consumption:

United Kingdom - Consumption by type for beer, wine & distilled spirits.

1950 - 72 - International Statistics on Alcoholic Beverages, 1950 - 72. Finnish Foundation for Alcohol Studies.

1973 - 75 - Hoeveel Alcoholhoudende Dranken Worden er in de Wereld Gedronken? Produktschap voor Gedistiller - de Dranken, Schiedam, Netherlands.

Past 1975 - Updates obtained by personal communication with the Distilled Spirits Council (DISCUS).

TABLE 9 B

ALCOHOL AND TOBACCO - (Continued)

Tobacco Consumption:

United Kingdom - Consumption per adult; number of cigaretts.
1950 - 74 - D.H. Beese, (Ed.). Tobacco Consumption in Various Countries, 4th edition. Tobacco Research Council, London.

past 1974 - Updates obtained by personal communication with the Tobacco Research Council and the Unit for the Study of Health Policy, Guy's Hospital, London, U.K.

OTHER

Average Monthly Temperature:

England & Wales, Scotland - "Mean daily air temperature at Sea Level." Annual Abstract of Statistics.

TABLE 10

REVISION IN WHO ICD CODE CLASSIFICATION
OF CAUSES OF DEATH

	1952	1965	1968
All causes (total mortality)	--	--	--
Cirrhosis of Liver	B 37	A 105	A 102
Motor Vehicle Accidents	BE 47	AE 138	AE 138
Suicide and Self-inflicted Injury	BE 49	AE 148	AE 147
Homicide and Injury Purposely Inflicted by Other Persons; Legal Intervention & Injury Resulting from Operations of War	BE 50	AE 149, 150	AE 148, 150
Cardiovascular Diseases	B 22, B 24-29	A 70, A 79-84	A 80-85
Heart Disease	B 24-29	A 79-84	A 80-85
Cerebrovascular Disease	B 22	A 70	A 70-A 85

TABLE 11
PREDICTIONS BASED ON EQUATIONS* FOR TOTAL MORTALITY RATES**
DURING 1955-1976

ENGLAND and WALES

FROM	TO	PERCENT ERROR	FROM	TO	PERCENT ERROR	FROM	TO	PERCENT ERROR	FROM	TO	PERCENT ERROR
1975	1976	1.0	1974	1975	0.1	1973	1974	6.5	1972	1973	0.3
1974	1976	0.8	1973	1975	0.1	1972	1974	6.4			
1973	1976	0.8	1972	1975	0.07						
1972	1976	1.0									

SCOTLAND

FROM	TO	PERCENT ERROR	FROM	TO	PERCENT ERROR	FROM	TO	PERCENT ERROR	FROM	TO	PERCENT ERROR
1975	1976	0.1	1974	1975	0.2	1973	1974	3.5	1972	1973	1.4
1974	1976	0.3	1973	1975	1.4	1972	1974	3.5			
1973	1976	0.5	1972								
1972	1976	0.4									

* See Table 1

** Age and Sex Adjusted

TABLE 12

Chow Tests Measuring Lack of Stability
Of Multiple Regression Equations of Age and Sex Adjusted
Mortality Rates on Economic and Health Risk Factors,
England and Wales, and Scotland, 1955-1976

Cause of Death	Region	Degrees of Freedom	Chow Statistic	F Value at p <.05	F Value at p <.01
Total Mortality	England and Wales (1)	(8,5)	1.20	4.82	10.3
	Scotland (1)	(9,3)	1.61	8.81	27.2
Cardiovascular Disease	England and Wales	(9,2)	17.4	19.4	99.4
	Scotland	(8,4)	2.67	6.04	14.8
Cerebrovascular Disease	England and Wales	(8,4)	4.22	6.04	14.8
	Scotland	(5,10)	1.93	3.33	5.64
Heart Disease	England and Wales	(9,2)	10.7	19.4	99.4
	Scotland	(8,4)	2.10	6.04	14.8
Cirrhosis of Liver	England and Wales	(8,4)	3.91	6.04	14.8
	Scotland	(9,2)	5.78	19.4	99.4
Suicide	England and Wales	(6,8)	2.29	3.58	6.37)
	Scotland	(7,6)	5.46*	4.21	8.26
Homicide	England and Wales	(6,8)	2.19	3.58	6.37
	Scotland	(8,4)	1.76	6.04	14.8
Motor Vehicle Accidents	England and Wales	(8,4)	2.42	6.04	14.8
	Scotland	(8,4)	2.43	6.04	14.8
Infant Mortality	England and Wales	(8,4)	2.34	6.04	14.8
	Scotland	(6,8)	2.02	3.58	6.37

(1) 1954-1976
* Only indication of significantly unstable relation.

TABLE 13

HYPOTHETICAL RELATIONS BETWEEN ECONOMIC CHANGES
AND MORTALITY RATES
(Lag Periods in Years)

Mortality Rates, Age and Sex Adjusted	Economic Development	Recession and Medium Term Economic Decline						
	Exp Trend Real PCI (-)	Unemployment Rate Short (+)	Med. (+)	Unemployment Male Under 20 Ratio (+)	Unemployment Male 20-40 Ratio (+)	Unemployment Female 20-40 Ratio (+)	Unemployment Male Over 40 Ratio (+)	Annual Change Real PCI (-)	Average Weekly Hours 'Cyclic Change' (-)
Total	0	<5	6-10	--	<5	--	<5	<1	<1
Infant	0	<2	--	--	<2	<2	--	<1	<1
Chronic Disease Causes									
Cardiovascular, Total	0	<5	6-10	--	<5	--	<5	<1	<1
Cerebrovascular	0	<5	6-10	--	<5	--	<5	<1	<1
Heart	0	<5	6-10	--	<5	--	<5	<1	<1
Cirrhosis of liver	0	<5	6-10	--	<5	--	<5	<1	<1
External Causes									
Suicide	0	<2	--	--	<2	--	<2	<1	<1
Homicide	0	<2	--	<2	<2	--	<2	<1	<1
Motor Vehicle Accidents	0	<2	--	<2	<2	--	<2	<1	<1

TABLE 14

RELATIONS BETWEEN ECONOMIC CHANGES AND MORTALITY RATES
ENGLAND AND WALES, 1955-1976

(Optimum Lag in Years)

	Economic Development		Recession and Medium Term Economic Decline						
Mortality Rates Age and Sex Adjusted	Exp Trend Real PCI (-)	Unemployment Rate Short (+) / Long (+)	Unemployment Male Under 20 Ratio (+)	Unemployment Male 20-40 Ratio (+)	Unemployment Female 20-40 Ratio (+)	Unemployment Male Over 40 Ratio (+)	Annual Change Real PCI (-)	Average Weekly Hours 'Cyclic Change' (-)
Total	0	1 10	-- --	2 --	-- --	2 --	0	--
Infant	0	1 --	-- --	-- --	0	-- --	--	0
Chronic Disease Causes								
Cardiovascular, Total	0	1 --	-- --	3 --	-- --	0 --	-- --	0
Cerebrovascular	0	1 --	-- --	3 --	-- --	-- --	-- --	--
Heart	0	1 --	-- --	3 --	-- --	-- 1	-- --	0
Cirrhosis of liver	0	1 --	-- --	1 --	-- --	1	-- --	0
External Causes								
Suicide	0	-- --	-- --	0 --	-- --	-- --	-1 --	-- --
Homicide	--	0 --	1 --	-- --	-- --	1 --	-1 --	-- --
Motor vehicle accidents	0	2 --	-- --	-- --	-- --	-- --	-- --	-- --

TABLE 15

RELATIONS BETWEEN ECONOMIC CHANGES AND MORTALITY RATES
SCOTLAND, 1955-1976
(Optimum Lag in Years)

Mortality Rates, Age and Sex Adjusted	Economic Development Exp Trend Real PCI (-)	Unemployment Rate Short (+)	Unemployment Rate Long (+)	Unemployment Male Under 20 Ratio (+)	Unemployment Male 20-40 Ratio (+)	Unemployment Female 20-40 Ratio (+)	Unemployment Male Over 40 Ratio (+)	Annual Change Real PCI (-)	Average Weekly Hours 'Cyclic Change' (-)
Total	0	--	6	--	1	--	1	--	0
Infant	0	--	--	--	--	0	--	--	--
Chronic Disease Causes									
Cardiovascular, Total	0	0	--	--	2	--	--	0	--
Cerebrovascular Heart	0 0	1 0	-- --	-- --	-- 2	-- --	-- --	0 --	-- --
Cirrhosis of liver	0	1	--	--	--	--	0	--	0
External Causes									
Suicide	0 --	-- 1	-- --	0 0.	3 --	-- --	-- 3	0 0	-- 0
Homicide	-- 0	1 --	-- --	-- --	-- 2	-- --	-- --	0 --	-- --
Motor Vehicle Accidents	0	--	--	--	--	--	--	--	--

Recession and Medium Term Economic Decline

71

TABLE 16

Hypothetical Relations Between Health Risk and Health
Service Factors, and Mortality Rates
(Lag Periods in Years)

Mortality Rates Age and Sex Adjusted	Heavy Alcohol Consumption (+)		Cigarette Consumption (+)		Health Services (−)		Winter Temperature (−)
	Short	Long	Short	Long	Short	Medium	Short
Total	<5	>10	<5	>10	0,1	5	0
Infant	<2	--	<2	--	<2	--	--
Chronic Disease Causes							
Cardiovascular, Total	<5	>10	<5	>10	<5	5	0
Cerebrovascular	<5	>10	<5	>10	<5	5	0
Heart	<5	>10	<5	>10	<5	5	0
Cirrhosis of liver	<5	>10	--	--	<5	5	0
External Causes							
Suicide	<5	--	--	--	--	--	--
Homicide	<5	--	--	--	--	--	--
Motor Vehicle Accidents	<5	--	--	--	<5	--	--

TABLE 17

RELATIONS BETWEEN HEALTH RISK AND HEALTH
SERVICE FACTORS, AND MORTALITY RATES
SCOTLAND, 1955-1976
(Optimum Lag in Years)

Mortality Rates Age and Sex Adjusted	Heavy Alcohol Consumption (+)	Cigarette Consumption (+)	Health Services (−)	Winter Temperature (−)
Total	0	2	0	0
Infant	2	2	0	--
Chronic Disease Causes				
Cardiovascular, Total	0	5	--	0
Cerebrovascular	0	5	0	--
Heart	0	5	--	0
Cirrhosis of liver	1-2	--	0	--
External Causes				
Suicide	0	--	--	--
Homocide	1	--	--	--
Motor Vehicle Accidents	3	--	--	--

TABLE 18

RELATIONS BETWEEN HEALTH RISK AND HEALTH
SERVICE FACTORS, AND MORTALITY RATES
ENGLAND AND WALES, 1955-1976

(Optimum Lag in Years)

Mortality Rates Age and Sex Adjusted	Heavy Alcohol Consumption (+)	Cigarette Consumption (+)	Health Services (-)	Winter Temperature (-)
Total	--	5	0	--
Infant	2	2	1	--
Chronic Disease Causes				
Cardiovascular, Total	1	5	1	0
Cerebrovascular	--	--	1	--
Heart	1	5	1	0
Cirrhosis of liver	1-3	--	--	--
External Causes				
Suicide	0	--	--	--
Homicide	0	--	--	--
Motor Vehicle Accidents	2			

TABLE 19

MULTIPLE REGRESSION OF TOTAL MORTALITY RATES** ON ECONOMIC AND HEALTH RISK FACTORS, ENGLAND AND WALES, AND SCOTLAND; 1955 - 1979

POOLED EQUATION (N = 50)

	Exp Trend Real PCI*	Regional Income Ratio (Region./U.K.)	Unemployment Rate	Unemployment Male 20-40 Ratio	Unemployment Male 40+ Ratio
ENGLAND & WALES AND SCOTLAND					
Coefficient	-0.0127	-3.328	0.0352	0.986	0.981
T Value	(-9.591)c	(-3.678)b	(2.824)a	(3.815)b	(2.148)a
Optimum Lag	0	0	2	1	2

TABLE 19 - continued

	Cigarette Consumption Per Capita*	National Health Service Exp & Govt Expenditures	Feb Temp	Constant	R^2	R^2 in Chgs	D.W.†	F
ENGLAND & WALES AND SCOTLAND								
Coefficient	0.00100	-4.526	-0.0158	15.417	.957	.714	2.081	109.583c
T Value	(2.953)a	(-2.565)a	(-1.868)a	(13.797)c				
Optimum Lag	5	1						

*United Kingdom (Other data are specific to England and Wales, and Scotland, respectively.)

**Age and sex adjusted

∅ T value near 0; variable subsequently omitted from the equation

† Cochrane-Orcutt technique used to minimize residual autocorrelation

a - p < .05
b - p < .01
c - p < .001

TABLE 20

MULTIPLE REGRESSION OF CARDIOVASCULAR MORTALITY RATES**
ON ECONOMIC AND HEALTH RISK FACTORS, ENGLAND AND
WALES, AND SCOTLAND: 1955-1979
POOLED EQUATIONS (N=50)

	Exp Trend Real PCI*	Annual Changes Real PCI*	Unemployment Rate	Unemployment Male 20-40 Ratio	Average Weekly Hours Mfg.*	Cigarette Consumption Per Capita*
ENGLAND & WALES AND SCOTLAND						
Coefficient	-0.00959	-0.00069	0.00552	0.180	-0.176	0.00047
T Value	(6.882)c	(-1.017)	(2.344)a	(2.137)a	(-4.025)b	(2.376)a
Optimum Lag	0	0	0,1	2,3	0	5

TABLE 20 - continued

	Spirits Consumption Ratio*	National Health Service Exp % Govt Expenditures	Feb Temp	Constant	R^2	R^2 in Chgs	D.W.†	F
ENGLAND & WALES AND SCOTLAND								
Coefficient	3.989	-5.912	-0.0183	17.636	.970	.678	2.176	137.117
T Value	(4.010)c	(-10.156)c	(-4.494)c	(6.882)c				
Optimum Lag	0	0,1	0					

*United Kingdom (Other data are specific to England and Wales, and Scotland, respectively.)

**Age and sex adjusted

∅ T value near 0; variable subsequently omitted from the equation

† Cochrane-Orcutt technique used to minimize residual autocorrelation

a - $p < .05$
b - $p < .01$
c - $p < .001$

TABLE 21

MULTIPLE REGRESSION OF TOTAL MORTALITY RATES**
ON ECONOMIC AND HEALTH RISK FACTORS,
GREAT BRITAIN: 1954 - 1979

	Exp Trend Real PCI*	Annual Changes Real PCI*	Unemployment Rate	Unemployment Male 20-40 Ratio	Unemployment Male 40+ Ratio
GREAT BRITAIN					
Coefficient	-0.02	-0.004	0.097	1.16	1.37
T Value	(-7.59)c	(-2.55)a	(4.56)b	(4.24)b	(2.96)b
Optimum Lag	0	0	2	1	2

TABLE 21 - continued

	Average Weekly Hours Mfg.*	Cigarette Consumption Per Capita*	National Health Service Exp & Govt Expenditures	Feb Temp
GREAT BRITAIN				
Coefficient	-0.34	0.001	-7.05	-0.02
T Value	(-3.06)b	(2.25)b	(-2.55)a	(-2.79)a
Optimum Lag		5	1	0

TABLE 21 - continued

	Constant	R^2	R^2 in Chgs	D.W.†	F
GREAT BRITAIN					
Coefficient	32.43	.971	.882	2.12	56.7c
T Value	(4.91)b				
Optimum Lag					

*United Kingdom (Other data are specific to England and Wales, and Scotland, respectively.)

**Age and sex adjusted

∅ T value near 0; variable subsequently omitted from the equation

† Cochrane-Orcutt technique used to minimize residual autocorrelation

a - $p < .05$
b - $p < .01$
c - $p < .001$

TABLE 22

MULTIPLE REGRESSION OF TOTAL CARDIOVASCULAR DISEASE MORTALITY RATES**
ON ECONOMIC AND HEALTH RISK FACTORS,
GREAT BRITAIN: 1955-1979

	Exp Trend Real PCI*	Annual Changes Real PCI*	Unemployment Rate	Unemployment Males 20-40 Ratio	Average Weekly Hours Mfg.*	Cigarette Consumption Per Capita*
GREAT BRITAIN						
Coefficient	-0.009	-0.001	0.009	0.18	-0.18	0.0006
T Value	(-9.56)c	(-1.66)	(4.01)b	(3.62)b	(-6.17)c	(3.52)b
Optimum Lag	0	0	0,1	2,3	0	5

TABLE 22 - continued

	Spirits Consumption Ratio*	National Health Service Exp & Govt Expenditures	Feb Temp	Constant	R^2	R^2 in Chgs	D.W.†	F
GREAT BRITAIN								
Coefficient	3.18	-7.24	-0.01	17.22	.979	.915	2.288	71.80c
T Value	(4.97)c	(-5.26)c	(-4.33)b	(8.26)c				
Optimum Lag	0	1	0					

*United Kingdom (Other data are specific to England and Wales, and Scotland, respectively.)

**Age and sex adjusted

ø T value near 0; variable subsequently omitted from the equation

† Cochrane-Orcutt technique used to minimize residual autocorrelation

a - p < .05
b - p < .01
c - p < .001

FIGURE 1

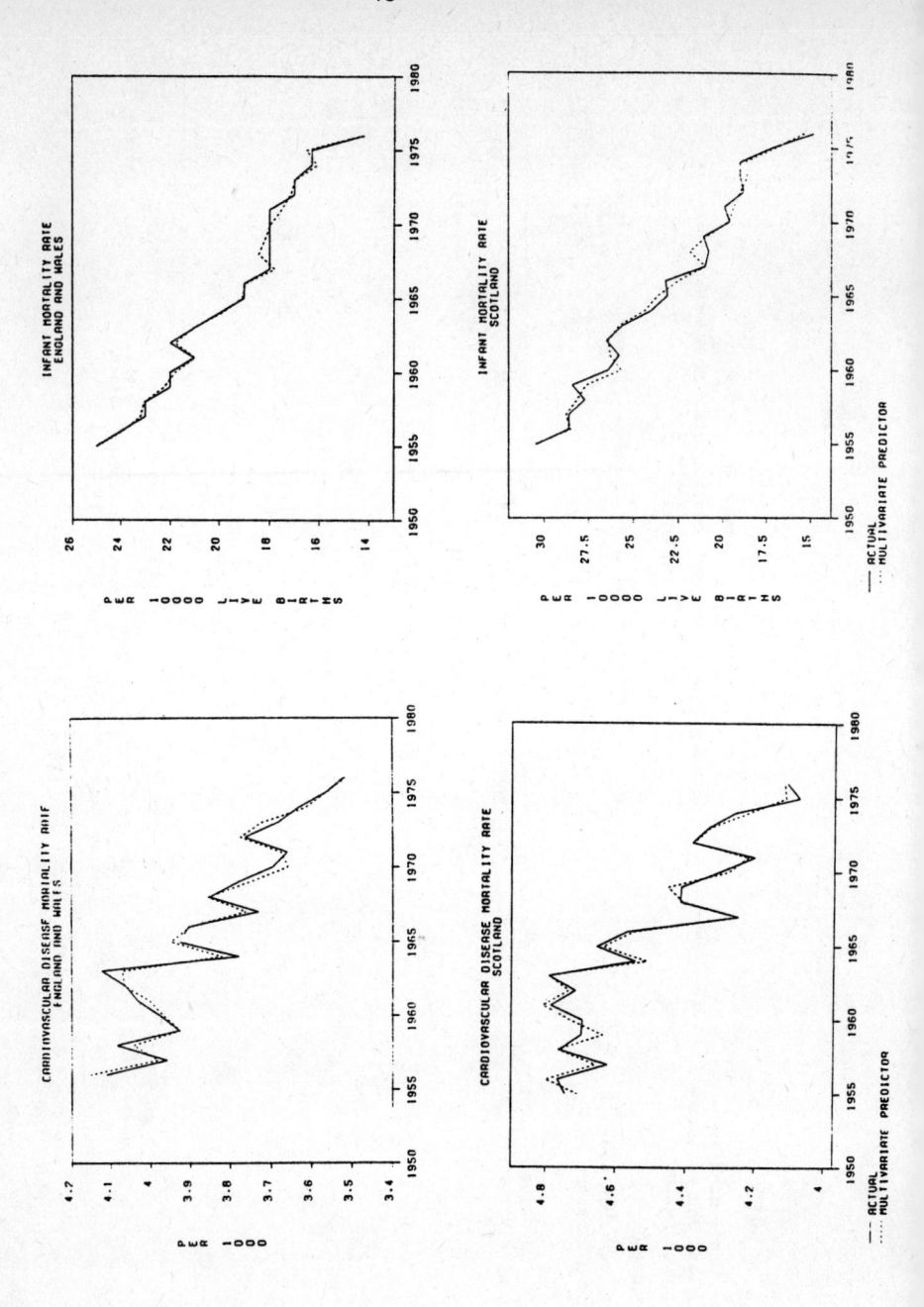

FIGURE 2

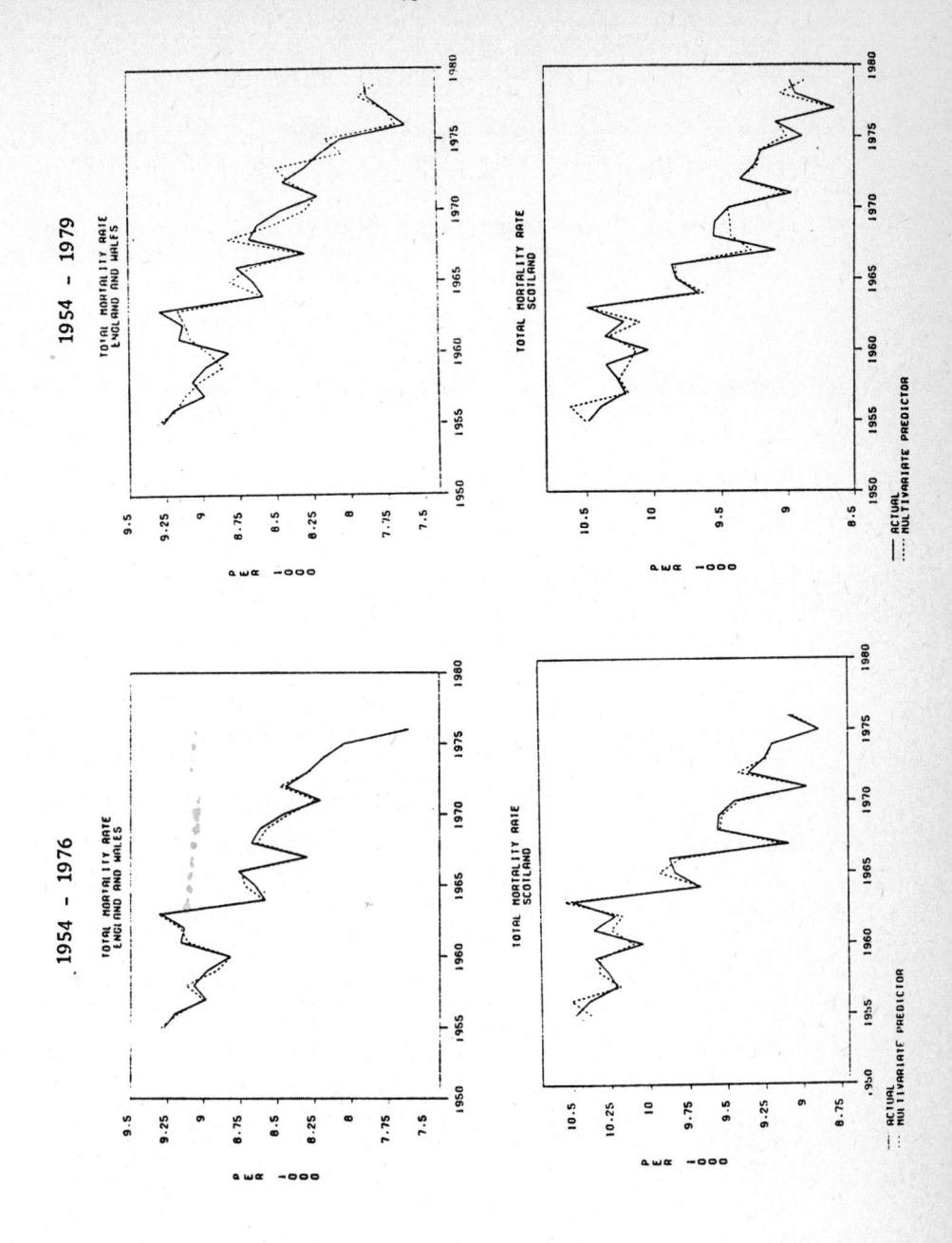

REFERENCES

(1) Occupational Mortality: The Registrar General's Decennial Supplement for England, 1970-72 London. London: H.M. Stationery Office (1976).

(2) COCHRANE, A., ST. LEGER, A.S., MOORE, F.: Health Services 'Input' and Mortality 'Output' in Developed Countries. Journal of Epidemiology and Community Health 32, 200-205 (1978).

(3) PRESTON, S.H.: Mortality Patterns in National Populations. New York: Academic Press (1976).

(4) BRENNER, M.H.: Mortality and the National Economy: A Review and the Experience of England and Wales, 1936-76. The Lancet, September 15, 568-573 (1979)

(5) GARDNER, M.J., CRAWFORD, M.D., MORRIS, J.N.: Patterns of Mortality in Middle and Early Old Age in the County Boroughs of England and Wales. British Journal of Preventive and Social Medicine 23, 133-40 (1964).

(6) BRENNER, M.H.: Industrialization and Economic Growth: Estimates of Their Effects on the Health of Populations. In: Assessing the Contributions of the Social Sciences to Health (Eds.: M.H. Brenner, A. Mooney, T. Nagy). Boulder, Colorado: Westview Press (1980).

(7) EEC COMMISSION: Report on the Development of the Social Situation in the Community in 1974. Brussels, Luxembourg: EEC 61-62 (1975).

(8) Ibid, p.7

(9) MORIYAMA, I.M., KRUEGER, D.E., STAMLER, J.: Cardiovascular Disease in the United States. Cambridge, Mass.: Harvard University Press (1971)

(10) Editorial: The Anomaly that Wouldn't Go Away. The Lancet, November 4, 978, (1978).

(11) ST. LEGER, A.S., COCHRANE, A.L., MOORE, F.: The Anomaly that Wouldn't Go Away. The Lancet, November 25, 1153 (1978).

(12) TOWNSEND, P.: Inequality and the Health Service. The Lancet, June 15 1179-1184 (1974).

(13) WOLFENDEN, H.W.: On the theoretical and practical considerations underlying the direct and indirect standardization of death rates. Population Studies 16, 188 (1962).

(14) GRAVELLE, H.S.E., HUTCHINSON, G., STERN, J.: Mortality and Unemployment: A Critique of Brenner's Time-Series Analysis. The Lancet, September 26, 675 (1981).

(15) BRENNER, M.H.: Unemployment and Health. The Lancet, October 17, 874 (1981).

REFERENCES PERTAINING TO SPECIFIC HYPOTHESES

GENERAL

1. Maxcy-Rosenau. Public Health and Preventive Medicine, 11th ed. (Edited by Last J.M.). Appleton-Century-Crofts, New York, 1980. Especially chapters 27,33,34, and 46.

2. LaPorte R.E., Cresanta J.L., and Kuller L.H. The relationship of alcohol consumption to atherosclerotic heart disease. Prev. Med. 9, 22, 1980.

3. U.S. Department of Health, Education, and Welfare. Proceedings of the Conference on the Decline of Coronary Heart Disease Mortality (Edited by Havlik R.J. and Feinleib M.). NIH Publication No. 79-1610, May 1979.

ALCOHOL

1. St. Leger A.S., Cochrane A.L., and Moore F. Factors associated with cardiac mortality in developed countries with particular reference to the consumption of wine. The Lancet 1, 1017, 1979.

2. Edwards G., Gross M.M., Keller M., Moser J., and Roam R. Alcohol-Related Disabilities. WHO Offset Publication No. 32. World Health Organization, Geneva, 1977.

3. U.S. Department of the Treasury and U.S. Department of Health and Human Services. Report to the President and Congress on Health Hazards Associated with Alcohol and Methods to Inform the General Public of These Hazards. November 1980.

4. Blackwelder W.C. et al. Alcohol and mortality: The Honolulu Heart Study. The Amer. J. Med. 68, 164, 1980.

CIGARETTES

1. Florey C. du V., Melia R.J.W., and Darby S.C. Changing mortality from ischaemic heart disease in Great Britain 1968-76. Br. Med. J. 1, 635, 1978.

2. Marmot M.G. et al. Changing social-class distribution of heart disease. Br. Med. J. 2, 1109, 1978.

3. Salonen J.T. Stopping smoking and long-term mortality after acute myocardial infarction. Br. Heart J. 43, 463, 1980.

4. U.S. Department of Health, Education and Welfare. The Women and Their Pregnancies. The Collaborative Perinatal Studies of the National Institute of Neurological Diseases and Stroke. DHEW Publication No. (NIH) 73-379, 1972.

5. Logan R.L. et al. Risk factors for ischaemic heart disease in normal men aged 40: Edinburgh-Stockholm Study. The Lancet 1, 949, 1978.

6. Dean G. et al. Factors related to respiratory and cardiovascular symptoms in the United Kingdom. J. Epi. Comm. Health 32, 86, 1978.

WINTER TEMPERATURE

1. Bainton D., Moore F., and Sweetnam P. Temperature and deaths from ischaemic heart disease. Br. J. Prev. Soc. Med. 31, 49, 1977.

HEALTH SERVICES

1. Cochrane A.L., St. Leger A.S., and Moore F. Health service "input" and mortality "output" in developed countries. J. Epi. Comm. Health 32, 200, 1978.

2. Chapman B.L. Effect of coronary care on myocardial infarct mortality. Br. Heart J. 42, 386, 1979.

3. Thom T.J. and Kannel W.B. Downward trends in cardiovascular mortality. Ann. Rev. Med. 32, 427, 1981.

SOCIAL STRESS

1. McKinlay J.B. Social networks influences on morbid episodes and the career of help seeking. In The Relevance of Social Science for Medicine (Edited by Eisenberg L. and Kleinman A.), p. 77. D. Reidel, Dordrecht, Holland, 1981.

2. Helsing K.J., Szklo M., and Comstock G.W. Factors associated with mortality after widowhood. Amer. J. Pub. Health 71, 802, 1981.

3. Theorell T. and Floderus-Myrhed B. "Workload" and risk of myocardial infarction: A prospective psychosocial analysis. Int. J. Epi. 6, 17, 1977.

4. Siegrist J. et al. Psychosocial risk constellations and first myocardial infarction. In Myocardial Infarction and Psychosocial Risks (Edited by Siegrist J. and Halhuber M.J.), p. 41. Springer-Verlag, Berlin, 1981.

5. Hinkle L.E.Jr. The effect of culture change, social change and changes in interpersonal relationships on health. In Stressful Life Events: Their Nature and Effects (Edited by Dohrenwend B.S. and Dohrenwend B.P.), p. 9. Wiley, New York, 1974.

6. Syme S.L., Borhani N.O., and Buechley R.W. Cultural mobility and coronary heart disease in an urban area. Am. J. Epi. 82, 334, 1965.

7. Scotch N.A. and Geiger H.J. The epidemiology of essential hypertension: A review with special attention to psychologic and sociocultural factors. II. Psychologic and sociocultural factors in etiology. J. Chron. Dis. 16, 1183, 1963.

8. Tyroler H.A. and Cassel J. Health consequences of culture change. II. The effect of urbanization on coronary heart mortality in rural residents. J. Chron. Dis. 17, 167, 1964.

9. Cassel J. Factors involving sociocultural incongruity and change: Appraisal and implications for theoretical development. Milbank Meml. Fund. Q. 45, 41, 1967.

10. Caplan R.D. Social support, person-environment fit, and coping. In Mental Health and the Economy (Edited by Ferman L.A. and Gordus J.P.), p. 89. The W.E. Upjohn Institute for Employment Research, Kalamazoo, Michigan, 1979.

11. Brenner M.H. Mental Illness and the Economy. Harvard University Press, Cambridge, Mass., 1973.

12. U.S. Department of Health, Education, and Welfare. Proceedings of the Forum on Coronary-Prone Behavior (Edited by Dembroski T.M.O. DHEW Publication no. (NIH) 78-1451, 1978.

13. Glass D.C. Type A behavior: Mechanisms linking behavioral and pathophysiologic processes. In Myocardial Infarction and Psychosocial Risks (Edited by Siegrist J. and Halhuber M.J.), p. 77. Springer-Verlag, Berlin, 1981.

14. Appels A. The syndrome of vital exhaustion and depression and its relationship to coronary heart disease. In Myocardial Infarction and Psychosocial Risks (Edited by Siegrist J. and Halhuber M.J.), p. 116. Springer-Verlag, Berlin, 1981.

15. Atkinson J.W. Motivational determinants of risk-taking behavior. Psych. Rev. 64, 359, 1957.

16. Brenner M.H. Time Series Analysis of the Relationships Between Selected Economic and Social Indicators, 2 vols. U.S. National Technical Information Service, Springfield, Va., March 1971.

17. Kasl S.V., Cobb S., and Gore S. Changes in reported illness behavior related to termination of employment: A preliminary report. Int. J. Epi. 1, 111, 1972.

18. Brenner M.H. Economic changes and heart disease mortality. Am. J. Pub. Health 61, 606, 1971.

19. Morris J.N. and Titmuss R.M. Health and social change. I. The recent history of rheumatic heart disease. The Medical Officer, p. 69, 26 August 1944.

20. Bunn A.R. Inschaemic heart disease mortality and the business cycle in Australia. Am.J. Pub. Health 69, 772, 1979.

21. Brenner M.H. Fetal, infant and maternal mortality during periods of economic instability. Int. J. Health Serv. 3, 145, 1973.

22. Brenner M.H. Trends in alcohol consumption and associated illnesses: Some effects of economic changes. Am. J. Pub. Health 65, 1279, 1975.

23. U.S. Congress. Joint Economic Committee. Estimating the Social Costs of National Economic Policy: Implications for Mental and Physical Health an Criminal Aggression (By Brenner M.H.). U.S. Government Printing Office, Washington, 26 October 1976.

24. Commission of the European Communities. Report on the Development of the Social Situation in the Community in 1974, p. 7. Brussels, March 1975.

25. Moriyama I.M., Krueger D.E., and Stamler J. Cardiovascular Diseases in the United States. Harvard University Press, Cambridge, Mass., 1971

26. Berkman L.F. and Syme S.L. Social networks, host resistance, and mortality: A nine-year follow-up of Alameda County residents. Am.J. Epi. 109, 186, 1979.

SOCIO-ECONOMIC CHANGE AND MORTALITY
A MULTIVARIATE COHERENCY ANALYSIS OF DANISH TIME SERIES

Jes Søgaard

Research Laboratory of Community Medicine and Health Economics
Odense University, Denmark

I   Introduction.

In this paper the socalled macro model of hypothesized relationships between socio-economic changes and mortality rates are discussed, in section II, and empirically evaluated using Danish time series, in section III.

The study of such macro relationships has a long tradition within the social sciences, from Ogurn and Thomas in the twenties (34, 35,41) to Brenner and Land in the seventies (1-7, 29). In these studies time series variables of aggregate measurements of social change and changes in health status of the population, usually indicated by mortality rates have been used to evaluate the hypothesis that changes in the economy, and the consequences these have for the social conditions, affect the general health status of the population of that economy. Usually the hypothesis is specified to deal with the direction of economic and social changes, so recessions in the economic cycles and ensuing worsened social condition, especially increased unemployment, are hypothesized to produce excess mortality, while periods of prosperity then logically must produce the opposite. There are, however, exceptions from this rule, e.g. (37), also the hypothesis are usually formulated to allow for negative effects on health of upturns in the economy, in problems of getting reintegrated in the labor market.

Results from the studies of Brenner, (1-7), most consistently indicate that the hypothesis of a negative impact of recessions in the economies on health status of the populations is reality. The studies of others have been less conclusive, e.g. (35), (41), and (9,10), and some studies have explicitly demonstrated that the hypothesis cannot be generalized to cover all causes of mortality, i.e. some cause specific mortality rates may be temporally, negatively correlated to recessions in the economy, (29), and (11), finally some studies have indicated that the relationships are very complex, one group of studies indicating this is (12-15), another is (19-20).

As some of these studies are based on the same population, spatially as well as in time period covered by the analyses, other matters must explain these differences in results of the analyses. This could be 1) the specification of the relationships subjected to statistical analysis, i.e. inclusion/exclusion of some variables, which may have a confounding or modification effect on the results, and/or 2) the specific statistical methods and techniques utilized in the analyses.

These 2 points are discussed in section II of this paper. It is concluded that variables indicating changes in consumption behavior, and in the case of suicide mortality a variable reflecting changes in cohesion of family networks, ought to be included in the models. Also modifying effects of changing levels of the rate of financial compensation to the unemployed for lost income might be included.

Concerning the second point, issues of model specification and especially control strategies in aggregate time series studies are discussed. It is suggested that explorative, more descriptive studies are done prior to parametric analysis, and in these studies effects of self explanatory elements of the single series should be controlled.

In section III, results from an explorative time series study on Danish time series indicators of socio-economic, and consumption behavioral variables, and 5 cause specific mortality rates are presented. These results do not support the findings of Dr. Brenner, that unemployment should have a strong positive effect on most indicators of mortality. On the contrary, this effect, if at all observable, changes in sign for various causes of death. An observation which has been made before, (29). The suggested inclusion of consumption behavioral indicators seems to be relevant for more of the mortality rates. These variables seem to be important mediators of effects from changes in the economy on health, suggesting other mechanisms than the stress-mechanisms.

II. Discussion of the Brenner type model and analysis.

II.1 Basic hypotheses of the Brenner Model.

The basic hypothesis of the Brenner model is that recessions in the economy account for the major part of short to medium range changes in health conditions. Two mechanisms are active. (1) Recessions of the economy result in disruption or even retrogression of the beenficial aspects of economic growth, and (2), indirectly, recessions are considered to be a major source of psychological stress.

Of these two mechanisms Brenner himself seems to rely most on the latter. It is especially the experience of unemployment, and/or insecure job conditions that increase the flow of stressful life events and changes during periods of economic recessions.

Brenner has in great detail described the stress mechanisms, from a sociological point of view in terms of disruption of micro social networks, and from a psychological point of view in terms of the effects of life events, such as dismissals, and life changes, such as being unemployed, on health.

These effects* are well known in the psychosomatic theories of illnesses, (17, 25, 38, 39).

The hypotheses of the Brenner model are usually expressed in terms of macro relations, but these macrorelations are clearly preconditioned by relations of micro level. Partly to make my own interpretation of the Brenner model clear, and partly to ease the subsequent criticisms of the (implicit) micro level assumptions, I have outlined the causal structure in the diagram of fig. II. 1.

---

* In most stress models , stress is assumed to reduce the general susceptibility. Life events - not necessarily of a negative sort, but any event or change requiring adjustment - are socalled coping mechanisms. These include changed consumption behaviors, e.g. increased smoking, see (32).

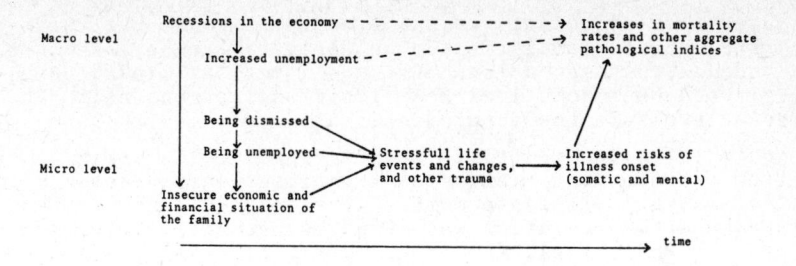

```
                    Recessions in the economy ─ ─ ─ ─ ─ ─ ─ ─ ─ ─ ─ →  Increases in mortality
Macro level                  │                              ─ ─ ─ ─ →  rates and other aggregate
                             ↓                                         pathological indices
                    Increased unemployment ─ ─ ─ ─ ─ ─ ─ ─ ┐
                             │                             │
                             ↓                             │
                    Being dismissed                        │
                             │                             │
                             ↓                             ↓
Micro level         Being unemployed ───────→ Stressfull life ──→ Increased risks of
                             │                events and changes,    illness onset
                             ↓                and other trauma       (somatic and mental)
                    Insecure economic and
                    financial situation of
                    the family
                    ────────────────────────────────────────────────→ time
```

Fig. II.1 Path diagram of the causal structure implicit in the Brenner model. Dashed lines represent the direct macro level hypotheses of the Brenner model.

I shall not raise any questions concerning the included variables and causal relations in the Brenner model. What is of concern are the variables and causal relations not included in the model. It seems to me that Brenner leaves out other relevant risk factors which are associated to the social and physical environment, risk factors which may also be associated to short to medium range changes in the economy. These include 1) hazards of the physical environment, e.g. connected to occupation, or traffic, 2) other 'stressors' than those associated to unemployment, e.g. work loads, migration, changed work conditions due to technological changes, 3) health behavior, including health counterproductive behaviors such as smoking, alcohol consumption, and overeating.

Inclusion of these other groups of risk factors has implications for the implicit micro level assumptions as well as the specification of the macro level relationships.

Concerning the former - the implied, micro level assumptions would be in better agreement with the findings from studies based on less controversial methods than is the case of the Brenner studies, (21, 27).

There are evidence that unemployment increases the risks of illness onset, so it is for the above mentioned factors, too. Combining results from time series analysis and results from micro level studies, Eyer, (20) found that unemployment accounted for only a tiny fraction of the short to medium range fluctuations of total mortality rates. Even though Eyer may underestimate the impact of unemployment, he demonstrates at least the necessity of inclusion of the other risk factors if we want to obtain results from macro analysis which in some way agree with results and known relations on micro levels.

Also concerning the micro level assumptions, the model would not have to rely so much on stress mechanisms, as is the case at the present stage. Less objective mechanisms, such as behavioral mechanisms could be included in the justification of the observed relationships over time.

In studies closely related to the Brenner studies, but where indicators of stress levels in the population have been included, the assumed stress mechanisms have had some weak links. Bunn, (9, 10), used Pharmaceutical Benefits Prescriptions as indicative of stress levels in the population.

This indicator was expected to mediate some of the estimated effect from unemployment changes on ischaimic heart disease mortality rates, (9) and all cause mortality rates (10). While a consistent and positive relation was found between the unemployment series and the PBP series, the expected relation between the PBP series and the mortality rates was not found. This may of course be due to invalidity of the PBP series as an indicator of stress levels, but it may also be due to real effects, namely that stress mechanisms are of limited importance concerning mortality.

In a series of studies, (12, 13, 15) Catalano and Dooley have examined the relationships between economic changes in a regional community, including unemployment, changes in the mix of industries, gross and net flows of jobs, inflation, and others, and survey measures of mental disorder, including measures of stressful life events, and measures of psycho-physiological symptoms and depressed mood. Unemployment and absolute structural changes in the regional economy were positively correlated with both the life events measures and the measures of weak mental disorder. However, the expected positive correlation between life events and mental disorders was not estimated. This may again indicate, that the stress mechanisms may not be that important in the models linking health and the economy. Therefore, inclusion of variables that makes evaluation of other mediating mechanisms possible would be relevant.

Concerning the specification of macro relations:
Changes in the underlying micro level assumptions of course influence the way hypotheses at the macro level are deduced. Hypotheses can no longer be restricted to cover negative impacts of recessions and unemployment on health, but should rather include hypotheses concerning the impacts of various cycles and various phases of these on health.

- It would be possible to specify specific models for specific causes of death. It is clearly a simplification, if not directly unrealistic to postulate a general model of the relation between the economy and various indicators of health.

In a study, (29), very similar in methodology to the Brenner studies, specific models were specified for specific causes of death. In this study it was also illustrated how various causes of death may be differently associated to unemployment. E.g. mortality rates due to diseases of the respiratory system and vehicle accident mortality rates were both related negatively to unemployment, while only circulatory disease mortality rates were related positively to unemployment. (And part of this relationship was mediated by increases in cigarette consumption in the recovery period of the business cycle).

The differences of sign simply reflect that different diseases respond differently to changes in the economic and social environment.

To sum up the discussion about the hypotheses of the Brenner model it has been suggested that the problem of relationships between short to medium range changes of the economy and health should be generalized, and not concentrated on impacts of recessions, and consequences of recessions, such as migration, work load problems, changes of consumption patterns, and perhaps also include other social consequence of economic change, e.g. changes in family net work cohesion.

II.2 Methodological issues.

Using aggregate time series measures of the involved variables of the model the analyst is able to describe the time structure of the possible relationships over a fairly long time range. This includes estimation of delays in effects from one variable to another, and even lag-distributed responses. Some times it may also be relevant to estimate on which cycles the relationships are strongest.

There are a number of problems involved due to the aggregate nature of the data. First the classic problem of fallacious interpretation, (see for instance 27 and 28); second, a low degree of reliability of the time series indicators, (see for instance 30 and 31); third, issues about the optimal level of spatial as well as time aggregation, (see for instance 12-14). These problems are all discussed in the literature and I shall not rediscuss them.

On the other hand, there seems to be some sort of agreement that aggregate time series analyses in this field may not be completely irrelevant when the results are interpreted with care. Therefore it would be appropriate to have a strategy for aggregate time series analysis in this field developed. This is not the purpose of this paper, but a few proposals will be made.

Briefly, during the last 10-20 years time series strategies have been developed by statisticians. Several issues of the proposed strategies separate them from standard econometric methods and analyses.

A main characteristic is a thorough explorative data analysis of the time series before a parametric regression analysis is performed. One of the purposes of this explorative analysis is to specify from the data the optimal structure of the equations, a specification of which is requisite to parametric analysis.

In the later Brenner studies, (5,7), and also in (29) parametric analyses are performed. In the former a specific polynomial structure and in the latter a specific, i.e. first order, rational structure are pre-assumed. There seems to be little evidence that it has been tested on the data, whether these specifications are optimal in some sense, and if they are not the results may be biased, and certainly inefficient.

Another main characteristic is the specific control strategy that is necessary in time series analysis on a set of time series. This is control for self explanatory components inherent in most single time series. In the extreme case, this component - or one of them - could be a trend in mean value, e.g. the series tends to increase or decrease with time. When this is the case some sort of detrending, preferably by taking differences, should be done before the series is correlated to some other series. However, even the detrended series may be dependent on its own past, and therefore a regression model for this internal dependency should be fitted. The residuals from this regression are assumed to represent the innovations of the original time series, i.e. the part of the series that cannot be explained by its own past behavior. Statistically the residual time series is white noise (completely random) if fitted univariate regression model is adequate. Therefore the procedure is called prewhitening.

This procedure is done on each time series, which means that the following cross correlation or regression* analysis is performed on innovations of each series. In this way the effects of self-explanatory components in the series are controlled for, hold constant, and one cause of spuriousness of coefficients of correlation or regression has been eliminated.

In the studies referred to above, (5, 7, 29), and indeed many others, detrending not to mention prewhitening has not been done prior to causal analysis. This of course does not necessarily imply that the results from these studies are biassed and/or spurious, but the possibility that they are have not been checked.

As indicated, very often cross correlation methods are used. That is, the detrended, - ideally the prewhitened - values of each pair of time series are correlated for different time lags between the two series. The crucial problem of this method is that it is extremely difficult to estimate partial correlations, i.e. to control for third group variables. Of course one could perform multivariate lagged regression, but if each regressor is included with many lags computational problems often occur and thus numerically instable estimates come out.

The problem may be circumvented by analysis in the frequency domain. In the frequency domain, the variance structure of each detrended series, - note that prewhitening is <u>not</u> required -, is decomposed on a set of frequencies, due to cycles of different periodicity in the series. Similarly the covariance structure between a pair of series is decomposed on frequencies, due to covariance between cyclic components on the same frequency for each of the two series. As the elements at different frequencies are linearly independent, one can construct the same measures of correlation - or coherency - at each frequency, including partial correlation measures, in the same way as is done in ordinary static analysis.

Correlation analysis in the frequency domain is usually called coherency analysis. In section III results are presented from a multivariate coherency analysis on detrended Danish time series indicators of some of the variables suggested for inclusion in the aggregate time series model of the influence of economic instability on health.

More details on that statistics used may be found in an appended section, A1.

III Results from time series analysis on Danish data.

III. 1 Introduction.

In this section the results from a time series analysis on Danish time series for indicators of the economy, 'counter health productive' consumption, and health, are summarized.

The results are not final or endproducts, rather the opposite, namely results from a preliminary, and explorative study.

The time series included in the analysis are defined in

---

* When the series have been prewhitened it is a matter of subjective preferences whether cross correlation methods or lagged regression methods are used.

table III.1. All series have been detrended for trend in mean and variance by taking 1. differences of the logtransforms of the original rates.

Abbreviation	Definition
G	Growth rates of the economy. Relative changes of deflated per capita income.
UN	Relative changes of the unemployment rates: percentage of work force unemployed. (36)
B	Relative changes of the ratio of unemployment benefits to lost wages. (36)
CIG	Relative changes of the consumption of cigarettes pr. 1000.
ALC	Relative changes of the consumption of alcohol, converted into litres of 100% spirits pr. inhabitant.
DM	Relative changes of the ratio of divorces pr. year to marriages pr. year.
HDM	Relative changes of the total rate of heart disease mortality. Males.
RM	Relative changes of the total rate of mortality caused by diseases of the respiratory system. Males.
IM	Relative changes of the ratio of infant mortality (less than 1 year old) to number of live borns.
AM	Relative changes of the total rate of mortality caused by accidents. Males.
SM	Relative changes of the rate of suicides. Males: 20-44 years old.

Table III.1. Abbreviation and definition of the 11 included time series. Denmark. 1921 thruogh 1978.

The quality of the mortality series are rather poor, as it has not been possible to make adjustments for changes in age structure. However, I believe this is a minor flaw when taking relative changes of the level series.

The purpose of the study was to test the Brenner findings on Danish series, when including some of the variables suggested in section I, they are cigarette consumption and alcohol consumption. Specifically for the analysis on suicide rates, an indicator of family network cohesion was included. Besides, the ratios of unemployment benefits to lost wages were included to control for modifying effects on the impacts of unemployment on health.

Five different types of mortality rates were analysed in order to examine whether the patterns of relationships to the economy were similar or not. I have not analysed the all cause mortality rate. The reason for this is that the underlying assumption of time invariance can be assumed violated, because the cause structure of deaths in society has changed so much over the period of analysis.

III.2 Summary statistics of bivariate squared correlation.

To get a first indication of the strength of linear association between the pairs of time series for a rather long range of lags, summary statistics of one-sided R_L^2 were computed and these are presented in table III.2. In the columns of table III.2. one may also identify the multivariate models which are treated in subsection III.3.

The one-sided, bivariate R_L^2 for L = 15, is computed in the following way. First the cross correlation between pair of vertical and horizontal variables, up to a lag of 15 for the vertical variables were computed. Second, these correlation coefficients were squared, and third, they were summed for all lags, including the zero-lag coefficients.

lagged	UN	CIG	ALC	HDM	RM	IM	AM	SM
G	.45(4)	.51(3)	.30	.45(5)	.36	.36	.34	.28
UN		.20	.37	.23	.18	.26	.26	.20
B*								
CIG				.48(3)	.37	.63(1)		
ALC				.33			.41(5)	
DM								.31

Significance levels: (1) 99,5%; (3) 97,5%; (4) 90.%

Table III.2 Estimated, one-sided R_{15}^2 measures of total, bivariate strength of association.

From these bivariate measures it is quite obvious that unemployment accounts for only a small part of the short to medium range changes in the 5 included, cause specific mortality rate series. None of the R_{15}^2 measures reach levels of significance.

The G series accounts for about ½ of the variance of the CIG series, and as either of these series appears to be account for almost ½ of the variance of the HDM series these two series may be

---

* As the B series is only included to control for modifying effects of unemployment benefits on the health impacts of unemployment - in the multivariate analysis - , it is not interpreted in this bivariate analysis.

good predictors of short to medium range changes of heart mortality rates. The multivariate analysis may describe this relationship more closely.

Besides the HDM series, the CIG series is also strongly correlated with the infant mortality series.

The ALC series is only correlated to one of the mortality rates, and only at a low significance level.

Finally, it is observed, that the DM series, assumed indicative of family network cohesion is not correlated with suicide rates.

It may be concluded from this bivariate analysis of over all strengths of associations, that the consumption variables account for a large part of the variances of 3 of the included mortality series, compared to the unemployment series.

III.3 Results from multivariate coherency analyses.

I have summarized the results from the multivariate coherency analyses in 'path'-type models at cyclic components.

The first three columns in table III.2 represent the 'internal' models* which describe how the input variables to the 'external' models are interrelated. The external models, (columns 4-8) then, are the models describing the relationships between the economy and consumption behavior and the mortality rates.

Throughout this subsection the simple, (bivariate), partial and multivariate squared coherency spectra will be presented in diagrams. Partial and bivariate K^2 spectra will be presented in the same diagram, the bivariate in dashed line and the partial in full line. Standard notation is used, that is the partial squared coherency spectrum between for instance the CIG and G series controlling for the UN series is denoted $K^2_{CIG,G \cdot UN}(f)$. The multivariate squared coherency spectrum between the CIG, G and UN series is denoted by $K^2_{CIG,G,UN}(f)$. 'f' is frequency and is with a time unit of one year read as cycles per year. The flat lines in the diagrams are the critical values of the null hypothesis of no coherency. That is when a part of the K^2 spectrum is above this flat test line, the possibility of coherency cannot be rejected at the 5% test level. The L values are the points at which the cross correlation functions were truncated, or in other words, the number of lags on both sides that were used to estimate the coherencies. The lower L the more degrees of freedom, and thus a smaller critical value. However, if L is too low the spectra may not resolve, and thus serious bias may come out. Either 10 or 15 lags have been used.

III.3.1 'Internal' models.

Results from the multivariate, 'internal' analyses, see fig. III.1-3, suggested three decomposed models. They are presented in fig. III.4.

---

* Initially the DM series was included in the 'internal' modeling, but no strong correlation between this series and the other input series was found.

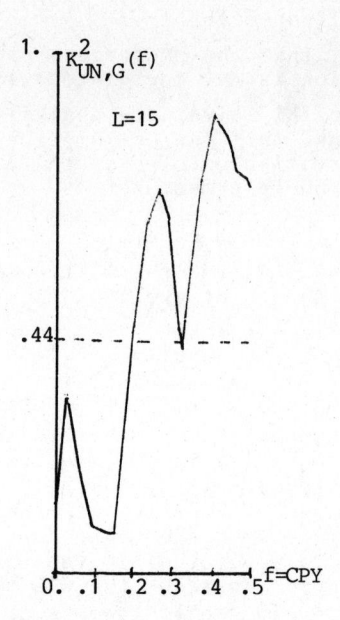

Fig. III.1. Squared bivariate coherency spectrum, K^2 between the G and UN series.

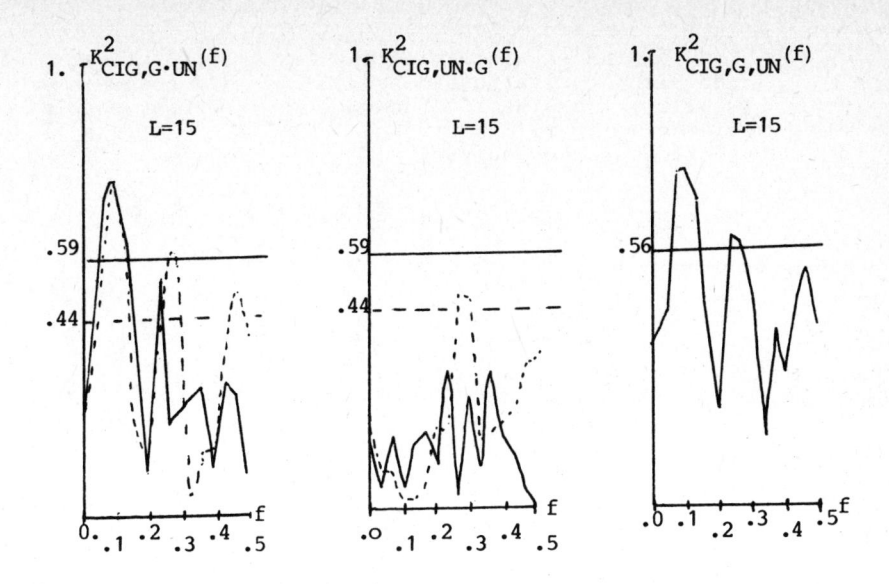

Fig. III.2. Simple, partial and multivariate squared coherency spectra of the CIG model.

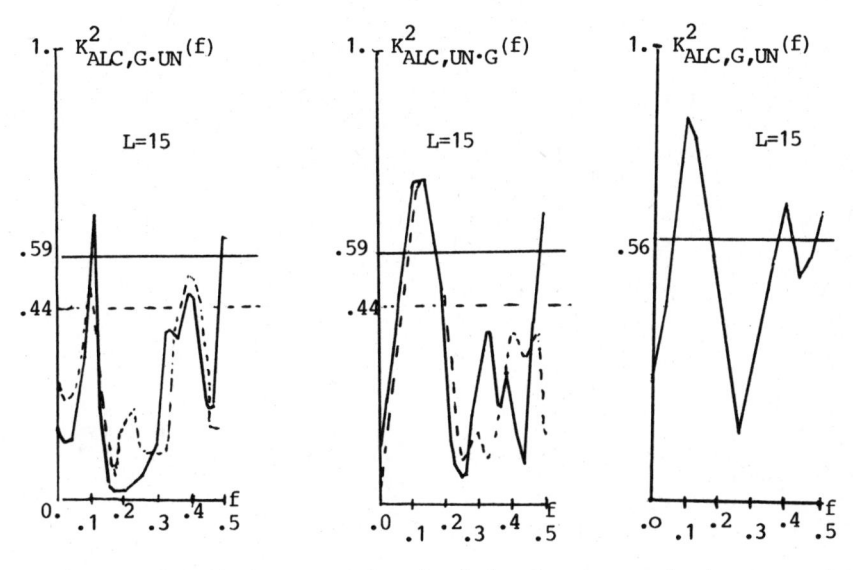

Fig. III.3. Simple, partial and multivariate squared coherency spectra of the ALC model.

The signs are based on interpretation of the phase statistics, and they all agree with expectations based on ordinary economic theory. The possibility that the two consumption variables should be positively related to unemployment, as a response to stress, could not be supported by the analyses.

6 to 12 years cyclic components.

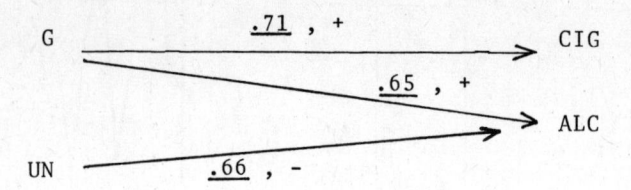

```
G ─────────── .71 , + ───────────► CIG
  ╲                .65 , +
   ╲─────────────────────────────► ALC
UN ──── .66 , - ────►
```

3 to 5 years cyclic components.

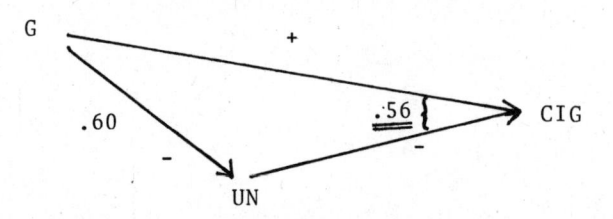

```
G ╲         +
   ╲         .56
    ╲.60        ╲──► CIG
      ╲    -
       ▼
       UN
```

Year to year fluctuations.

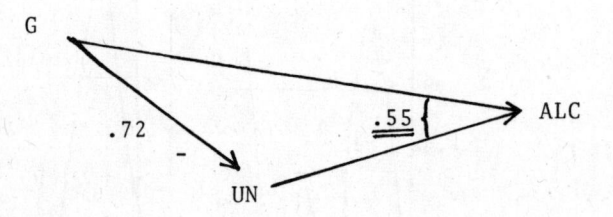

```
G ╲
   ╲         .55
    ╲.72        ╲──► ALC
      ╲    -
       ▼
       UN
```

Fig. III.4. Suggested 'path' models, decomposed on three cyclic components. The numerical values refer to mean K^2 coefficients. No underlining: bivariate, single underlining: partial, and double underlining: multiple. Signs are estimated from phase statistics.

III.3.2. 'External' models.

III.3.2.1. Heart disease mortality.

Based on fig. III.6 two models are suggested.

1. Long range cycles (15-∞)

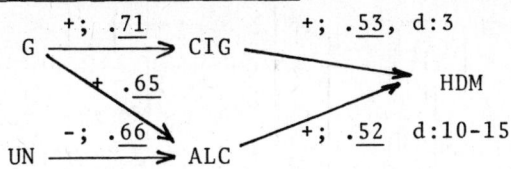

```
        +; .71              +; .53, d:3
   G ─────────► CIG ─────────────────┐
      ╲  .65                          ▼
       ╲                             HDM
        ╲                             ▲
     -; .66 ╲     +; .52  d:10-15    │
   UN ─────────► ALC ────────────────┘
```

2. Short/medium range cycles (4-8 years)

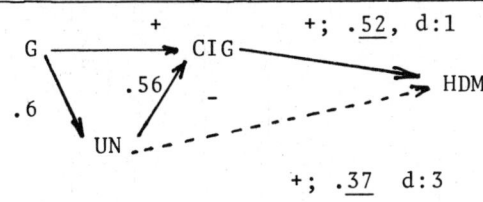

```
          +                +; .52, d:1
   G ─────────► CIG ──────────────────┐
    ╲         ▲                        ▼
     ╲   .56 ╱    -                  ─► HDM
   .6 ╲    ╱   ─ ─ ─ ─ ─ ─ ─ ─ ─ ─ ─
       ╲  ╱
        UN ─ ─ ─ ─ ─ ─ ─ ─ ─ ─ ─ ─ ─
              +; .37   d:3
```

Fig. III.5. Path diagrams of suggested pattern between socio-economic, behavioral variables and HDM. The numbers indicate mean, squared coherencies, simple, partial or multiple, the d-values indicate delay in years.

The two models suggest that on the long range relationship, no direct effect exist between the two socioeconomic variables and HDM, but indirect mediated by increased consumption of cigarettes and alcohol in periods with high growth rates. Indirectly, mediated by the positive, long lagged effect of alcohol consumption, unemployment has a negative impact on heart disease mortality rates.

On the short to medium range cycles, the possibility of an direct positive impact from unemployment on HDM cannot be totally rejected. However, the positive effect from cigarettes, peaking with growth peaks, and unemployment through , on HDM is stronger. Thus the possible direct and positive from UN on HDM, may be outweighed by an indirect and negative effect from UN on HDM through cigarette consumption.

III.3.2.2. Respiratory disease mortality.

Three decomposed 'path' models for RM mortality, fig. III.7 are very similar in structure. However, they must be interpreted only with reservations.

From the R^2 measures it was seen that the RM mortality rate series was only weakly related to the input series. The significant K^2 coefficients of G and CIG are due to highly concentrated and narrow peaks, see fig. III.8., and these are always to be handled carefully. They may be spurious, and due to instability of the spectra. However, for the sake of completion, the models are

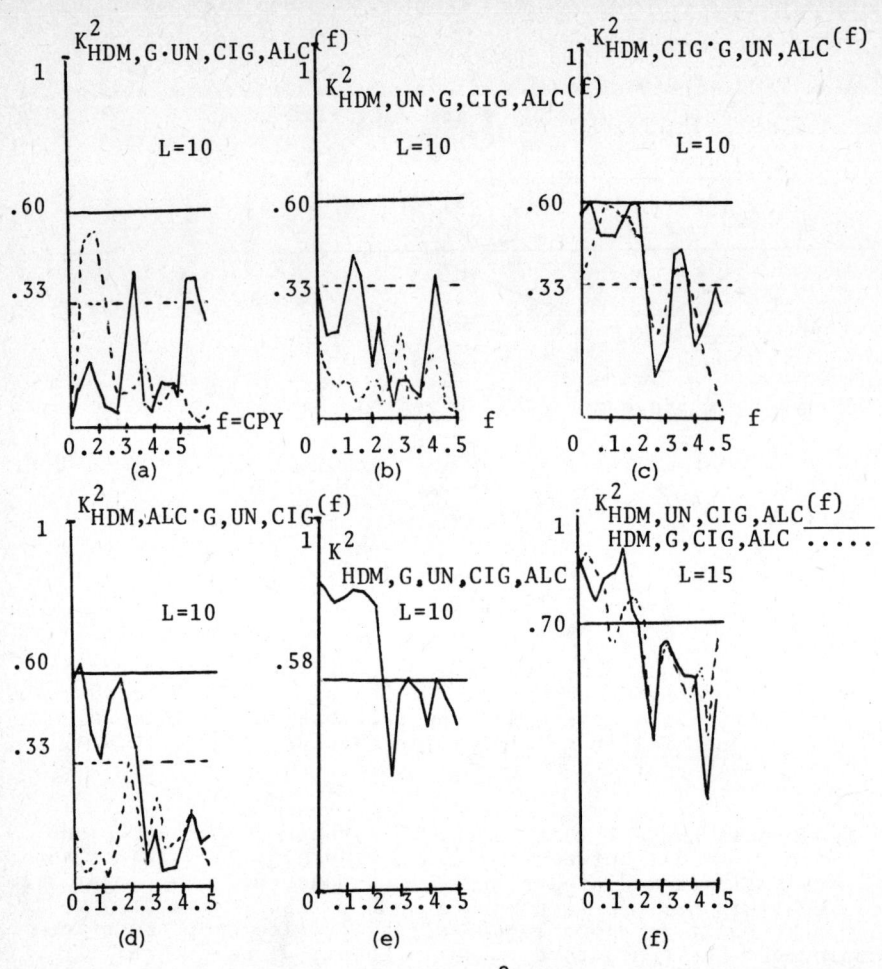

Fig. III.6. Partial and bivariate K^2 spectra in (a)-(d) of the HDM model. In (e) the multivariate K^2 spectrum including all 'input' variables, in (f) full line: G excluced, and dashed line: Un excluded.

reported without further comments.

Trend and long range cycles. 15 to ∞ years.

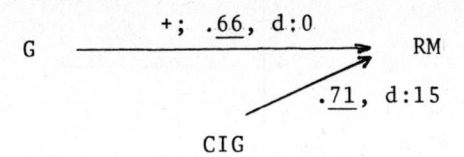

```
           +; .66, d:0
  G ─────────────────► RM
                    ↗
                .71, d:15
              ↗
            CIG
```

Medium range cycles. 6 to 12 years.

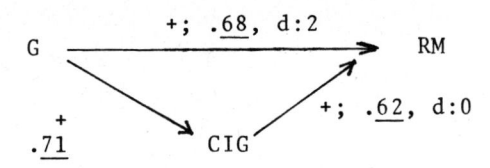

```
           +; .68, d:2
  G ─────────────────► RM
      ↘           ↗
        ↘     +; .62, d:0
   +      ↘ ↗
  .71      CIG
```

Short range cycles. 2 to 3 years.

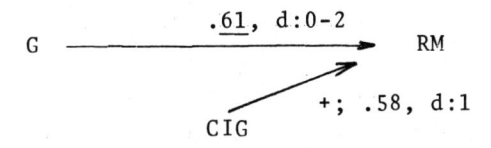

```
           .61, d:0-2
  G ─────────────────► RM
                    ↗
                +; .58, d:1
              ↗
            CIG
```

Fig III.7. 'Path' models for RM mortality.

III.3.2.3. Infant mortality.

For the K^2 spectra of the IM series on the G, UN, B, and CIG series, see fig III.9., the opposite phenomena are observed, especially for the IM and CIG K^2-spectra. This is spread out on a large part of the spectrum, the middle part, covering 3 to 5 years cycles.

Only one model, on 3 to 5 years cycles, is suggested from the estimations on this series.

Short to medium range cycles. 3 to 5 years.

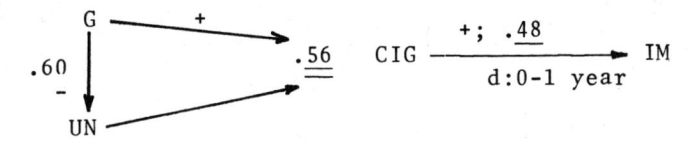

```
       G ──────+───►
              ↘          +; .48
  .60          .56  CIG ────────► IM
   -          ↗         d:0-1 year
       UN ───►
```

Fig. III.10. 'Path' model of IM mortality.

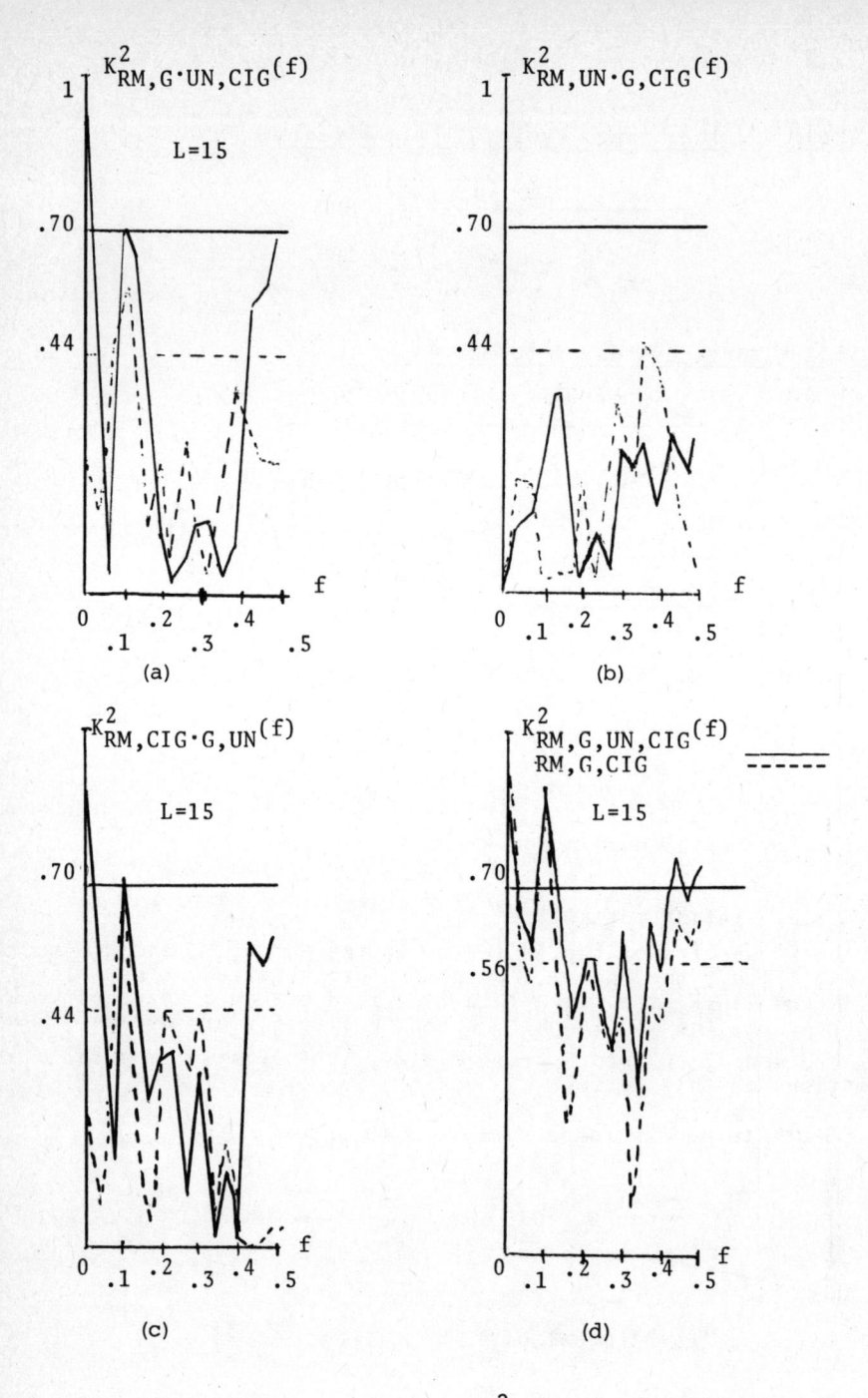

Fig. III.8 Partial and bivariate K^2 spectra in (a)-(c) of the RM model. In (d) the multivariate including all three input variables, full line, and dashed line:only the G and CIG series.

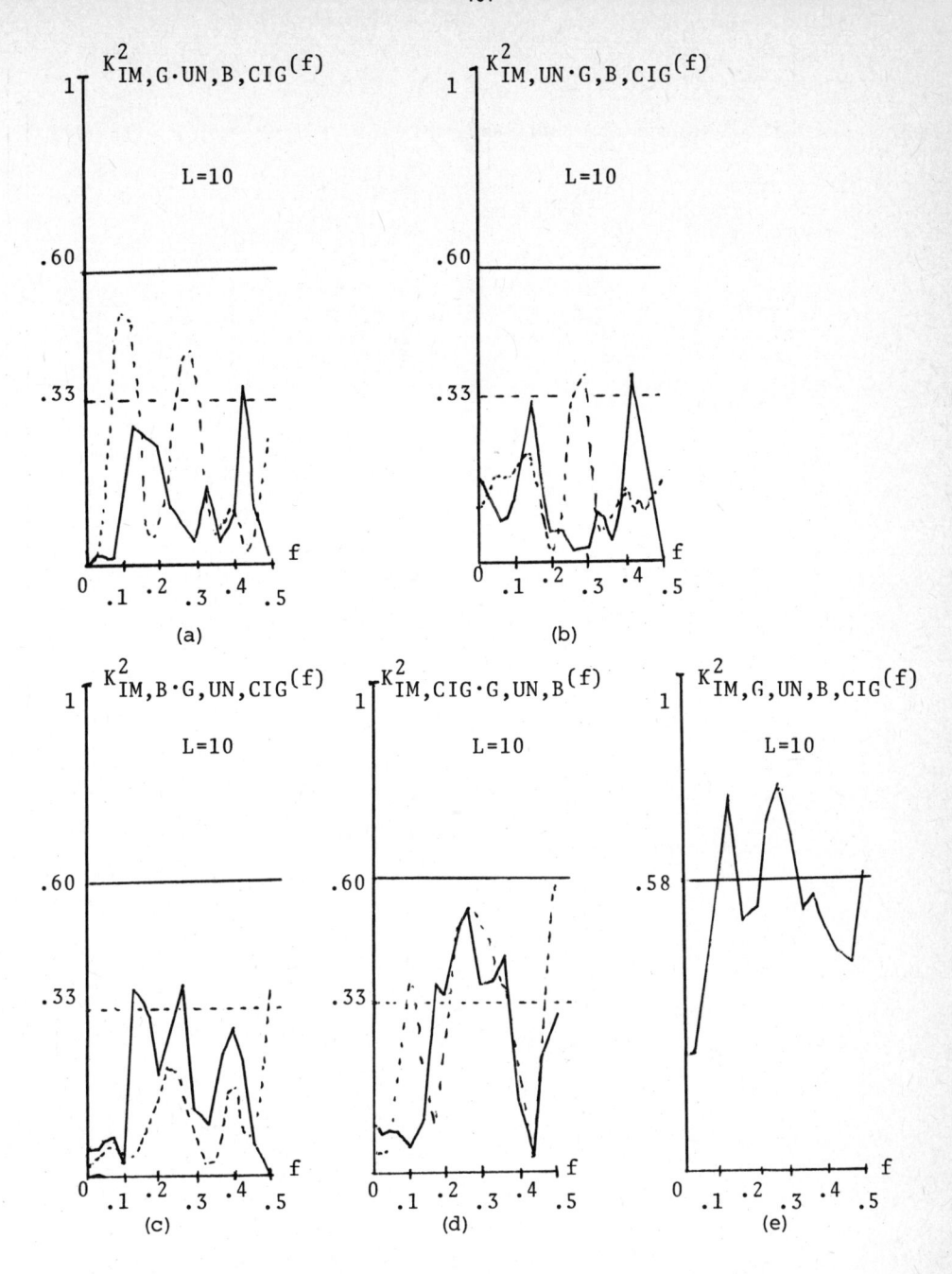

Fig. III.9 Partial and bivariate K^2 spectra in (a)-(d) of the IM model. In (e) the multivariate K^2 spectrum including all 4 input variables.

It is first to be mentioned that the direct 'path' between the CIG series and the IM series is not significant in a statistical sense. However, the peak is broad, and it is obvious, that the large R^2 value between the two series is due to coherency within these cycles.

No direct, (from the Brenner studies, expected positive) relation between unemployment and infant mortality was found, when controlling for growth rates, cigarette smoking, and unemployment benefits*.

Infant mortality may on the contrary be indirectly, but <u>negatively</u> related to high levels of unemployment, mediated through decreases of (maternal) cigarette consumption in periods of high levels of unemployment and short term decreases of income.

III.3.2.4. Accident mortality

Two decomposed 'path' models could be extracted from the results of the multivariate coherency analysis of accident mortality rates on growth rates, unemployment rates, and alcohol consumption rates.

As observed from the table of the bivariate R^2 measures, accident mortality rates are only weakly related to the three series, and only significantly, at a low level, with the alcohol consumption rates. However, due to concentration of these over all measures of associations in rather narrow bands of frequencies, significant, or close to significant, coherencies are estimated, see fig III.11.

15 to ∞ years relations.

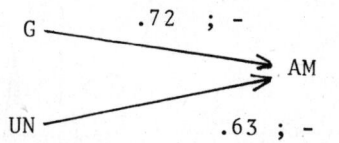

```
        .72 ; -
G ─────────────┐
               ▼
               AM
               ▲
UN ────────────┘
        .63 ; -
```

4 to 6 years relations.

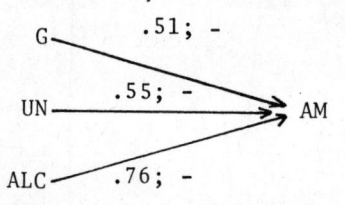

```
        .51; -
G ─────────────┐
        .55; - │
UN ────────────┼──► AM
        .76; - │
ALC ───────────┘
```

Fig. III.12. Two decomposed 'path' models for accident mortality rates.

---

* This was actually the only case, in which the B series could be observed to have a modifying effect on unemployment. (Modifying the indirect, negative impact on infant mortality).

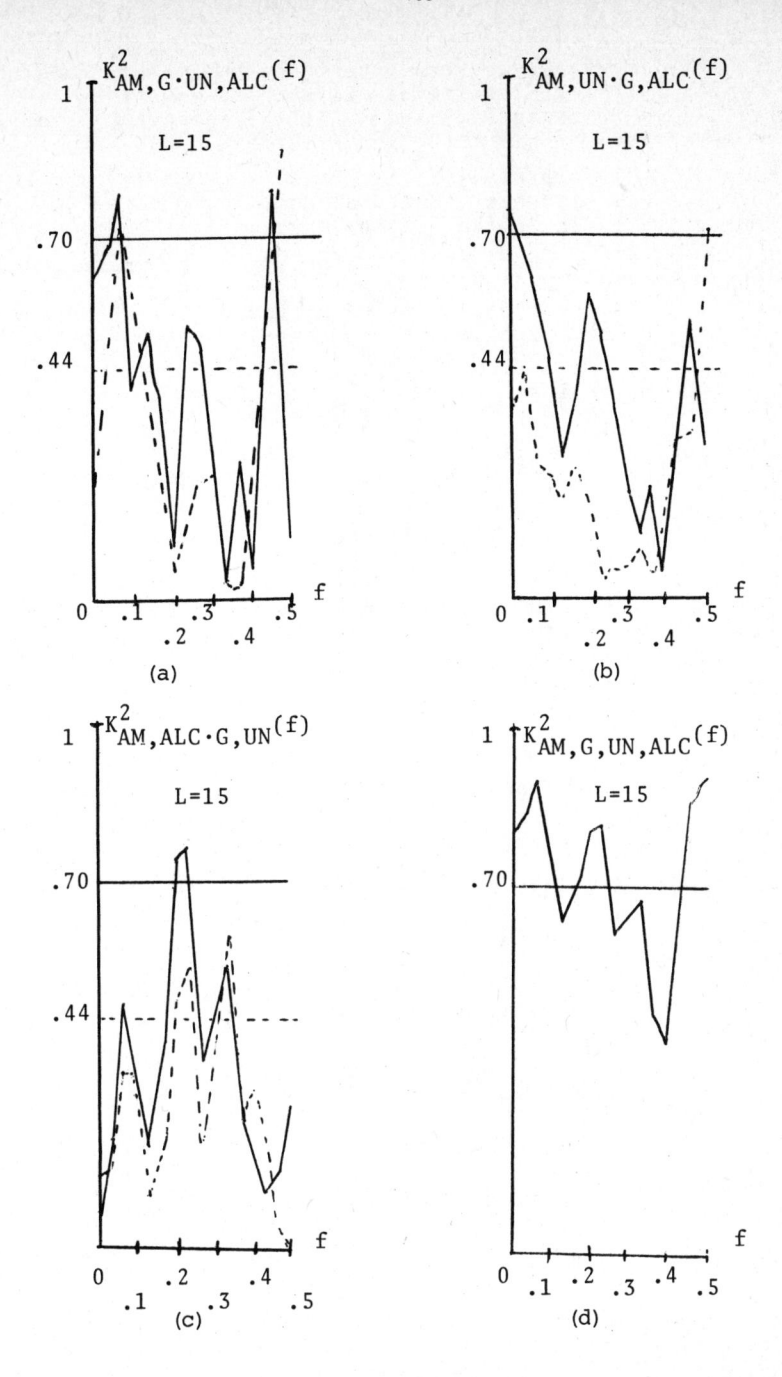

Fig. III.11 Partial and bivariate in (a)-(c) of the AM model. In (d) multivariate K^2 spectrum including all 3 input variables.

Accidents mortality rates were expected to be negatively related to unemployment rates, and positively related to the other two input series. As is observed from fig. III.12., however, negative signs were estimated for all three input series.

This anomaly makes interpretation difficult, especially concerning the negative relationship between alcohol consumption and accident mortality rates on the 4 to 6 years cyclic component.

As with the RM model, I shall sustain from further comments, and the model has only been included for principal reasons, that is to present all estimated models, including those, for which the analyses do not produce expected or intuitively reasonable results.

III.3.2.5. Suicide mortality.

Suicide is probably the cause of death which has attracted most attention from social scientists. Based on Durkheim's theory of suicide, (18), suicide rates have been related to a number of indicators of the economy or the business cycle, e.g. (24, 37, 42).

It has been argued that the Durkheim theory of anomie, and thus suicides in society could be related to the short term changes of the economy, such as business cycles. This is also the basic points of the above mentioned studies. I am not too sure, that it was this kind of fluctuations in the economy which Durkheim thought of, but rather a more profound type of changes, which also appear in the economy and society with some kind of regularity.

The analysis on suicide rates also showed that this may be the case. At least it was clear that the relationship between the economy and suicide rates do not appear on short to medium range cycles, but rather long cycles, about 8 to 15 years, see fig. III.13.

Medium to long range cycles. 8 to 15 years.

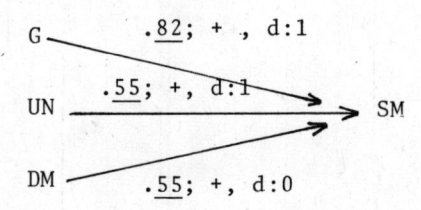

```
G ──────── .82; + , d:1 ─────┐
                             ↓
UN ─────── .55; +, d:1 ────→ SM
                             ↑
DM ─────── .55; +, d:0 ──────┘
```

Fig. III.14. Path model for suicide mortality rates. (Males, 20-44 years old).

The SM series is positively related to all three input series, for the two economic series with an estimated delay of 1 year. In a preceeding analysis the B series was included, but it apparently did not influence the relation between unemployment and suicide rates, males 20-44 years old.

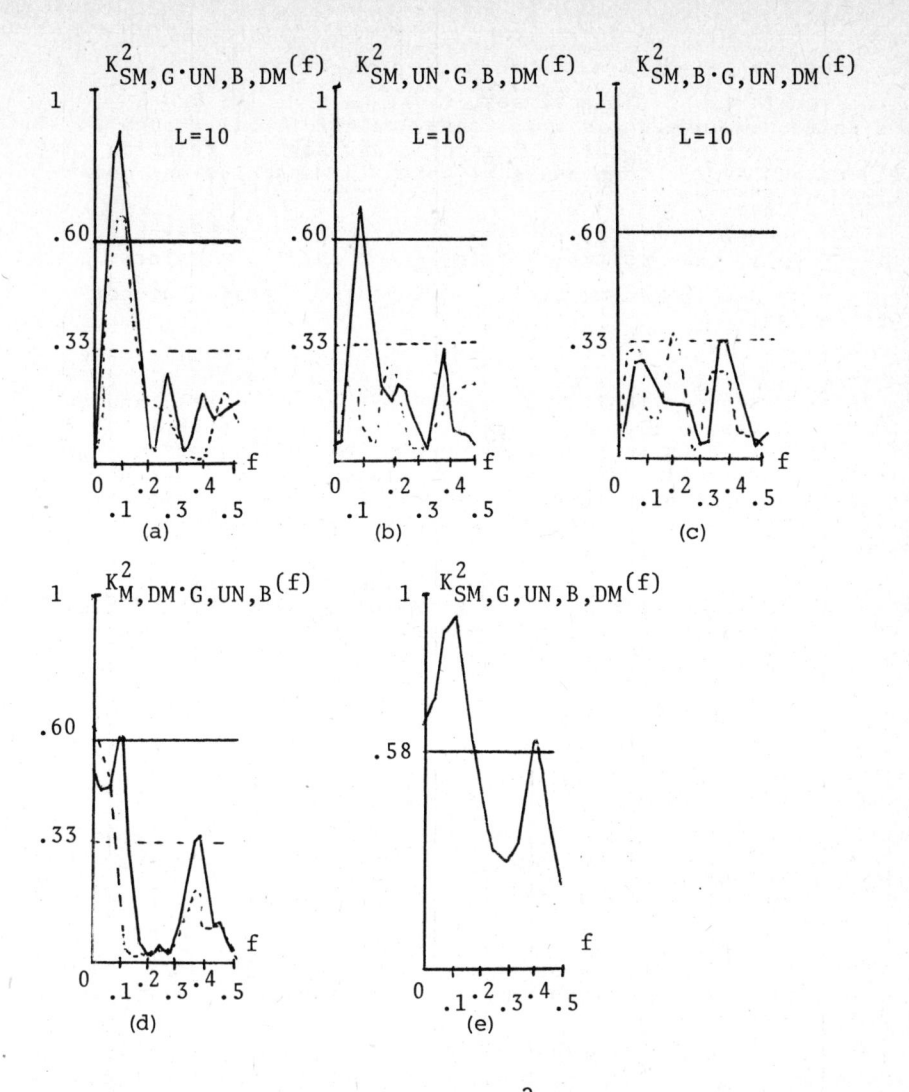

Fig. III.13. Partial and bivariate K^2 spectra in (a) - (d) of the SM model. In (e) the multivariate K^2 spectrum including all 4 input variables.

III.4. Summary

Results from three of the analyses, those on HDM, IM, and SM showed that unemployment is differently related to different causespecific mortality rates. This concerns sign of relation as well as the cyclic components at which the associations concentrate.

Generally, unemployment is only weakly correlated to health indicators, at least when mortality rates are used as indicators.

However, when decomposed on cyclic components, significant correlations appear.

Three types of relation between unemployment and mortality rates have been illustrated. (1) HDM was directly, and positively related to unemployment (only weakly, and not significant), and at the same time indirectly, but negatively related to unemployment, as unemployment seems to decrease consumption of cigarettes. (2) IM was only indirectly and negatively related to unemployment, again mediated by cigarette consumption. (3) The only case of a direct positive relation, not weakened by other mechanisms, was observed for the SM series.

These results are taken as evidence for the suggestions made in section II, that the relationships between unemployment and health may vary for different aspects of health, that there are other mechanisms at work than the stress mechanisms. It was quite clear that the relations between the consumption variables and health indicators were much stronger than those between unemployment and health.

Appendix 1. Definition of the coherency spectrum based on the covariance generating functions.

In this appendix, A1, the coherency spectrum between the two processes $X(t)$ and $Y(t)$, is defined.

The variance structure of a stochastic process, e.g. $X(t)$, may be described by its autocovariance function, $c_{xx}(k)$. Assuming that the process is stationary of second order, i.e. no trend in mean and variance, and without loss of generalization also that this constant mean is zero, we can define $c_{xx}(k) = E\{X(t), X(t+k)\}$ for k running from zero to ∞.

Given a realization, a sample, of the process, the sample time series being denoted by x_t, $t = 1, 2, \ldots T$, we can estimate the sample autocovariance function by (a1),

(a1) $$\hat{c}_{xx}(k) = (T^{-1}) \sum_{t=1}^{T-k} x_t x_{t+k}, \quad k=0,1,2,\ldots T-1.$$

Normalizing $c_{xx}(k)$ by the variance, which is $c_{xx}(o)$, we obtain the autocorrelation function, $r_{xx}(k)$. This function describes the dependence on the past behavior of the series itself. Note that $c(k)=c(-k)$ under the assumption of stationarity.

Using the shift operator, B, defined by the operation, $B^j x_t = x_{t-j}$, the information of the autocovariance function may be summarized in the associated autocovariance generating function, $C_{xx}(B)$, defined in (a2),

(a2) $$C_{xx}(B) = \sum_{k=-\infty}^{\infty} c_{xx}(k) B^k$$

Similar functions may be defined for the process $Y(t)$, and estimated, if the sample time series y_t is given.

The covariance structure between the two processes may be described by the cross covariance function, defined $c_{xy}(k) = E\{X(t), Y(t+k)\}$, for k running from $-\infty$ to ∞. Based on the two sample series, the sample cross covariance function may be estimated following (a3),

(a3) $\qquad \hat{c}_{xy}(k) = (T^{-1}) \sum_{t=1}^{t-k} x_t y_{t+k}$, $k=-T+1,\ldots,-1,0,1,\ldots,T-1$.

Normalizing by $(c_{xx}(0)c_{yy}(0))^{-\frac{1}{2}}$ we obtain the cross correlation function, $r_{xy}(k)$. This function describes the linear dependency between the two processes, or series, at various lags. Note that $c_{xy}(k)$, and $r_{xy}(k)$ are not even functions of lag, but $c_{xy}(k) \neq c_{xy}(-k) = c_{yx}(k)$.

In the same way as with $c_{xx}(k)$ we may summarize the information of the covariance structure between the two processes in the cross covariance generating function, defined in (a4),

(a4) $\qquad C_{xy}(B) = \sum_{k=-\infty}^{\infty} c_{xy}(k) B^k$

The cross correlation function is of course only normalized by the zero lag variance of the two processes. We have not accounted for effects from the autocorrelation in either of the two series. If one or both are actually autocorrelated it may be shown, see for instance (26), that the sample cross correlation function may be seriously biased, often inflationarily. Therefore, it is necessary to account for, or control for, autocorrelation in either series before estimating the two series. This is done by a transformation which transforms the two series cross correlated into white noise, i.e. non-autocorrelated series. This transformation is most often taking residuals of a univariate autoregressive and/or moving average regression, that models the auto-dependency in each series.

When each series are white noise, the $c_{xx}(k) = c_{yy}(k) = 0$ for all non-zero lags.

Another way of accounting for autocorrelation in each series would be to define the cross correlation generating function, i.e.

(a5) $\qquad R_{xy}(B) = \dfrac{C_{xy}(B)}{(C_{xx}(B)C_{yy}(B))^{\frac{1}{2}}}$

and use the $r'_{xy}(k)$ from this definition rather than those from the usual one. Note that they will be identical when the two series are white noise, because then $C_{xx}(B) = c_{xx}(0)$, and $C_{yy}(B) = c_{yy}(0)$.

However the series need not be white noise, only stationary in (a5), to obtain unbiased estimates of $r_{xy}(k)$, because we 'normalize' by the whole variance structure of the two series, and thus directly control for autocorrelation in both series.

Now, in practice we cannot obtain the $r'_{xy}(k)$ from (a5), but this

is easily done in the frequency domain, which means that we evaluate the polynomial functions in (a5) on the unit circle.
Thus we substitute B by $e^{-i\omega}$, where i is the imaginary unit, $(\pm 1)^{\frac{1}{2}} = i$, and ω is the angular frequency.

Doing this for ω running from $-\pi$ to $+\pi$ we obtain the two spectra, $S_{xx}(f)$ and $S_{yy}(f)$, and the cross spectrum between the two processes, or series, $S_{xy}(f)$. Based on (a2) and (a4) and the substitution of B by $e^{-i\omega}$ these are defined in (a6),

(a6)
$$S_{xx}(f) = \sum_{\text{all } k} c_{xx}(k)e^{-i\omega k}$$
$$S_{yy}(f) = \sum_{\text{all } k} c_{yy}(k)e^{-i\omega k} \quad , \text{ for } -\pi \leq \omega \leq +\pi$$
$$S_{xy}(f) = \sum_{\text{all } k} c_{xy}(k)e^{-i\omega k}$$

where f, is frequency in cycles per time unit. f and ω are related by the equation: $\omega = 2\pi f$. From f the period of cycle is obtained by $P = 1/f$, where P denotes the period of the cycle. It is seen that the spectra are defined for f in the interval $-\frac{1}{2}$ to $+\frac{1}{2}$. Also $S_{xx}(f)$ and $S_{yy}(f)$ are real and even functions of f, while $S_{xy}(f)$ is a complex function, and $S_{xy}(f) \neq S_{xy}(-f) = S_{yx}(f)$.

Having Fourier transformed the auto and cross covariance functions to spectra and the cross spectrum, we may on each frequency, f, put these values into (a5) instead of the generating functions. Then we obtain a complex function called the coherency function, K(f), that on each frequency measures the correlation between the two series on that frequency.

Note that this measure of correlation is not affected by autocorrelation in the two series, as we have on each frequency normalized by the variance of each series attributable to that cycle. Formally, K(f) is defined

(a7)
$$K(f) = \frac{S_{xy}(f)}{(S_{xx}(f)S_{yy}(f))^{\frac{1}{2}}} \quad \text{ for } -\frac{1}{2} \leq f \leq \frac{1}{2}$$

From (a7) we may go back to the time domain, i.e. lagged function, or stay in the frequency domain, i.e. functions of cycle frequencies. In this paper, it was decided to stay in the frequency domain, as much of the discussion about the relationship between economic conditions and health status of the population has dealt with relationships on certain cycles, i.e. usually the business cycle.

In section III partial and multiple (squared) coherency spectra are reported in diagrams. These are easily obtained in a way quite similar to the way partial and multivariate (squared) zero-lag coefficients of correlation are obtained.

How do we interpret the coherency as a measure of temporal correlation. Actually it is the most natural measure of temporal correlation that we have. Not only does it make us able to control directly for autocorrelation in each series, but it tells us something about the stability of the cyclic covariance between the two series. If the two series have a fixed temporal time-relationship on a frequency, i.e. the period is fixed for all time intervals, and the time lag (phase) between the two series on that frequency is also fixed, then we will have the top limit of the cross spectrum of the two series, and this top limit is the geometric mean of the two single spectra. Thus nominator and denominator in (a7) will be identical, and we have a coherency with modulus = 1. On the other hand if the period and the phase relationship change randomly across subintervals of the time span we will have a cross spectrum of zero, and thus a coherency of 0 on that frequency.

In interpreting the coherency spectrum we usually take the argument and the square of the modulus of $K(f)$. The former is called the phase difference of the two series on each frequency, and it measures in radians or time units the mean of the optimal lag between the two series on each mean frequency. The phase statistic may often be indicative of signs of the relationship. This is the way it is interpreted in section III, and the phase statistics are not directly reported.

Taking the square of the modulus of $K(f)$ we get a measure of the linear temporal relationship across frequencies. However, in the interpretation we usually want to examine relationships across a sub-band of frequencies. Doing this we minimize the risk of over-interpretation of a single high coefficient of coherency. If the spectrum of the 'dependent' variable, for instance y_t, fluctuates across frequencies, which it does if y_t is autocorrelated, then we cannot simply integrate the squared coherency spectrum in the sub-band of frequencies, but weight by the spectrum of y_t in that sub-band. Therefore the mean squared coherency coefficients reported in the text are defined,

(a8)
$$\bar{K}^2_{f_1-f_2} = \frac{\int_{f_2}^{f_1} (K^2(f) S_{yy}(f)) df}{\int_{f_2}^{f_1} S_{yy}(f) df}$$

where f_1 to f_2 defines the subband of frequencies.

More information of the statistics defined above is given in econometric textbooks, e.g. (16), or special books on spectral analysis, e.g. (22, 26).

References:

(1) M.H. Brenner, 1971, "Economic Changes and Heart Disease Mortality", AJPH, pp. 606-611.

(2) M.H. Brenner, 1973a, "Mental Illness and the Economy". Cambridge, Mass.

(3) M.H. Brenner, 1973b, "Fetal, Infant, and Maternal Mortality During Periods of Economic Instability", IJHS, pp. 145-159.

(4) M.H. Brenner, 1975, "Trends in Alcohol Consumption and Associated Illness. Some Effects of Economic Change", AJPH, pp. 1279-1292.

(5) M.H. Brenner, 1976, "Estimating the Social Costs of National Economic Policy: Implications for Mental and Physical Health, and Criminal Aggression". Washington D.C.

(6) M.H. Brenner, 1977, "Personal Stability and Economic Security", Social Policy, pp. 2-5.

(7) M.H. Brenner, 1979, "Mortality and the National Economy", Lancet, pp. 568-573.

(8) G.E.P. Box and G.M. Jenkins, 1976, "Time series analysis: Forecasting and Control". San Francisco.

(9) A.R. Bunn, 1979, "Ischaemic Heart Disease Mortality and the Business Cycle in Australia", AJPH, pp. 772-781.

(10) A.R. Bunn, 1980, "II. IHD Mortality and the Business Cycle in Australia". AJPH, pp. 409-411.

(11) R. Catalano, 1979, "Health costs of economic expansion: The case of manufactoring accident injuries", AJPH, pp. 789-794.

(12) R. Catalano & C.D. Dooley, 1977, "Economic Predictors of Depressed Mood and Stressfull Life Events in a Metropolitan Community", JHSB, pp. 292-307.

(13) R. Catalano and C.D. Dooley, 1979a, "Economic, life, and disorder changes: time series analysis." American Journal of Community Psychology, pp. 381-396.

(14) R. Catalano & D. Dooley, 1980, "Economic Change as a Cause of Behavioral Disorder", Psychological Bulletin, pp. 450.

(15) R. Catalano et al., 1981, "Economic, life, and symptom changes in a nonmetropolitan community", JHSB, pp. 144-154.

(16) PH.J. Dhrymes, 1970, "Econometrics - statistical foundations and applications." New York.

(17) B.S. Dohrenwend and B.P. Dohrenwend, 1978,"Some Issues in Research on Stressfull Life Events." The Journal of Nervous and Mental Disease, pp. 7-15.

(18) E. Durkheim, 1978, "Selvmordet", Norsk oversættelse, København.

(19) J. Eyer, 1977a, "Prosperity as a cause of death." IJHS, pp. 125-150.

(20) J. Eyer, 1977b, "Does Unemployment Cause the Death Rate Peak in Each Business Cycle?", IJHS, pp. 625-662.

(21) J. Eyer & M.H. Brenner, 1976, "Debate on Mental Illness and the Economy", IJHS, pp. 139-168.

(22) G.S. Fishman, 1969, "Spectral methods of econometrics." Cambridge, Mass.

(23) D.S. Hammermesh & N.M. Soss, 1974, "An Economic Theory of Suicide," Journal of Political Economy, pp. 83-98.

(24) A.F. Henry & J.F. Short, 1954, "Suicide and Homicide." New York.

(25) J.S. House, 1974, "Occupational stress and coronary heart disease: A Review and theoretical integration." JHSB, pp. 12-27.

(26) G.M. Jenkins and D.G. Watts, 1968, "Spectral Analysis and its application". San Francisco.

(27) S.V. Kasl, 1979, "Mortality and the Business Cycle: Some questions about research strategies when utilizing macro-social and ecological data." AJPH, pp. 784-788.

(28) S.V. Kasl, 1980, "Problems in the analysis and interpretation of ecological data." AJPH, pp. 413-414.

(29) K.C. Land and M.M. McMillen, 1980, "A Macrodynamic Analysis of Changes in Mortality Indexes in the United States 1946-75: Some Priliminary Results", Social Indicator Research, pp. 1-46.

(30) E.A. Lew, 1979, "Mortality and the Business Cycle: How far can we push an association." AJPH, pp. 782-783.

(31) E.A. Lew, 1980, "Heart disease mortality: Changing terminology, Diagnostic fashions, and capabilities." AJPH, pp. 411-412.

(32) J.J. Lindenthal et al, 1972, "Smoking, psychological status and stress." Social Science and Medicine. pp. 583-591.

(33) J.R. Marshall and D.P. Funch, 1979, "Mental illness and the Economy: A Critique and Partial Replication." JHSB, pp. 282-289.

(34) W.F. Ogburn, 1964, "The Fluctuations of Business as Social Forces", pp. 235-246 in "On Culture and Social Change", Chicago, reprint from: Journal of Social Forces, 1923.

(35) W.F. Ogburn & D.S. Thomas, 1923, "The Influence of the Business Cycle on Certain Social Conditions," American Statistical Association pp. 324-34.

(36) P.J. Pedersen, 1979, "Aspekter af fagbevægelsens vækst i Danmark. 1911-1976". Memo. Aarhus.

(37) A. Pierce, 1967, "The Economic Cycle and the Social Suicide Rate", American Sociological Review, pp. 457-462.

(38) R.H. Rahe et al., 1964, "Social Stress and Illness Onset", Journal of Psychosomatic Research, pp. 35-44.

(39) R.H. Rahe and R.J. Arthur, 1978, "Life change and illness studies: Past history and future directions." Journal of Human Stress, pp. 3-15.

(40) J.L. Simon, 1968, "The effect of Income on Suicide Rates: A Paradox Resolved." American Journal of Sociology, pp. 302-303.

(41) D.S. Thomas, 1927, "Social Aspects of the Business Cycle", London.

(42) G. Vigderhous & G. Fishman, 1978, "The Impact of Unemployment and Familial Integration on Changing Suicide Rates in the U.S.A., 1920-1969", Social Psychiatry, 239-248.

Sources of data.

The time series for per capita income$^{*)}$ male population cigarettes and alcohol consumption rates, and incidences of marriages and divorces have been obtained from the Statistical Yearbook of Denmark, through the years.
The mortality rates$^{**)}$ were obtained from the "Causes of Death in the Kingdom of Denmark", published by the National Health Service of Denmark, through the years of analysis.

*) Based on disposable national income at current market prices. This series was deflated, 1929 prices, and finally divided by total population pr. year.

**) The male suicide rates, 20 to 44 years aged, were kindly made disposable to me by lic.med. Lisbet Kolmos, the Hospital of Odense.

AJPH: American Journal of Public Health
IJHS: International Journal of Health Services
JHSB: Journal of Health and Social Behavior

ECONOMIC INSTABILITY AND MORTALITY
IN THE FEDERAL REPUBLIC OF GERMANY

Problems of Macroanalytical Approach with Special Reference
to Migration

Jürgen John

Gesellschaft für Strahlen- und Umweltforschung (GSF)
Institut für Medizinische Informatik und Systemforschung (MEDIS)
Neuherberg, Federal Republic of Germany

The following paper gives a short survey on the preliminary work for a study on the influence of economic instability on health which we have done up to now, stimulated in the first place by the WHO Planning Meeting for an international comparative study on the influence of economic development on health, held in Copenhagen, November 1980. In accordance with the recommendations of this meeting, the proposal was taken up to reestimate and test the model developed by Brenner on the data base for countries other than the United States or England and Wales.

The decision to reestimate Brenner's model for the Federal Republic of Germany, despite many objections against his approach, was mainly based on the consideration that it could be useful to evaluate the results presented by Brenner in the light of independent empirical evidence.

The first section of the paper reports on this test. The second section deals with the problem that the model is specified for a spatially stationary population, whereas the data used for the estimation of the model stem from a population which is not spatially stationary. In the third section the problem of model specification and of the quantitative foundations of the regression models estimated will be discussed.

1. Models and estimation results

The models we have estimated do not reflect in full the statistical analyses of Harvey Brenner. So far, we have restricted ourselves to an investigation into the overall mortality. For only from 1968 onwards, the West German statistics on causes-of-death are in harmony with the I.C.D. code; before then, a classification system was in use here that renders impossible the calculation of consistently classified cause-of-death specific death rates for some groups of diseases analysed by Brenner. Likewise, some of the controlling variables, which are supposed to reflect the influence of the classical risk factors on mortality and which Brenner has most recently incorporated in his study, could not yet be taken into consideration. For this, the data situation has still to be clarified.

For these reasons, the model versions so far estimated have been confined to the connection between overall death rates (by sex as well as by age), unemployment and rapid economic change. Area of research is the Federal Republic of Germany, including West Berlin. The total period of analysis ranges from 1950 to 1979; the periods of estimation vary for the different models, according to the supposed distributed lag, between 1951 to 1979 and 1955 to 1979.

Before going to present the specifications of the model and some estimation results, the essential features of the development of mortality, unemployment and economic growth in the F.R.G., shall be characterized.

The usual age classification was applied at the computation of death rates specific to age groups: under 1 year, 1 to under 5 years, 5 to under 10 years, etc. up to the age group of 75 to under 80 years. The age group which is open in upward direction was not included in the statistical analysis. The development of mortality, based on this age classification, is as follows:
- The death rates for the female resident population are in all age groups lower at the end of the period of analysis than at its beginning. The decrease of the rates ranges between 75% and 30%. A continuous downward trend can be observed during the whole period for most age groups. There appear to be breaches in the trend of that development for only two age groups: The mortality rates of the 15 to 19 year old show a declining trend only up to the mid-sixties and afterwards an increasing trend with strong oscillations. Likewise, the death rates of the 20 to 24 year old show a decreasing trend until the mid-sixties but afterwards keep oscillating around a constant figure.

- The death rates for the male population have been much less uniform in their development over the years. For several age groups (20-25, 50-55, 60-80), the death rates in the year 1979 are about the same as the ones in 1950 or even higher. In all age groups between 15 and 55, the development of death rates shows extremely strong and erratic oscillations. For the age groups of 60 to 74, there is an upward trend to be seen till the mid- or late sixties, changing into a downward trend later on. As compared to the mortality of women, the development for men has been - in all age groups above 15 - remarkably less favourable.

Brenner's model, therefore, has - when being applied to the data on West Germany - to face an extraordinarily great variability of the time series of death rates in question.

The pre-conditions for a rigid test on the statistical explanation power of the model are hence rather favourable.

Glancing at the economic development of West Germany with particular reference to unemployment and the gross national product, one should mention that the rapid growth of the economy during the reconstruction phase has led to a swift reduction of unemployment, which used to be very high in the early fifties. Full employment was reached at the beginning of the sixties and could be stabilised up until 1966. In 1967, for the first time in the history of the F.R.G., the GNP dropped and the rate of unemployment went up. Whereas it was possible, even on the labour market, to overcome the recession of 1967 very quickly, the second recession of the year 1975 was followed by a rather slow recovery of the employment figures.

The first model which we have re-estimated with German data is essentially identical with Brenner's model described in his well-known article in "Lancet"[1]. Dependent variables of the regression equations are the indices of the (sex- and age-specific) death rates (1952=100); this transformation of the death rates was carried out to facilitate comparisons between the estimation results for different age groups. Current and/or lagged unemployment rates, the growth trend values of real GNP, and - as indicators of "rapid economic change" - the growth trend residuals of GNP, and the change of growth rates of GNP are included in the regression model as independent variables.

The model estimated by us differs from Brenner's model in two aspects:
- Due to the small number of observations instead of a 0-10 year period only a 0-5 year lag was specified for the unemployment variable. If should be mentioned that in Brenner's study on influence of economic instability on mortality in U.S.A.[2] the assumption of a 0-5 year lag has proved to be very successful.
- Instead of an exponential growth trend we assume a linear growth trend of GNP; of course, this assumption may be crucial for the estimation results. But the data show very clearly that an exponential growth

trend is a poor description of the development of GNP over time.

The regression equations were estimated with use of OLS procedure; Brenner made use of the standard finite distributed lag model. It is true, that the application of Almon techniques is a very efficient way to handle the problem of high multicollinearity between the lagged variables; on the other hand, the use of Almon techniques has the disadvantage that <u>any</u> form of incorrect specification of the lag period results in biased and inconsistent estimators and limited value of the classical statistical tests, as well.

The estimation results are recorded in table 1. In the case of male death rates the findings are completely negative: A significant influence on death rates can be demonstrated neither for the unemployment variables nor for the variables representing rapid economic change. The findings for the female death rates are not much better: Only 3 regression coefficients of unemployment variables (one of them with the 'false' sign) and two regression coefficients of variables representing rapid economic change are significantly different from 0.

The interpretation of the estimation results for model 1 leads to two problems. The first problem arises from the intercorrelation of the independent variables. The correlation matrix of the independent variables of this model (see table 5) shows that especially the lagged unemployment variables are highly intercorrelated. Therefore we cannot exclude that with regard to these variables the poor results are caused by multicollinearity. To check this, F-tests for the subset of unemployment variables were carried on; the results of these tests are recorded in table 2. The tests indicate that the inclusion of unemployment variables is connected with a significant reduction of unexplained variance of death rates
- in the case of the male population: for infants and the age groups between 55 to 69 years,
- in the case of female population: for infants and the age groups between 20 and 34 years.

It should be pointed to the fact that significant results supporting Brenner's hypothesis are only the findings for male and female infants, and for the female age group between 20 to 24 years, whereas in the case of male death rates for the age groups between 55 to 69 years the total influence of unemployment is negative.

To overcome the problem of multicollinearity we have specified a second model in which only one unemployment variable was included, namely the cumulated value of unemployment rates in the 2-4 lag period. This variable was used by Brenner in a model the results of which were presented at the 1st Planning Meeting for the Study on Influence of Economic Development on Health. [3)] Due to the small number of observations the second unemployment variable controlling for the long term impact of unemployment could not be included into the regression model.

The estimation results for this model are recorded in table 3. With respect to the variables representing rapid economic change the findings are negative again. With regard to the unemployment variable the results demonstrate
- in the case of the male population: a significant influence of unemployment on mortality supporting the hypothesis for infants, and the age groups between 1-4, 20-24, 25-29, and 45-49 years, significant influence contradicting the hypothesis for all age groups between 55 and 74 years;
- in the case of the female population: significant influence of unemployment on mortality supporting the hypothesis for infants, for the age group between 1 to 4 years, and for all age groups between 20 to 34 years, significant influence contradicting the hypothesis for the age group between 60 to 64 years.

The second problem concerns the autocorrelation of the residuals. The results of the Durbin Watson test prove for the majority of the estimation equations of model 1 as well as of model 2 that the residuals follow a first-order autoregressive scheme; therefore the tests of significance are invalid. A re-estimation of both models with the aid of other estimation procedures was not carried out because of the uncertainty whether "true" autocorrelation exists or whether the serial correlation of the residuals results from mis-specification. It should be also remembered that the OLS-estimators although they are not efficient in the case of autocorrelation they are unbiased; the estimation results which do not correspond to the theoretical expectations therefore cannot be caused by the serial correlation of residuals.

These preliminary findings can hardly be regarded as strong additional support for Brenner's suggestion that increasing unemployment has a positive impact on death rates. However, we should mention, that the findings for infants and the female population between 20 to 34 years are in accordance with the results of Brenner's study on infant and maternal mortality in periods of economic instability.[4] If we accept Brenner's conclusion, we should assume a very short reaction period. Therefore we have estimated a third model with a 0-1 time lag period. The results are recorded in table 4. In all cases we find a highly significant influence of unemployment on mortality. The findings also demonstrate the difficulty to filter out the "true lag" on the basis of estimation results in the case of a close collinearity. Moreover, a comparison of the findings of model 1, 2,and 3 shows that - due to the multicollinearity of unemployment variables as well - the "long run equilibrium" effects of a change of unemployment are fairly similar.

The Durbin Watson test also indicates an autocorrelation for some estimation equations of model 3. We therefore estimated model 3 by applying GLS with appropriate weights. OLS - and GLS- estimators differ only slightly, and comparable results were obtained by the significance tests. For this reason the GLS estimation results are not included here.

2. Problems of migration movements

To give an explanation to the fact that the empirical findings do not seem to confirm conclusively Brenner's hypotheses for the F.R.G., there are many thinkable reasons - just to mention some:
- the lag structures of the tested model versions may be misspecified,
- possibly relevant variables are not included in the equations,
- the used independent variables may be invalid indicators of the population's psychic, social, and economic burden, caused by economic instability,
- last but not least it cannot be excluded that the population's strain on health related to the fluctuations of economic activity is, in fact, not weighty enough to influence the development of the death rates, e.g. because the West German system of social security has been developed to a far wider extent than in the United States or in the United Kingdom.

These or similar reasons shall now not be entered into more closely; but a special problem of model specification shall be dealt with. This problem does not catch one's eye at once, however, it can be of signifi-

cance for the application of the model to the F.R.G.: I mean the problem of migration movements. Brenner's model is specified for a spatially stationary population. When applied to an area with border-crossing migration movements the model implicates - due to the postulated reaction lag of death rates on changes of economic conditions - that
- the investigated population includes, at any observation time, part of the population that was exposed to economic conditions other than those described in the model variables (immigration),
- part of the population that was exposed to the economic state as described is no longer included in the investigated population at the time of observation (emigration).

Since the F.R.G. was established in 1949, an above-average degree of migration entanglements compared with other countries has existed: The annual immigration number fluctuates between 0,3 and 1,1 million persons during the observation period (this corresponds to 0,6-1,8% of the resident population at the time in question); the number of migrations amounts to 0,15 to 0,66 million persons (which corresponds to 0,3-1,1% of the resident population at the time in question). The immigration streams had been mainly fed from German Democratic Republic refugees until the erection of the wall in Berlin in 1961; afterwards foreign workers (Gastarbeiter = "guest workers") and their families from the mediterranean area, i.e. Turkey, Yugoslavia, Italy, Greece, and Spain, have been predominating. The emigration movement is mainly composed of the foreign workers' return to their native countries.

Judging by the theoretical considerations underlying Brenner's model, the migration movements of the foreign workers and their families are especially important on the grounds that
1. the potential of foreign workers represents, to a certain degree, a cyclical buffer-function for the West German labour market; the risk to lose one's job in a period of recession is bigger for foreign workers than for their German co-workers. Therefore one could expect that health effects of economic instability would be traceable especially in the foreign population. In addition, a great number of the foreign population falls within the discriminated fringe groups of our society, apart from the labour situation with its chances and The accumulation of stress in different compasses of a life-time may increase the probability that loss of employment or other forms of economic deprivation cause serious effects on health.

Unfortunately, in view of the foreign population in the F.R.G. the models tested are not quite adequate to show a connection possibly existing between economic instability and mortality. The foreign population is characterized by a large share of immigrants and emigrants: The immigration quota has fluctuated between 9 and 47%, the emigration quota between 10 and 19%, since 1967. The numbers point to considerable divergencies between the model population and the investigated population that in fact was recorded. These divergencies are a problem especially in view of the great follow-up loss. Above all, in case of recession it scarcely can be imputed that the foreign workers who are remaining in the F.R.G. as well as those returning to their native countries will be subjected to a deterioration in the labour market situation to the same extent. It rather must be assumed that loss of employment and limited chances for a soon re-employment will be the deciding factor to return home.

2. The considerable intensity of migration entanglements does not only confront us with the problem that a population group that is exposed to the risks of economic instability very strongly, evades, to a large extent, the analysis within the scope of the tested models. Parallel to this problem, the question must be asked whether the death rates computed on the resident's population plan draw a sufficiently correct picture of the development of the death rates as far as the stationary part of resident population is concerned. The migration movements of the foreign workers and their families let us doubt this again. If health checks, carried out officially and by employers, to which foreign workers are subjected upon entry into West Germany and at the beginning of their employment, are effective, if personnel policy of enterprises tends to increase the risk of losing one's job in case of ill-health and to decrease the possibility of re-employment, but at the same time, loss of employment and a small chance only for a new job cause emigration movements, then it may happen that these filters of selecting health will be reflected in lower death rates of the foreigners residing in the F.R.G. The fact that the foreign portion of the resident population has increased rapidly since the early sixties (1961: 0,69 millions = 1,3%; 1970: 2,98 millions = 4,9% 1980: 4,45 millions = 7,2%) would imply that the development of the death rates of the total population would increasingly underestimate the death rates of the stationary part of the resident population.

Furthermore, taking into account that the volume of migration streams is mainly determined by the situation of the domestic labour market and assuming that processes of health selection become tenser in recession phases, it may occur that the difference between the death rates of the resident population and those of the stationary population fluctuates corresponding to the national labour market conditions. Therefore, we cannot exclude a connection existing between economic instability and mortality of the stationary population which is, however, hidden by measurement errors of systematic nature.

While the question of possibly exported health effects of economic instability in the F.R.G. cannot be answered with the data available for us, we can, at least, attempt to investigate the validity of death rates of the resident population as indicators for the death rates of the spatially stationary population by comparing the death rates of the foreigners with those of the Germans.

It was not possible to compute the death rates by nationalities for the F.R.G. in the years preceding 1974. Therefore we decided to work with the data of the Free State of Bavaria which have been available since 1971. This procedure has the advantage that the analysis period includes a phase of full-employment. The German population can be regarded as stationary in the sense of the model (since 1967 the immigration and emigration quotas of the German population have fluctuated by 0,2 respectively 0,1% with slight deviations only). A computation of the death rates of foreigners which differentiates according to the duration of their stay is not feasible.

The results of the computations are described in short as follows:
- The infant mortality of the two sexes is higher among foreigners than in the German population.
- The death rates of male and female children between 1 to 15 years do not show any systematic difference between foreigners and Germans.
- The death rates of the grown-ups are, without exception, lower for male foreigners that for the German male population of Bavaria in all age groups and in all years under observation.
- The death rates of the grown-ups are, almost without exception, lower for the female foreigners than for the German population of Bavaria. The discrepancies between the death rates are smaller in most cases compared to the male population.

- In comparing the ratio of death rates of the foreigners with those of Germans in 1971, a year of full-employment, and in the recession year of 1975, it can be observed that these ratios drop sharply in all age groups for men and women as well. However, if one compares the development of the year 1975 with 1978, in which year a slight recovery in the labour market could be archieved, the development is not homogenous.

These findings are essentially consistent with our hypothesis that migration movements are also the results of selection processes of health, and that these selection processes are intensified considerably during a recession phase. The fact that differences in death rates are smaller in the case of women than in men could be explained within the scope of our hypothesis that the female labour supply is smaller than that of the male population among foreigners, too. In addition, due to sex-specific differences of income, a women's loss of employment might not exert the same economic pressure on the families of the foreign workers as in the case of the man's loss of job.

The following test supports the assumption that the decrease of the ratio of death rates of foreigners and Germans in the year 1975, compared to 1971, is influenced by the deterioration of the labour market conditions. The accidental deaths were eliminated in all age groups, in which accidents as cause of death play a main role, from the total number of deaths of the male grown-ups. As the accidental death is not related to previous ill-health, which would allow a selection upon the entry into Germany or a return to the native country, it can be expected according to the hypothesis that the ratio of the death rates of foreigners and Germans, excluding the accidental deaths, will still decrease on a larger scale. The results show that this proves to be true for the most age groups. Judged by the standardized death rates (based on the resident population in 1975), the relation of death rates receded by 30% including accidental deaths, and by 39% excluding accidental deaths.

On the one hand, the results of our computations prove quite significantly that Brenner's model is not very suitable for the purpose to show a possible connection between economic instability and mortality in the foreign population: Ill health is especially exported into foreign countries during phases of recession. The liberal orthodoxy likes to describe economic crises as "cleaning crises" during which the economy frees itself from the ballast of "sick" enterprises. Due to the opening of the German labour market for foreign workers, economic crises will include this function with respect to a number of sick employees, too.

On the other hand, the findings confirm our suspicion that the death rates of the total population are a rather poor indicator for the mortality of the spatially stationary population: Considerable differences in the mortality between foreigners and Germans form a picture, drawn too favourably, of the trend in the development of death rates because of the growing numbers of foreigners; moreover, the extent of the measurement error is obviously dependent on the labour market conditions. The following numbers offer an illustrative example of the differences between the death rates for two age groups covering the male population between 40 to 44 years and between 45 to 49 years and the corresponding death rates for the male population of German nationality. The computations are based on the assumption that mortality differences between foreigners and Germans in Bavaria are representative for those of the F.R.G. The value for the year 1961 was estimated by assuming that the mortality differences in 1961 correspond to those in 1971 (both years are years of full-employment. In order to make the comparison more transparent the death rates are also listed as indices.

Age group		Numer of deaths per 100.000 of population								
		1961	1971	1972	1973	1974	1975	1976	1977	1978
40-44 years	(1)	332.9	379.6	380.2	379.4	361.5	385.8	367.9	346.8	352.1
	(2)	335.8	394.1	400.5	402.1	381.5	411.3	387.2	361.1	365.9
	(1)	87.7	100.0	100.2	99.9	95.2	101.6	96.9	91.4	92.8
	(2)	85.2	100.0	101.6	102.0	96.8	104.4	98.3	91.6	92.9
45-49 years	(1)	550.8	567.8	572.7	570.8	566.4	592.3	591.9	575.9	598.5
	(2)	552.8	576.9	586.9	591.7	586.7	615.9	612.2	595.4	621.2
	(1)	97.0	100.0	100.9	100.5	99.8	104.3	104.2	101.4	105.4
	(2)	95.8	100.0	101.7	102.6	101.7	106.8	106.1	103.2	107.7

(1) Total resident population
(2) German resident population

A comparison shows that the measured values of the two series do, indeed, not well conform. In each of the two age groups it can be even observed that in one case the two death rates develop in different directions. We should not be misled by the apparent smallness of these differences: if, in the true model, the variance of death rates explained by the indicators of economic instability constitutes only a small share of their total variance, minor measurement errors of systematic nature might suffice to blur the whole context.

Let us sum up these considerations by saying that it is probably premature to reject the hypothesis which claims a relationship between mortality rates, unemployment and fluctuations of economic growth, although the different model versions tested so far, could not satisfy the expectations. Against a rejection on this ground it is to be said, first, that the mortality of foreigners is necessarily beyond the analytical reach of the model and, second, that the mortality rates of the resident population - used as indicators for the mortality of the (in accordance with the model) stationary population - are of a weak validity.

Whether, in the framework of an aggregate-level analysis, the competence of Brenner's hypothesis for the foreign population can be studied at all, is to be doubted. On the basis of macro-statistical data from the home countries of the "guest workers", one is, at best, able to show that the migration movements to and from these countries have also some influence on the death rates of people living there. It seems almost impossible to find out whether this influence is anything other than a mere reflexion of the processes of health-specific selection as described above; for that purpose, rather differentiated statistical data would have to be at hand - and those are certainly not available. The only way to proceed in this case, might be to study the life careers of the re-migrating foreigners.

As for the possibilities to investigate more deeply the potential ratio between economic instability and mortality in the stationary resident population of West Germany, the most simple method - that is a calculation of death rates of the stationary population - is not viable due to a lack of adequate data. Even auxiliary constructs, like the introduction of migration movements as additional controlling variables, are not very promising since the number of degrees of freedom is small enough and the multicollinearity between migration movements and the unemployment rate is rather high.

A feasible approach to the subject, however, could be to examine the basic hypothesis by way of a cross-sectional analysis. At least, when using more recent cross-sectional data, it would be possible to eliminate all foreigner-related information from the mortality statistics,

and by doing so, to approximate to the concept of stationary population.
True, the price for this will be that, in the framework of a cross-sectional analysis, one is confronted with the problem of interregional
migration of German people. Whether it will be possible to define a
sufficiently big number of study regions with a sufficiently great variability of economic states in a way so that the migration movements
can be held within acceptable proportions, will still have to be explored.

3. Methodological Considerations

The final remarks concern two problems which are of a rather methodological nature. They usually come about when regression techniques are
employed and they are of particular importance when these techniques
are being used for the testing of Brenner's model.

The first problem concerns the specification of the model and the model
selection respectively. Over the years, Brenner has - in line with a
widely accepted practice in econometrics - formulated a number of models
of the relation between economic instability and mortality and he has
tested them within the same space-time segments - a practice which, as
you have just seen, has been followed, too.

It is held, though, that of several competing models with regard to the
same space-time segment only one, at the utmost, can be specified correctly: n or n-1 models must be mis-specified, that is they either contain
irrelevant variables or they fail to contain relevant one.

We should, therefore, remember that - apart from the rather rare case of
orthogonality between included and excluded variables - the exclusion of
relevant variables leads to biased and, usually, inconsistent estimators
of the parameters of the included variables; in addition, it also leads
to an over-estimation of the variance of residuals. Hence, in such a
situation, the classic statistical tests are only of a very limited value.
On the other hand, the inclusion of irrelevant variables in the regression
equation does not, to be sure, affect the properties of unbiasedness and
consistency of OLS-estimators; yet, the resulting loss of efficiency will
lead to a comparably unprecise estimation of the influence the relevant
variables exert. Furthermore, an increasing number of independent variables intensifies, as a rule, the problem of multi-collinearity.

The decision about how many and exactly which variables are - in a specific case - to be included in the regression is particularly difficult under circumstances where the theoretical foundation of the model is weak and/or the lack of empirical a priori information is considerable. In such a situation the econometric practices prefer a procedure of model selection that discriminates between the competing models according to the best-fit criterion. This implies, amongst other things, that the adjusted coefficient of multiple determination or of the respective residual sum of squares becomes the point of orientation. The theoretical reasoning for this sort of selection procedure is such that, under (rather) general conditions, the residual sum of squares - after having been adjusted by the number of degrees of freedom - of the false model specification is, <u>on average</u>, bigger than the corresponding sum of squares of the correctly specified model.

When applying this selection strategy (which is sometimes referred to as the application of the Theil-criterion), one should however not forget that this procedure is purposeful only when the "true model" is in fact one of the competing models in question. The criterion, moreover, fails whenever a comparison is made between the correctly specified model and models which include irrelevant variables since, in this case, for all specifications the same adjusted residual sum of squares will, on average, be reached. As to models with lag structures - the case that interests us most -, two additional problems are to be considered:
- The application of the criterion is controversial whenever the competing models are special cases of a more comprehensive model (that is when, for instance, models are compared with each other which only differ with regard to the size of the lag interval). For in such a case, even the addition of variables which do not fulfill the requirements of the significance level, may increase the adjusted coefficient of determination.
- This approach, after all, produces clear distinctions only when, on the one hand, the expected values differ remarkably and, on the other hand, the probability distributions of the adjusted sums of squares group closely round their expected values. Since, particularly with regression models having alternative distributed lags, the residual sums of squares frequently tend to differ very slightly, the chance to be able to select the correct model should not be over-estimated. This is impressively demonstrated by a more recent Monte Carlo study which analyses the problem of specification of distributed lags.[5]

Given these constraints, it does not appear very useful to mainly base the model selection - especially with regard to the "optimal lag" - on the Theil-criterion. As long as empirical a priori information on the structure of lags in the relationship between stress and illness or even death is not more secure than hitherto, it is highly recommendable to perform supplementary tests on specification errors; just recently those test procedures have been substantially improved.[6]

The second, even more serious problem concerns the relationship between the models tested and Brenner's crucial hypothesis (which underlies these models), namely that "economic instability and insecurity increase the likelihood of immoderate and unstable life habits, disruption of basic social networks, and major life stresses"[7] and that these consequences of economic instability and insecurity are a major source of higher mortality rates.[8]

Now, the validity of econometric estimation and statistical test of significance presupposes that the numerical values of the time series used validly respresent magnitudes of quantities. When we look at the regression equations and ask whether the real numbers we use for our computations really represent magnitudes of quantities, then we might answer this question in a positive manner (although some doubt may be appropriate as to whether the real GNP should be regarded as a quantity!). When, however, the econometric estimation and statistical tests of significance have also to be seen as a verification of the hypothesis underlying the regression models, further questions should be asked:
- Is there any quantitative foundation of Brenner's hypothesis which permits us to regard unstable life habits, disruption of basic social network, or life stresses in a population as variable properties that are quantities?
- Which are the arguments that support the assumption that the variables of the model actually are valid indicators of these quantities?

Certainly, the second question can only be answered when the answer to the first question is known. If the variable to be represented by an indicator is no quantity, then an indicator of this variable which ensures the validity of econometric estimation does not exist.

My impression is that a well-confirmed quantitative foundation for a quantitative representation of Brenner's hypothesis is still lacking. While this is so, it must remain uncertain how the results of model estimations can be interpreted in relation to the underlying hypothesis. It is to be apprehended that, in consequence of this uncertainty, a never-ending debate will commence, first, on the probability of the occurrence of statistical artefacts, secondly, on the indicator validity of the variables used - a debate which will be useless as long as we do not know whether indicators which are valid for the application of regression analysis, or any other econometric techniques, do exist at all.

List of variables and symbols

M01T = Index of male age-specific death rates, age group < 1 year
M05T = Index of male age-specific death rates, age group 1-< 5 years
M10T = Index of male age-specific death rates, age group 5-<10 years
.
.
.
M80T = Index of male age-specific death rates, age group 75-<80 years

F01T = Index of female age-specific death rates, age group < 1 year
F05T = Index of female age-specific death rates, age group 1-< 5 years
F10T = Index of female age-specific death rates, age group 5-<10 years
.
.
.
F80T = Index of female age-specific death rates, age group 75-<80 years

GT = Growth trend value of real GNP p.c.
GTR = Residual of GT (absolute values)
CGR = Change of growth rates of real GNP p.c.
UR0 = Unemployment rate in the year t
UR1 = Unemployment rate in the year t-1
.
.
.
UR5 = Unemployment rate in the year t-5
UR(2-4) = Sum of unemployment rates in the years t-2 to t-4

R^2 = Coefficient of determination
$\bar{R}^2$ = Corrected coefficient of determination
F = F Statistic
DW = Durbin Watson Statistic

Results of regression analysis: Model 1
Table 1
(t-values in parentheses, sign omitted)

Dep. var.	C	URO	UR1	UR2	UR3	UR4	UR5	GT	GTR	CGR	$R^2(\bar{R}^2)$	F	DW
M01T	80.65	0.02 (0.00)	-2.04 (0.94)	0.59 (0.29)	0.70 (0.37)	-0.15 (0.08)	2.09 (1.66)	-0.0037[+] (4.21)	0.0068 (1.08)	0.8988 (1.66)	0.9682 (0.9491)	50.76[+]	0.97
M05T	103.43	-0.85 (0.90)	-0.86 (0.45)	1.89 (1.37)	-0.57 (0.44)	0.49 (0.41)	0.13 (0.16)	-0.0050[+] (8.41)	0.0036 (0.84)	0.3063 (0.83)	0.9913 (0.9723)	94.55[+]	2.54
M10T	114.58	-2.66 (1.65)	-0.32 (0.13)	0.39 (0.16)	1.07 (0.49)	0.44 (0.22)	-0.87 (0.60)	-0.0039[+] (3.92)	0.0158 (1.30)	0.7804 (1.25)	0.9565 (0.8639)	17.92[+]	1.09
M15T	111.79	-1.91 (0.98)	0.61 (0.20)	-0.99 (0.35)	2.22 (0.83)	-0.79 (0.32)	-0.77 (0.44)	-0.0037[+] (3.02)	0.0073 (0.82)	0.6310 (0.84)	0.9078 (0.7185)	7.81[+]	0.97
M20T	77.21	-1.24 (0.38)	-0.30 (0.06)	-1.37 (0.29)	2.56 (0.57)	-2.47 (0.60)	2.21 (0.75)	0.0025 (1.24)	0.0129 (0.87)	0.6473 (0.51)	0.5076 (-.1878)	0.58	1.00
M25T	84.71	-0.60 (0.28)	0.21 (0.06)	-1.75 (0.55)	1.60 (0.53)	0.01 (0.00)	2.31 (1.18)	0.0001 (0.09)	-0.0010 (0.10)	0.0419 (0.05)	0.8788 (0.6356)	5.65[+]	2.37
M30T	102.61	-2.04 (1.46)	0.40 (0.18)	0.44 (0.22)	1.32 (0.69)	-0.25 (0.15)	0.34 (0.27)	-0.0023[o] (2.56)	0.0091 (1.43)	0.0053 (0.00)	0.9501 (0.8442)	15.45[+]	1.34
M35T	101.33	0.84 (0.66)	-0.45 (0.23)	-0.99 (0.53)	1.41 (0.81)	-1.33 (0.84)	0.92 (0.80)	-0.0016[o] (1.99)	0.0002 (0.05)	-0.0447 (0.09)	0.8730 (0.6195)	5.34[+]	0.85
M40T	91.58	-0.69 (0.70)	0.18 (0.12)	-0.22 (0.15)	0.70 (0.53)	-1.18 (0.97)	0.80 (0.91)	-0.0002 (0.36)	0.0043 (0.97)	0.3110 (0.82)	0.6130 (0.0012)	1.00	1.19
M45T	77.91	0.25 (0.16)	-0.88 (0.35)	-0.001 (0.00)	-0.41 (0.18)	-0.24 (0.12)	1.33 (0.91)	0.0015 (1.47)	0.0088 (1.20)	0.2240 (0.36)	0.5697 (-.0807)	0.80	0.82
M50T	87.92	-0.26 (0.24)	0.92 (0.55)	-0.61 (0.39)	1.38 (0.93)	-1.10 (0.82)	0.32 (0.33)	0.0007 (1.01)	0.0028 (0.57)	0.0462 (0.11)	0.6752 (0.1295)	1.40	1.25
M55T	107.64	0.40 (0.44)	0.01 (0.00)	0.26 (0.19)	-0.18 (0.15)	-0.63 (0.55)	0.23 (0.27)	-0.0014[o] (2.43)	0.0051 (1.22)	-0.0253 (0.07)	0.8194 (0.4742)	3.41[o]	1.53
M60T	121.27	-1.21 (1.67)	0.11 (0.10)	-0.56 (0.53)	-0.05 (0.05)	0.18 (0.20)	0.40 (0.61)	-0.0018[+] (3.86)	0.0041 (1.22)	-0.2167 (0.77)	0.9683 (0.9001)	25.02[+]	1.72
M65T	143.47	-1.81 (1.94)	1.88 (1.29)	-2.29 (1.67)	2.16 (1.68)	-2.03 (1.74)	-0.32 (0.38)	-0.0028[+] (4.84)	0.0046 (1.09)	-0.1617 (0.45)	0.9505 (0.8454)	15.58[+]	2.12
M70T	134.73	-1.69 (0.88)	0.19 (0.06)	0.63 (0.22)	-0.64 (0.25)	-1.07 (0.45)	-0.38 (0.22)	-0.0017 (1.39)	0.0124 (1.43)	0.0742 (0.10)	0.8147 (0.4621)	3.29[o]	1.01
M75T	110.17	-1.58 (0.77)	1.00 (0.31)	0.22 (0.07)	-0.33 (0.11)	-1.03 (0.40)	0.34 (0.18)	0.0001 (0.07)	0.0106 (1.13)	0.0049 (0.00)	0.5993 (-.0253)	0.93	0.98
M80T	96.39	-0.85 (0.55)	0.52 (0.22)	0.07 (0.03)	-0.43 (0.21)	-0.42 (0.22)	1.06 (0.76)	0.0004 (0.40)	0.0098 (1.41)	0.0937 (0.16)	0.3929 (-.3530)	0.30	1.49
F01T	84.30	0.63 (0.50)	-1.91 (0.98)	1.33 (0.73)	-1.48 (0.86)	1.39 (0.89)	1.66 (1.47)	-0.0041[+] (5.38)	0.0030 (0.53)	0.7164 (1.48)	0.9881 (0.9662)	68.79[+]	1.22
F05T	113.43	-1.24 (1.26)	1.69 (1.11)	-1.41 (0.98)	2.13 (1.59)	-0.43 (0.35)	-0.17 (0.19)	-0.0058[+] (9.42)	0.0041 (0.93)	0.0564 (0.15)	0.9919 (0.9742)	101.72[+]	2.29
F10T	116.43	-1.42 (0.60)	-0.93 (0.25)	1.15 (0.33)	-0.27 (0.08)	1.19 (0.40)	-1.02 (0.48)	-0.0039[+] (2.63)	0.0104 (0.97)	0.4407 (0.48)	0.9001 (0.6963)	7.11[+]	1.04
F15T	116.68	-3.22 (1.43)	3.70 (1.05)	-3.34 (1.01)	3.76 (1.21)	-1.24 (0.44)	-0.77 (0.38)	-0.0034[o] (2.38)	-0.0019 (0.19)	0.1513 (0.17)	0.8765 (0.6293)	5.53[+]	1.56
F20T	73.69	-1.99 (0.66)	3.81 (0.82)	-2.29 (0.52)	1.45 (0.35)	-0.60 (0.16)	0.09 (0.03)	0.0008 (0.41)	0.0093 (0.68)	-0.5136 (0.44)	0.3915 (-.3547)	0.30	1.19
F25T	68.99	-0.46 (0.35)	0.85 (0.42)	-1.41 (0.75)	2.99 (1.69)	-0.42 (0.26)	-0.34 (0.29)	-0.0012 (1.51)	0.0054 (0.92)	0.6080 (1.21)	0.9092 (0.7226)	7.95[+]	1.35
F30T	83.43	-0.33 (0.47)	0.61 (0.55)	0.29 (0.28)	1.08 (1.11)	-0.35 (0.39)	0.75 (1.16)	-0.0028[+] (6.34)	0.0029 (0.89)	-0.2246 (0.81)	0.9914 (0.9726)	95.51[+]	2.04
F35T	108.20	1.67[o] (1.93)	-0.02 (0.00)	-0.29 (0.23)	1.25 (1.05)	-0.74 (0.68)	0.07 (0.10)	-0.0041[+] (7.54)	-0.0066 (1.68)	-0.2428 (0.72)	0.9868 (0.9580)	61.79[+]	2.00
F40T	109.02	-2.17[+] (2.75)	2.34[o] (1.91)	-0.29 (0.26)	-0.48 (0.44)	0.39 (0.40)	-0.51 (0.72)	-0.0038[+] (7.61)	0.0056 (1.56)	-0.2767 (0.90)	0.9853 (0.9533)	55.45[+]	1.91
F45T	107.78	0.83 (0.72)	-1.83 (1.02)	1.18 (0.69)	-1.02 (0.64)	0.06 (0.03)	0.57 (0.54)	-0.0028[+] (3.88)	0.0017 (0.32)	0.2904 (0.65)	0.9544 (0.8574)	17.03[+]	0.87
F50T	107.07	-1.10 (0.89)	-0.13 (0.06)	0.86 (0.48)	-0.03 (0.00)	0.04 (0.03)	-0.47 (0.42)	-0.0021[+] (2.76)	0.0039 (0.69)	0.1537 (0.32)	0.8940 (0.6789)	6.64[+]	1.22
F55T	104.58	0.35 (0.29)	-0.84 (0.45)	0.39 (0.22)	-0.21 (0.12)	0.18 (0.12)	-0.34 (0.31)	-0.0022[+] (2.84)	0.0046 (0.85)	0.5053 (1.08)	0.8847 (0.6523)	6.00[+]	0.89
F60T	101.29	-1.10 (1.50)	0.67 (0.59)	0.001 (0.00)	-0.60 (0.59)	0.54 (0.59)	0.21 (0.31)	-0.0019[+] (4.16)	0.0057 (1.71)	-0.0365 (0.13)	0.9687 (0.9014)	25.39[+]	0.93
F65T	120.72	-0.47 (0.54)	0.38 (0.29)	0.47 (0.37)	0.07 (0.06)	-0.56 (0.52)	-0.32 (0.41)	-0.0037[+] (6.79)	0.0034 (0.86)	-0.1833 (0.55)	0.9748 (0.9203)	31.77[+]	1.26
F70T	112.90	-1.10 (0.97)	0.32 (0.18)	-0.05 (0.03)	0.53 (0.34)	-0.49 (0.34)	0.23 (0.23)	-0.0033[+] (4.66)	0.0091[o] (1.78)	0.2953 (0.67)	0.9664 (0.8943)	23.56[+]	1.29
F75T	117.76	-0.56 (0.40)	0.57 (0.26)	-0.28 (0.14)	-0.02 (0.00)	0.61 (0.35)	-0.43 (0.34)	-0.0037[+] (4.23)	0.0054 (0.85)	-0.0799 (0.15)	0.9550 (0.8592)	17.27[+]	1.41
F80T	109.45	-0.80 (0.66)	0.55 (0.29)	-0.15 (0.08)	0.26 (0.15)	-0.47 (0.31)	0.88 (0.80)	-0.0030[+] (3.89)	0.0097[o] (1.76)	0.2152 (0.46)	0.9651 (0.8901)	22.60[+]	1.63

o) significant at the .05-level
+) significant at the .01-level

Table 2

Hierarchical tests for subsets of variables
(model 1)

(1) Growth
(2) Growth + Unemployment
(3) Growth + Unemployment + Rapid Economic Change

Dependent Variable		F_T	F_A	$\bar{R}^2$	$\Sigma \hat{b}_i$ (UR)	Partial correlation UR 0 1 2 3 4 5	GTR
M01T	(1)	275.32		.9196		+ + + + + +	+
	(2)	58.84	2.70°⁾	.9440	1.53		+
	(3)	50.76	1.86	.9491	1.22		
M05T	(1)	675.75		.9657		+ + + + + +	−
	(2)	126.44	2.09	.9734	.55		+
	(3)	94.55	.58	.9723	.43		
M10T	(1)	107.83		.8166		− − − − − −	+
	(2)	18.01	1.36	.8323	−1.61		+
	(3)	17.92	2.98°⁾	.8639	−1.96		
M15T	(1)	64.89		.7383		− − − − − −	+
	(2)	10.28	1.05	.7302	−1.15		+
	(3)	7.81	.65	.7185	−1.63		
M20T	(1)	4.47		.1265		− − − − − −	+
	(2)	.65	.17	−.1150	− .32		+
	(3)	.58	.48	−.1878	− .30		
M25T	(1)	29.84		.5458		+ + + + + +	−
	(2)	8.23	2.58	.6782	1.79		−
	(3)	5.65	.01	.6356	1.79		
M30T	(1)	117.06		.8287		+ + + + + +	+
	(2)	18.54	1.57	.8539	.20		+
	(3)	15.45	.00	.8442	.20		
M35T	(1)	61.20		.7150		+ + + + + +	+
	(2)	7.78	.42	.6641	.39		+
	(3)	5.34	.01	.6195	.40		
M40T	(1)	6.11		.1754		− − − − − −	+
	(2)	1.10	.93	.0293	− .28		+
	(3)	1.00	.76	.0012	− .40		
M45T	(1)	5.07		.1450		+ − − − − +	+
	(2)	.84	.29	−.0500	.16		+
	(3)	.80	.76	−.0807	.05		
M50T	(1)	6.78		.1942		+ + + + + +	+
	(2)	1.94	1.10	.2150	.61		+
	(3)	1.40	.17	.1295	.65		
M55T	(1)	33.11		.5722		+ − − − − −	+
	(2)	4.29	.38	.4896	.11		+
	(3)	3.41	.75	.4742	.08		
M60T	(1)	94.07		.7950		− − − − − −	+
	(2)	28.81	4.63⁺⁾	.9026	− .89		+
	(3)	25.02	.30	.9001	−1.13		

Table 2 (continued)

Hierarchical tests for subsets of variables
(model 1)

(1) Growth
(2) Growth + Unemployment
(3) Growth + Unemployment + Rapid Economic Change

Dependent variable		F_T	F_A	$\bar{R}^2$	$\Sigma \hat{b}_i$ (UR)	Partial correlation UR 0 1 2 3 4 5	GTR
M65T	(1)	13.42		.3411		− − − − − −	+
	(2)	20.48	14.06+)	.8504	−2.43		+
	(3)	15.58	.62	.8454	−2.42		
M70T	(1)	.09		−.0396		− − − − − −	+
	(2)	3.93	4.55+)	.4605	−2.85		+
	(3)	3.29	1.03	.4621	−2.97		
M75T	(1)	2.16	.98	.0462		− − − − − −	+
	(2)	1.12	.98	.0388	−1.39		+
	(3)	.93	.00	−.0253	−1.39		
M80T	(1)	.47		−.0226		− − − − − +	+
	(2)	.11	.07	−.3515	.04		+
	(3)	.30	.99	−.3530	− .06		
F01T	(1)	293.25		.9241		+ + + + + +	+
	(2)	86.20	4.70+)	.9613	2.47		+
	(3)	68.79	1.18	.9622	1.62		
F05T	(1)	671.25		.9654		+ + + + + +	+
	(2)	139.99	2.68	.9759	.63		+
	(3)	101.71	.44	.9742	.59		
F10T	(1)	76.28		.7583		− − − − − −	+
	(2)	9.47	.38	.7119	−1.09		+
	(3)	7.11	.56	.6963	−1.30		
F15T	(1)	51.44		.6776		− − − − − −	−
	(2)	8.01	.93	.6714	−1.09		−
	(3)	5.53	.04	.6293	−1.12		
F20T	(1)	1.55		.0223		+ + + + + +	+
	(2)	.33	.21	−.2865	.32		+
	(3)	.30	.19	−.3547	.47		
F25T	(1)	27.18		.5217		+ + + + + +	+
	(2)	9.80	3.70o)	.7195	1.43		+
	(3)	7.95	1.09	.7226	1.22		
F30T	(1)	128.24		.8413		+ + + + + +	−
	(2)	109.70	17.12+)	.9731	1.98		+
	(3)	95.51	.67	.9726	2.05		
F35T	(1)	177.99		.8806		+ + + + + +	−
	(2)	73.73	7.32+)	.9550	1.84		−
	(3)	61.79	1.61	.9580	1.96		

Table 2 (continued)

Hierarchical tests for subsets of variables
(model 1)

(1) Growth
(2) Growth + Unemployment
(3) Growth + Unemployment + Rapid Economic Change

Dependent variable		F_T	F_A	$\bar{R}^2$	$\Sigma \hat{b}_i$(UR)	Partial correlation UR 0 1 2 3 4 5	GTR
F40T	(1)	391.70		.9421		+ + + + + +	+
	(2)	65.22	1.55	.9493	-.18		+
	(3)	55.45	1.72	.9533	-.14		
F45T	(1)	188.91		.8868		- - - - - -	+
	(2)	23.95	.51	.8700	-.12		+
	(3)	17.03	.25	.8574	-.22		
F50T	(1)	65.79		.7297		- - - - - -	+
	(2)	9.59	.80	.7147	-.77		+
	(3)	6.64	.11	.6789	-.81		
F55T	(1)	60.25		.7117		- - - - - -	+
	(2)	6.78	.49	.6584	-.43		+
	(3)	6.00	.72	.6523	-.47		
F60T	(1)	251.56		.9126		- - - - - -	+
	(2)	30.43	.82	.9075	-.30		+
	(3)	25.39	.02	.9014	-.28		
F65T	(1)	311.64		.9283		- - - - - -	+
	(2)	42.95	.81	.9244	-.46		+
	(3)	31.77	.55	.9203	-.43		
F70T	(1)	238.24		.9081		- - - - - -	+
	(2)	27.42	.23	.8851	-.41		+
	(3)	23.56	1.74	.8943	-.56		
F75T	(1)	218.10		.9005		- - - + + -	+
	(2)	25.13	.11	.8756	-.10		+
	(3)	17.27	.41	.8592	-.11		
F80T	(1)	232.67		.9061		+ + + + + +	+
	(2)	26.70	.23	.8823	.40		+
	(3)	22.60	1.61	.8901	.27		

F_T : F-value for the entire regression equation

F_A : F-value for the additionally included variables (UR0, UR1, UR2, UR3, and UR4, UR5 resp. GTR, and CGR)

    o) significant at the .05-level
    +) significant at the .01-level

$\Sigma \hat{b}_i$(UR) : Sum of regression coefficients of unemployment variables

Partial correlation: Sign of partial correlation coefficients of variables not included in the regression equation

Table 3

Results of regression analysis: Model 2
(t-values in parentheses, sign omitted)

Dep. var.	C	UR(2-4)	GT	GTR	CGR	$R^2(\bar{R}^2)$	F	DW
M01T	101.10	0.4735[+] (4.31)	-0.0055[+] (14.69)	0.0052 (0.90)	0.2732 (0.67)	0.9809 (0.9550)	50.76[+]	0.97
M05T	107.74	0.2757[+] (3.96)	-0.0054[+] (22.90)	0.0008 (0.22)	0.0414 (0.16)	0.9908 (0.9782)	94.55[+]	2.54
M10T	122.76	-0.2085 (1.52)	-0.0047[+] (10.24)	0.0109 (1.50)	-0.0280 (0.06)	0.9342 (0.8486)	36.03[+]	0.71
M15T	113.08	-0.2147 (1.45)	-0.0039[+] (7.70)	0.0045 (0.57)	0.1165 (0.21)	0.8897 (0.7519)	19.94[+]	1.02
M20T	94.97	-0.1498 (0.61)	0.0010 (1.30)	0.0099 (0.84)	0.2522 (0.30)	0.5005 (0.1077)	1.75	0.88
M25T	105.86	0.5253[+] (3.26)	-0.0017[+] (3.20)	-0.0017 (0.19)	-0.1394 (0.23)	0.8589 (0.6878)	14.77[+]	1.94
M30T	110.53	0.2291[o] (2.16)	-0.0030[+] (8.28)	0.0051 (0.91)	-0.2555 (0.65)	0.9400 (0.8614)	39.83[+]	1.16
M35T	103.98	0.0635 (0.71)	-0.0018[+] (5.89)	0.0016 (0.34)	-0.1053 (0.32)	0.8745 (0.7648)	17.08[+]	0.91
M40T	96.57	-0.0686 (0.99)	-0.0007[+] (2.81)	0.0025 (0.67)	0.1611 (0.63)	0.5556 (0.1771)	2.35	1.17
M45T	88.94	-0.0104 (0.10)	0.0006 (1.45)	0.0083 (1.41)	0.0185 (0.05)	0.5123 (0.1219)	1.87	0.63
M50T	85.48	0.1901[+] (2.58)	0.0009[+] (3.59)	0.0026 (0.66)	0.1930 (0.71)	0.6413 (0.2991)	3.67[o]	1.49
M55T	104.91	-0.0530 (0.84)	-0.0011[+] (5.36)	0.0054 (1.62)	0.1432 (0.61)	0.8075 (0.5858)	9.84[+]	1.62
M60T	131.04	-0.3093[+] (4.71)	-0.0026[+] (11.92)	0.0021 (0.60)	-0.3924 (1.61)	0.9395 (0.8603)	39.48[+]	1.54
M65T	141.43	-0.7210[+] (8.36)	-0.0027[+] (9.30)	0.0028 (0.61)	-0.0637 (0.20)	0.9072 (0.7892)	24.40[+]	1.83
M70T	135.11	-0.8274[+] (6.14)	-0.0017[+] (3.78)	0.0087 (1.21)	-0.0669 (0.13)	0.8128 (0.5960)	10.22[+]	0.91
M75T	112.43	-0.3925[+] (2.82)	-0.0001 (0.27)	0.0072 (0.98)	0.0536 (0.11)	0.6377 (0.2937)	3.60[o]	1.01
M80T	104.00	-0.0563 (0.53)	-0.0003 (0.79)	0.0077 (1.38)	0.1672 (0.42)	0.3261 (-.0639)	0.63	1.49

Table 3 (continued)

Results of regression analysis: Model 2
(t-values in parentheses, sign omitted)

Dep. var.	C	UR(2-4)	GT	GTR	CGR	$R^2(\bar{R}^2)$	F	DW
F01T	101.35	0.5208[+] (5.09)	-0.0056[+] (16.13)	0.0025 (0.47)	0.3230 (0.85)	0.9847 (0.9638)	167.45[+]	0.57
F05T	112.63	0.2525[+] (3.44)	-0.0058[+] (23.24)	0.0032 (0.84)	0.1392 (0.51)	0.9907 (0.9780)	278.75[+]	2.30
F10T	120.79	-0.2109 (1.27)	-0.0043[+] (7.72)	0.0077 (0.88)	0.0021 (0.00)	0.8910 (0.7546)	22.22[+]	0.95
F15T	115.08	-0.0736 (0.43)	-0.0034[+] (5.83)	-0.0051 (0.56)	0.0495 (0.08)	0.8528 (0.6752)	13.99[+]	1.59
F20T	71.35	0.3013 (1.43)	0.0009 (1.25)	0.0073 (0.66)	-0.3374 (0.43)	0.3515 (-.0434)	0.74	1.25
F25T	65.90	0.4985[+] (5.33)	-0.0011[+] (3.40)	0.0059 (1.18)	0.4829 (1.39)	0.9140 (0.8039)	26.63[+]	1.54
F30T	85.28	0.6140[+] (11.39)	-0.0030[+] (16.44)	0.0021 (0.74)	-0.0694 (0.35)	0.9904 (0.9773)	270.46[+]	1.98
F35T	99.34	0.5118[+] (6.74)	-0.0023[+] (12.83)	-0.0035 (0.86)	-0.0112 (0.05)	0.9818 (0.9571)	140.36[+]	1.57
F40T	106.23	0.0523 (0.74)	-0.0036[+] (15.01)	0.0022 (0.59)	-0.0331 (0.13)	0.9752 (0.9417)	101.97[+]	1.98
F45T	112.96	-0.1049 (1.30)	-0.0032[+] (11.84)	0.0018 (0.42)	0.0822 (0.27)	0.9532 (0.8913)	52.24[+]	0.90
F50T	107.62	-0.1398 (1.59)	-0.0022[+] (7.38)	0.0015 (0.33)	-0.0196 (0.06)	0.8790 (0.7293)	17.84[+]	1.14
F55T	104.01	-0.0741 (0.86)	-0.0021[+] (7.20)	0.0049 (1.07)	0.2646 (0.83)	0.8841 (0.7401)	18.80[+]	0.80
F60T	106.65	-0.0199 (0.37)	-0.0024[+] (13.37)	0.0037 (1.32)	-0.1045 (0.53)	0.9654 (0.9189)	71.85[+]	1.06
F65T	116.46	-0.1167[o] (1.90)	-0.0033[+] (15.92)	0.0023 (0.71)	-0.0951 (0.42)	0.9728 (0.9361)	92.53[+]	1.23
F70T	116.99	-0.0873 (1.11)	-0.0037[+] (13.88)	0.0069 (1.67)	0.1415 (0.49)	0.9657 (0.9197)	72.56[+]	1.24
F75T	117.59	-0.0060 (0.06)	-0.0037[+] (11.70)	0.0050 (1.01)	-0.0503 (0.15)	0.9568 (0.8994)	56.87[+]	1.51
F80T	115.69	0.0664 (0.78)	-0.0035[+] (12.21)	0.0081[o] (1.78)	0.2638 (0.83)	0.9632 (0.9139)	67.32[+]	1.61

o) significant at the .05-level;
+) significant at the .01-level;

Table 4

Results of regression analysis: Model 3
(t-values in parentheses, sign omitted)

Dep. var.		C	UR0	UR1	GT	$R^2(\bar{R}^2)$	F_T	F_A	DW	$\Sigma \hat{b}_i$(UR) in model 3	2	1
M01T	(1)	111.05			$-0.0062^{+)}$ (6.76)	0.9229 (0.9196)	$275.32^{+)}$					
	(2)	111.56	$1.3922^{+)}$ (2.81)		$-0.0063^{+)}$ (19.00)	0.9433 (0.9381)	$182.98^{+)}$					
	(3)	109.49		$1.2097^{+)}$ (2.84)	$-0.0060^{+)}$ (18.30)	0.9436 (0.9385)	$183.98^{+)}$				(2)	1.53
	(4)	110.29	0.6567 (0.49)	0.6842 (0.59)	$-0.0061^{+)}$ (15.35)	0.9442 (0.9363)	$118.49^{+)}$	$3.96^{o)}$	0.41	1.34	0.47	(3) 1.22
M05T	(1)	114.73			$-0.0058^{+)}$ (26.50)	0.9671 (0.9657)	$675.75^{+)}$					
	(2)	113.61	$0.6225^{o)}$ (1.94)		$-0.0059^{+)}$ (27.91)	0.9719 (0.9694)	$380.58^{+)}$					
	(3)	112.04		$0.7121^{+)}$ (2.76)	$-0.0057^{+)}$ (28.65)	0.9758 (0.9733)	$439.19^{+)}$				(2)	0.55
	(4)	110.79	-1.0239 (1.30)	$1.5314^{o)}$ (2.26)	$-0.0056^{+)}$ (24.22)	0.9774 (0.9742)	$302.59^{+)}$	$4.73^{o)}$	2.39	0.51	0.28	(3) 0.43
F01T	(1)	115.67			$-0.0064^{+)}$ (16.95)	0.9273 (0.9241)	$293.25^{+)}$					
	(2)	112.53	$1.7474^{+)}$ (3.92)		$-0.0065^{+)}$ (21.77)	0.9571 (0.9532)	$245.65^{+)}$					
	(3)	110.02		$1.4954^{+)}$ (3.86)	$-0.0062^{+)}$ (20.80)	0.9567 (0.9527)	$242.81^{+)}$				(2)	2.47
	(4)	111.25	1.0000 (0.83)	0.6952 (0.66)	$-0.0064^{+)}$ (17.78)	0.9580 (0.9520)	$159.77^{+)}$	$7.70^{+)}$	0.52	1.69	0.52	(3) 1.62
F05T	(1)	120.56			$-0.0062^{+)}$ (25.96)	0.9669 (0.9654)	$671.25^{+)}$					
	(2)	119.18	$0.7675^{o)}$ (2.30)		$-0.0063^{+)}$ (28.55)	0.9733 (0.9708)	$400.57^{+)}$					
	(3)	117.46		$0.8214^{+)}$ (3.05)	$-0.0061^{+)}$ (29.05)	0.9767 (0.9746)	$461.58^{+)}$				(2)	0.63
	(4)	116.45	-0.8269 (0.99)	$1.4831^{o)}$ (2.06)	$-0.0060^{+)}$ (24.00)	0.9778 (0.9746)	$307.78^{+)}$	$5.00^{o)}$	2.10	0.60	0.25	(3) 0.59
F25T	(1)	80.34			$-0.0019^{+)}$ (5.22)	0.5417 (0.5217)	$27.18^{+)}$					
	(2)	77.50	$1.5847^{+)}$ (3.57)		$-0.0020^{+)}$ (6.79)	0.7100 (0.6836)	$26.93^{+)}$					
	(3)	74.59	-0.1101 (0.10)	1.5765 (1.59)	$-0.0017^{+)}$ (4.91)	0.7412 (0.7043)	$20.05^{+)}$	$81.14^{+)}$	1.30	1.47	0.50	(2) 1.43 (3) 1.22
F30T	(1)	102.10			$-0.0041^{+)}$ (11.44)	0.8479 (0.8413)	$128.24^{+)}$					
	(2)	98.41	$2.0538^{+)}$ (5.80)		$-0.0042^{+)}$ (18.44)	0.9399 (0.9341)	$171.94^{+)}$					
	(3)	94.58	-0.1747 (0.21)	$2.0729^{+)}$ (2.95)	$-0.0039^{+)}$ (16.04)	0.9575 (0.9514)	$157.54^{+)}$	$27.40^{+)}$	1.43	1.90	0.61	(2) 1.98 (3) 2.05
F35T	(1)	111.54			$-0.0041^{+)}$ (13.36)	0.8856 (0.8806)	$177.99^{+)}$					
	(2)	108.25	$1.8303^{+)}$ (6.53)		$-0.0043^{+)}$ (22.37)	0.9611 (0.9575)	$271.45^{+)}$					
	(3)	107.02	1.1121 (1.03)	0.6681 (1.49)	$-0.0041^{+)}$ (18.73)	0.9629 (0.9577)	$181.90^{+)}$	$21.50^{+)}$	2.18	1.78	0.51	(2) 1.84 (3) 1.96

F_T : F-value for the entire regression equation
F_A : F-value for the subset of unemployment variables
    o) significant at the .05-level
    +) significant at the .01-level
$\Sigma \hat{b}_i$(UR) : Sum of regression coefficients of unemployment variables.
    Model 1 (2): regression equation without variables representing "rapid economic change"
    Model 1 (3): regression equation with all variables included

Table 5

Correlation matrices of independent variables

Model 1

	URO	UR1	UR2	UR3	UR4	UR5	GT	GTR	CGR
URO	1.0000	0.8976	0.7465	0.6193	0.5149	0.4001	0.0833	0.0979	0.3000
UR1		1.0000	0.9243	0.8133	0.7233	0.6188	-0.1660	-0.0910	0.3596
UR2			1.0000	0.9437	0.8632	0.7800	-0.3796	-0.1742	0.2048
UR3				1.0000	0.9589	0.8889	-0.5560	-0.1682	0.1283
UR4					1.0000	0.9619	-0.6961	-0.1853	0.1246
UR5						1.0000	-0.8112	-0.2289	0.1480
GT							1.0000	0.2203	-0.1258
GTR								1.0000	-0.0793
CGR									1.0000

Model 2

	UR(2-4)	GT	GTR	CGR
UR(2-4)	1.0000	-0.6383	-0.2159	0.0499
GT		1.0000	0.2461	-0.0607
GTR			1.0000	-0.0574
CGR				1.0000

Model 3

	URO	UR1	GT
URO	1.0000	0.8976	0.0833
UR1		1.0000	-0.1660
GT			1.0000

NOTES

1) BRENNER, M.H.: Mortality and the National Economy. A Review, and the Experience of England and Wales, 1936-76. The Lancet, September 15, 1979, 568-573 (1979)

2) BRENNER, M.H.: Health Costs and Benefits of Economic Policy. International Journal of Health Services, 7, 4, 581-623 (1977)

3) BRENNER, M.H.: Estimates of the Impact of Economic Change on Health: A Refined Model Including Life Style and Environmental Factors (Tables), presented at the 1st Planning Meeting for Study on Influence of Economic Development on Health, WHO, Copenhagen, November 1980

4) BRENNER, M.H.: Fetal, Infant, and Maternal Mortality during Periods of Economic Instability. International Journal of Health Services, 3,2,145-159 (1973)

5) PETIT, H.: Die Spezifikation von Modellen mit verteilten Verzögerungen. Ökonomische Theorie, ökonometrische Ansätze, empirische Analysen (The Specification of Distributed Lag Models. Economic Theory, Econometric Approaches, Empirical Analyses), Munich (1979)

6) see e.g. RAMSEY, J.B.: Classical Model Selection through Specification Error Tests. In: Frontiers in Econometrics (Ed.: P. Zarembka) New York-London-San Francisco, 13-47 (1974)

7) BRENNER, M.H.: Mortality and the National Economy ..., p. 568

8) BRENNER, M.H.: Mortality and the National Economy ..., p. 568

AN ATTEMPT TO ANALYSE SOME DEPENDENCES
BETWEEN ECONOMIC AND HEALTH STATUS
IN POLAND IN THE YEARS 1959 - 1979

Włodzimierz Cezary Włodarczyk
Zuzanna Szubert
Marek Bryła

Institute of Occupational Medicine
Łódź, Poland

Theoretical Background

It is useful for the analysis of every phenomenon to locate it within the defined discipline. Such an assignation, especially when it is related to the discipline which has its own tradition allows to establish relatively unequivocal criteria of importance and value of the problem and to determine correct methods for its solution. Traditional investigative disciplines have a developed terminological and theoretical apparatus just enough for precise description, explanation and prediction of phenomena.

Analysis of relationships and dependences between social and economic phenomena on the one hand and health status of population on the other, cannot be univocally related to one traditional scientific discipline. It is a typical multi-/interdisciplinary problem with all its methodological advantages but also with many obvious disadvantages which result from the fact that it is not rooted in one determined scientific discipline. The lack of explicit theoretical frameworks for analysing the relationships between socioeconomic phenomena and health might be resolved in two ways.

1. The first appeals to establishing our own tradition of analysis of the relationships between socioeconomic and health phenomena. For a few decades now, immense - and growing - scientific efforts have been made to explore the field. At the macro level, first of all the works by M.H. Brenner should be mentioned.[1] The results obtained by S. Kasl have enriched the knowledge at the micro level.[2] Also contributions by A.R. Bunn, J. Eyer, A.L. Cochrane, A. Pierce, S. Cobb, R. Catalano, D. Dooley and many others research workers are to be appreciated.[3] Though art has been remarkably developed it can hardly be

said that the findings gathered enable an attempt to develop a proper theoretical base with its terminology, assumptions and methodology.

The second - and more promising - way to resolve the problem calls for some practical scientific discipline. In a practical discipline a question need not be related to a theory. It is enough if the question is claimed to be relevant from the point of view of social values. In our analyses those socially important problems apply to three areas:

- possibility of affecting the health of population, i.e. its improvement or at least prevention of its degradation through positive action on socioeconomic phenomena;

- possibility of anticipating the trend and intensity of the changes in health of population which result from not fully controlled processes occurring in the sphere of socioeconomic phenomena;

- possibility of changing and forming the social consciousness through pointing to the relationships between some aspects of socioeconomic activities and their health consequences.

If it is assumed that the majority of economic activities is treated as activities of instrumental type, the value of which is justified by the value of goals to which they lead, that the possibility of health deterioration may alter the axiological evaluation of those social and economic activities.

If those areas of application of relationships between socioeconomic phenomena and health are soundly defined then one may presume that the results of our analysis of this type will be interesting first of all for decision-makers formulating social policy and for those groups and institutions which are interested in this policy formulation. However, political expectations and the missing link with particular scientific discipline causes that our problem must be formulated in every-day language, and not in the language of science. In this situation definition of the problem inherits, in an inevitable way, all disadvantages of using in science the every-day language, where dullness, ambiguity and emotional tinge of the expressions is obvious and natural. However what adds grace to common parlance is an obstacle in putting scientific problems. One can note that the effect of emotional attitude on the way of putting the discussed problem is visible in the manner in which the titles of the two conferences devoted to this problem are formulated. In the optimistic version the title of the conference in Copenhagen was:"The influence of economic <u>development</u> on health", in a pessimistic version the title of the Conference in Munich is: "The influence of economic <u>instability</u> on health".

It seems that the essential point of view and the topical range of both conferences is the same. Putting it into other words, economic development and economic instability denote the same empirical sphere of social phenomena. The emotional load of both expressions is that what differs significantly. It testifies to the fact that the way of defining serves not only to describe the given group of problems but it positively fulfils a persuasive type of functions. Using the expressions of persuasive type we reveal our attitudes to politics, at least to social politics.

Since we placed our analysis in the context of a practical framework, another important point should be stressed. We mean here obvious expectations of decision-makers that the analysis like ours will reveal relationships of causal type. Only such type of dependences is fully useful for practical applications.

Hence one may observe a tendency to undertake causal interpretation even if findings would not reliably support this. Assertions from many different disciplines (sociology, social psychology, antropology, epidemiology) may be borrowed to make such an interpretation more reliable. But there is a risk that the only guide in singling out proper assertions happens to be a common sense. This is not a very solid base for scientific analysis.

2. The factor which affects the form of analysis of relationships between socioeconomic phenomena and health, is the way of interpretation of the term "health". The starting point is here the definition adopted by WHO in which three aspects of the status determined as health are distinguished: somatic, psychical and social wellbeing.

If the so defined term is treated from methodological viewpoint as a theoretical term (concept), it is indisputable that any use of that term in the investigative procedure calls for its operationalization. To this end the term "health" is rendered into a number of indicators which may be subject to empirical measurement. It may be acknowledged that it is a specific case of the manipulation called partial defining.[4] Selection of indicators which are used in such cases affects, to some extent, the way of interpretation and meaning of the defined term. Therefore in practice a difficult situation may occur in which in spite of common acceptance of the definition of the principal theoretical term, its detailed interpretation takes a divergent course. At operationalization of the term "health" we observe as a rule an unanimity regarding selection of indicators determining somatic health aspects. The remaining aspects, if they are included into operative interpretation of the term, are characterized by using the differing parameters. As an example let us show the differences occurring in two recent and important documents. In "Goals for the Nation" prepared by U.S. Department of Health and Social Services the term "health" includes the following non-somatic aspects as: smoking, excessive use of alcohol, stress, use of violence.[5] In the well-known document: "Regional strategy for attaining health for all by the year 2000" there is a statement that principal health phenomena of Europe, among non-somatic aspects, are: alcoholism, smoking and suicides.[6]

In both mentioned examples the selection of indicators depends, in principle, on the importance or rank of the group of phenomena for the respective country or continent i.e. in compliance with the principles of building up partial definition. In the partial definition we select what is considered to be important, however, one may doubt whether common semantic feelings univocally allow to include in the concept of health such phenomena as violent behaviour or suicides and treat them as health indicators. Perhaps it would be more convenient to link them with other theoretical terms such as e.g. social pathology.

Various factors cause difficulties in interpretation of the term "health". It seems that only some shortcomings may be overcome through the researchers' theoretical and methodological effort.

The first point which seems to be inevitably linked with the attempts of making the term "health" explicit results from its links with philosophic and ethical problems. If e.g. in the previously

quoted document of WHO Regional Office it is stated that:
> "... the main social target ... should be the attainment ... of a level of health that will permit them to lead a socially and economically productive life"[7]

or at another that:
> "... health in its widest sense" includes such elements as a sense of community and meaningful life,[8]

then undoubtedly we are in the investigation area characteristic for philosophy or ethics but not for sciences. Although we do not doubt that sciences refer to various valuations especially where they participate in formation of social changes, we should become aware of their weakness and incompetence in judging and resolving such problems.

The second reason is connected with complexity and heterogeneity of relationships between these phenomena which are treated as indicators of health in its theoretical sense. Empirical dependences between these indicators - irrespective of the obvious linkage of definition type - may assume one of the following forms if we take into consideration only pairs of indicators:

1) Phenomenon A brings about - with a defined probability - the phenomenon B (causality)
2) phenomenon A coexists (with a defined frequency) with phenomenon B (statistical relation)
3) occurrence of phenomenon A decreases probability of occurrence of phenomenon B (causality and/or statistical relation)
4) occurrence of phenomenon A increases probability of occurrence of phenomenon B (causality and/or statistical relation)
5) phenomenon A occurs irrespective of phenomenon B (definitional relation).

Each of the above presented types of dependences may occur in each of the three aspects mentioned in the WHO definition of health. And so these relationships occur in the sphere of somatic, psychic and social phenomena and also among phenomena belonging to each of these spheres. Moreover taking into account the fact that the above indicated dependences occur in practice not only between pairs of indicators but also in sets of more indicators it may be ascertained that we have to do with indicators in a very complex structure. In this connexion a very important question may be put, i.e. whether an attempt of unequivocal evaluation of health status or aspiration after building up synthetic indicators is justified from the viewpoint of logical analysis of the term "health".

It may be assumed that such efforts are justified only in cases when positive causality occurs between specific indicators. Then speaking about improvement or deterioration of health status, we give an account of the changes running in the convergent direction. In all remaining cases and therefore in the cases when, from the character of relationships between particular indicators, their discordance is observed - wishing to remain on scientific ground - we should be satisfied with the statement, that improvement of health in one respect is accompanied by deteriorations in the other.[9] Admitting that one of the aspects is of special importance and forms the basis for synthetic measure we leave the scientific ground and move into philosophical regions.

Characterizing the possible relationships between various indicators of health we have assumed that deterioration of the character of relationship between them is established. In practice, significant controversy may occur very frequently, concerning the direction of causal dependences, the level of probability and susceptibility to other factors.

3. The problem of relationships between characteristics of economic and health status should be located within a larger theory which could be used to explain a mechanism of population health determinants. It is undoubtful that socioeconomic factors constitute only one of the groups of factors on which health status depends. Consideration of this group of factors if separated from the other determinants of health - at least on the level of the theoretical model - would lead to quite unjustified conclusions.

At the same time the investigative reasons may recommend the (purposely omitted) inclusion of the excessive number of variables for building up the designed model. The explanatory power of a simple model is obviously greater. However, in such a case one should indicate the phenomena which are not taken into account from a set of these phenomena which are known, on the basis of the available knowledge, to affect health.

It seems that topical degree of development of sciences dealing

with the analysis of factors affecting health in its broad sense
does not offer too rich suggestions enabling reconstruction of
theoretical frames for analysis of the problem of health determinants. In the most general sense it may be assumed that two
orientations may be used to this end:

- epidemiological orientation
- systems approach orientation.

In epidemiological orientation a number of characteristics of the
individual or population is considered, of which it is diagnosed
that they differentiate health. The most frequently mentioned factors are: age, sex, ethnic group, marital status, family structure,
kind of job, socioeconomic status, place and geographical disposal,
migrations.[10] In epidemiological orientation, carrying out, classification of factors affecting health is not oriented on building
up integrated models determining the effect of some groups of
factors on synthetically understood health.

This concerns rather the specification of detailed dependences between the selected measures of health and the groups of sometimes
significantly correlated factors - treated as their determinants.[11]

Systems approach linked first of all with the IIASA work aims at
establishing internal relations between different factors considered to be health determinants.[12]

In the known Venediktov's model, the collection (subsystem) of socio-economic factors occurring along with natural conditions and health
care system includes the following elements: population characteristics, the status of industry, agriculture and transport, the level
of knowledge and technology, capital outlay, quality of nutrition,
living standard, services, education and culture.[13] Each of these
elements may be treated in its static aspect as the collection of
parameters obtained or as an institutional system or - in dynamic
aspect - as a system of activities and functions.

In the other model elaborated by IIASA health is related to the
following groups of factors: incomes, education, the range of the
possessed knowledge, level of nutrition, tobacco and alcohol consumption, sanitary and living conditions, age, place of habitation,

climate, industrial structure, working capacity, transport, hazards in natural environment, supply of and demand for health services.[14] In this model some hypotheses and assertions describing the direction and character of dependences between various elements treated as health determinants are assumed. And thus the influence of age on the magnitude of supply of and demand for health services is indicated. This influence may be felt both directly and indirectly through the relationships between age and incomes. It also points out to the indirect character of the effect of industrial structure through forming the hazardous level of natural environment.

Systems approach orientation, which should be regarded rather as complementary than as competitive with regard to epidemiological orientation, is promising from both the theoretical and practical viewpoint.

Reconstruction of an overall multielemental dependence chain allows to make a richer interpretation of the phenomena and to bring the seeming dependences to light. At the same time empirical verification and confirmation allows the identification of those socioeconomic factors whose intentional formation may lead to the intended changes in health.

It seems, however, that the topically available elaborations may meet only in part the ambitious expectations of social policy practice. Only in some cases they may use the sufficiently confirmed statements about health determinants.

Analytical scheme

1. Taking into account the results of our previous considerations we locate our problem in the framework of the analyses specific for social policy. We mean by this the practical sense of questions regarding health determinants on the one hand and - on the other - the necessity of borrowing information from the results of different scientific disciplines for interpretation of the answers to be formulated.

2. In our analytical scheme, on the level of theoretical ideas, health of population, at the defined period, is regarded as a dependent variable. This variable is regarded as a complex of two componential

variables: health in somatic aspect and health in psychosocial aspect. The final element explained in our scheme of analysis is somatic health. The characteristic economic situation is treated as our independent variable. We use the neutral term "situation" to avoid an emotional load of other terms such as development or crisis. The state of the health care system determined by its resources is regarded as an intermediary variable. The adapted analytical scheme assumes an unidirectional system of dependences consciously omitting the possibility of multidirectional interpretation.

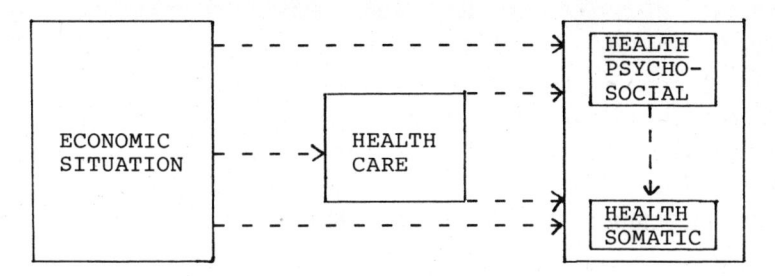

Fig. Analytical scheme

We think, that at the present stage of analysis it is indispensable to employ a system of dependences as simple as possible. Taking into account this reservation we assume that the following system of dependences may be subject of the analysis:

- somatic health, as a result of:
  a) psychosocial aspect of health,
  b) direct effect of economic status,
  c) indirect effect of economic status through its impact on health care

- psychosocial aspect of health as a result of:
  a) direct effect of economic status,
  b) indirect effect of economic status through its impact on health care.

By adopting this system of dependences in the analysis scheme we avoid a priori decisions in the dilemma signalized earlier regarding convergence or divergence of measures between various aspects of health or at least between somatic and psychosocial aspects.

The scheme proposed here leaves the problem of these levels - as well as a problem of territorial range – open to further analysis. Such dependences may regard the phenomena on different levels of generalization: individuals (persons), social or territorial groups, nation, these levels reveal different faces of the problem as well.

Presenting the list of dependences we outline the scope of questions which may be deduced from our research scheme. This paper, however, is not aimed at finding answers to all questions. Our aims are much simpler. We limit ourselves to an attempt of interpretation and elucidation of relationships between selected phenomena occurring on the macro-level. First of all we wish to check to what extent the use of some methods allows to carry out causal interpretation of relationships between economic and health status in order to receive answers to practical questions. It is to be stressed that this method was developed and used in a social context quite different from the one in which we have applied it.

3. The foregoing characteristics of our analytical scheme was carried out on the level of theoretical concepts, the measurement and direct empirical interpretation of which is not possible. Hence it is necessary to present operationalized indicators of each of the theoretical terms mentioned in the scheme.

The list of selected indicators is not exclusively due to our theoretical preferences. It is a consequence of a compromise between our eagerness after reliable interpretation of theoretical concepts and accessibility and range of information (and quality of software of our computer facilities).

The list of our indicators resulting from that compromise is as follows:

1. Indicators of somatic health

   Y_1 total mortality rate (per 1000 population)
   Y_2 mortality rate due to malignant neoplasms (per 10000 popul.)
   Y_3 infant mortality rate (per 1000 live births occurring in the year)
   Y_4 incidence rate of virus hepatitis (per 10000 population)
   Y_5 incidence rate of sexually transmitted diseases (per 10000 population)

Y_6 incidence rate of malignant neoplasms
Y_7 natural abortion rate (per 100 women aged 15 - 49)
Y_8 total absenteeism rate due to diseases and accidents
Y_9 absenteeism rate due to malignant neoplasms
Y_{10} absenteeism rate due to nervous and psychiatric diseases
Y_{11} absenteeism rate due to cardiovascular diseases

2. Indicators of psychosocial aspects of health

S_1 divorces rate (per 1000 population)
S_2 migrations
S_3 alcohol consumption rate per capita
S_4 total suicide rate
S_5 tobacco consumption rate per capita
S_6 artificial abortion rate (per 100 women aged 15 - 49)

3. Indicators of economic status

X_1 national income per capita
X_2 health expenditures as a proportion of state budget
X_3 investment expenditures per capita
X_4 investment expenditures as a proportion of state budget
X_5 health and social welfare as a proportion of overall investment expenditures

4. Indicators of resources of the health care system

Z_1 physicians (per 10000 population)
Z_2 nurses (per 10000 population)
Z_3 hospital beds (per 10000 population)

It seems that the presented list of indicators is worthy of comment. Firstly: The group of indicators of health somatic aspects was divided into two subgroups: somatic indicators in the strict sense and somatic indicators in a broad sense related to absenteeism. Distinction of the latter is based on the assumption that although absenteeism is a health status indicator, the impact of non-somatic factors is very significant here. Perhaps in our model this group of indicators is a middle stage between somatic and psychosocial aspects of health. Secondly: The indicators exemplifying the magnitude of expenditure for health care have been included into economic indicators, while the indicators illustrating the obtained level of resources are included into health care indicators. This is consistent with the established scheme of our analysis in which health care is regarded as an intermediary variable. Thirdly: Numerical values of all indicators were gathered from official statistical data published by Chief Census Bureau and Ministry of Health and Social Welfare.

Methods of analysis

In the first part of our paper we emphasized many difficulties with regard to the selection of an adequate theoretical framework for the analysis of relationships between economic and health status. Researcher's decision is incomparably easier as far as the choice of methods is concerned because a set of analytical techniques developed by Professor Brenner is offered.[15] In our paper we use his suggestions.

In the first stage the investigations of dependences between pairs of variables with the help of correlation coefficients were carried out. The analysis was concerned with the impact of the selected indicators of the economic situation as independent variables and indicators of health care as intermediary variables on indicators of health seen as dependent variables. The same type of analysis was carried out to test dependences between indicators of one variable, i.e. between indicators of somatic health and separately between indicators of psychosocial aspects of health.

Analysis of correlation diagrams allowed to treat the relationships between variables in the form of linear function. Therefore the analysis of these relationships was based on the following theoretical models:

(1) $Y = f(S,X,Z) + \varepsilon$
(2) $S = f(X,Z) + \zeta$

with:

Y - indicators of somatic health
S - indicators of psychosocial aspects of health
X - indicators of economic status
Z - indicators of resources of health care system
ε, ζ - random components

The presented models were assessed with the least squares method using standard programmes on the computer "Odra 1305".

Both models (1) and (2) were formulated generally (in a theoretical way). In practice, estimation of the model for each coefficient of somatic health $(Y_1...Y_{11})$ was carried out.
According to the method of the set of best explanatory variables we selected the best fitted coefficients from the set of coefficients $S_1..., X_1...,$ and $Z_1....$ In the same way models for indicators of psychosocial aspects of health were estimated.

The criterion for the selection of explanatory variables was both the significance of parameters of particular variables measured with the T-Student test at the level of significance = 0,05 and the multiple correlation coefficient value - R^2. In consideration of the used long-term series of empirical data for estimation of model parameters, the occurrence of autocorrelation of random components was studied with the Durbin-Watson's test.

Moreover a considerable problem in the estimation of the models of that type is a danger of collinearity of explanatory variables. The indicators we had at our disposal did not offer great possibilities for the selection of specified variables as almost all of them were highly intercorrelated. It seems, however, that this has not interfered with the results, as in many trials estimating several variants of the models the standard errors of coefficients were not too high.

Nevertheless the results of the estimation of the models should be treated with great caution, first of all due to the fact that studying such complex social phenomena one cannot be convinced of the fulfillment of the basic assumptions of the classic model of linear regression. The more so, as the used method of estimation is too simple to result in good parameters estimation in case the assumptions of linear regression model were ignored. The use of more complicated estimation methods was impeded due to the limited possibilities of computer programmes and other constraints we previously mentioned.

One of the elements of analysis of relationships between the variables was finding out the period of time lag with which one of the variables S, X, and Z affects the variable Y. Such an analysis was carried out on the basis of the standarized variables pairs presented in the respective figures.

Results

According to our previous statements, the first stage of analysis is to consider the dependences between pairs of variables.

1. Somatic health indicators

The dependences between the indicators of somatic health are presented in Table 1. The results confirm the hypothesis formulated earlier on the divergency of the direction and strength of dependence between particular parameters characterizing somatic health.

In the strict "somatic" set of indicators we find - among others - a highly positive dependence between incidence rate and mortality rate due to malignant neoplasms, between total mortality rate and mortality rate due to malignant neoplasms. It is undoubtful, that these dependences are relations of causal type (incidence and mortality) as well as relations of definitional type occurring between particular measures (total mortality rate and specific mortality rates). At the same time in this group of indicators, very high negative dependences occur, as for example between infant mortality rate and mortality rate due to malignant neoplasms.
It seems that in each of these cases we cannot find - at least based on the confirmed knowledge - dependences of causal type, which would consist in this that one nosologic unit (health phenomenon) forces out another nosologic unit. The disaccords observed are rather consequences of complexity of phenomena included by the term "health", already on the level of purely somatic indicators, among which multi-directional trends are to be found.

The previous conclusions will be confirmed if we take into consideration the remaining indicators of somatic health. Here we see high positive dependences between total mortality rate and different sickness absenteeism rates. High positive dependences can be seen also when we analyse the relation between mortality rate and sickness absenteeism rate due to the same reason (e.g. neoplasms). Therefore the conclusion may be drawn, that regarding absenteeism measures as indicators of somatic health is, at least to a certain extent, justified. Nevertheless a negative relationship between all sickness absenteeism rates and the infant mortality rate should be pointed out, as this measure is widely used as one of the most convenient general indicator of health.

2. Indicators of psychosocial aspects of health

The dependences between the indicators of psychosocial aspects of health are presented in Table 2.

In this group of indicators an interesting phenomenon occurs. All indicators selected by us reveal strong positive correlation except one indicator - artificial abortion rate. If we assume that the information on abortion is fully reliable then we should state that the indicator illustrating artificial abortion rate is related to some other phenomenon than the remaining indicators of psychosocial aspects of health. Therefore if we took only the remaining indicators into consideration we would speak about a relatively coherent syndrom of phenomena regarded as a psychosocial aspect of health.

3. Indicators of somatic and psychosocial aspects of health

The dependences between the indicators of somatic and psychosocial aspects of health are presented in Table 3.

In general the dependences between indicators of somatic and psychosocial aspects of health have a positive and strong character. It is more perceptible in the case of dependences between sickness absenteeism rates, regarded as an element of characterization of somatic health, and psychosocial indicators than in the case of relationships of the latter with strict somatic indicators. This phenomenon may be explained if it is assumed that the level of sickness absenteeism is formed by somatic health through total collection of psychosocial factors. The correlations between the purely somatic indicators of health and indicators of psychosocial aspects of health are also highly positive except for the infant mortality rate and natural abortion rate. The result is not surprising inasmuch as the trends which lead to these two rates were discordant also with the trends of the majority of strict somatic indicators of health.

Hence a conclusion may be drawn that convergence of trends takes a course not according to the distribution into strict somatic and psychosocial aspects of health. It seems that there are groups of phenomena which comprise indicators included in different categories in our analytical scheme.

4. Determinants of health

Within the general scheme of explanation presented earlier, in this part of the paper we wish to find out more detailed dependences between particular indicators of health and indicators of economic status. According to this, both the results of statistical analysis and a set of assumptions on empirical dependences between specific phenomena will be interpreted. The former are presented in Table 4.

4.1 Determinants of psychosocial aspects of health

S_4 Total suicide rate

This indicator of psychosocial aspects of health is positively related to one economic indicator, i.e. national income, and negatively to another one, i.e. proportion of investment in the national budget. According to our interpretation the latter reflects the relative magnitude of expenditure for the non-productive sphere of economy. Our results confirm this direction of dependences in which the increase of the suicide rate is related to the decrease of expenditure for these economic sectors in which values and social norms are transmitted, i.e. where the sense of existence of an individual is formed. The second factor present in the model - national income - can be understood as a general indicator reflecting various changes taking place in a society along with economic development. Since these changes are not identified here, more detailed conclusions cannot be drawn, apart from the stipulation to extend investigations on different determinants of the problem.

S_6 Artificial abortion rate (ambulatory and social) in proportion to the number of women aged 15 - 49

The magnitude of the artificial abortion rate is usually regarded as a consequence of two groups of causes. Firstly: the general line of social changes in the sphere of moral values and, related to this, patterns of conduct. Secondly: the health policy tries to regulate the intensity of the phenomenon, i.e. by methods used to explain the facts of life, by making available contraceptives and by control of the accessibility to artificial abortions.

Our results partly confirm the hypothesis, if it is assumed, that changes (increase) in the level of national per capita income is related - to a certain degree in causal relation - to general changes in the sphere of moral changes. The second part of the hypothesis was confirmed as well. Since if we assume, that explaining the facts of life and rendering contraceptives accessible is included first of all in the scope of activities of nurses, so the increase of their number should lead to an increase of activity in that field. In consequence a decrease in the level of artificial abortion rates can be expected. Also the alternative model based on the same hypothesis in which the increase in the level of investment expenditures occurs instead of the increase in the national income, confirms the assumed direction of dependences.

4.2 Determinants of somatic health

Y_1 Total mortality rate

Total mortality rate in our model is negatively related to the level of expenditures for health care and positively to the intensity of migration processes (from villages to towns).
Migration and stress breaking existing interpersonal bonds may be simply related to health in causal interpretation. It is especially impressive, as in this case, migration is not only a change of the place of residence but also parting with the traditional local community still functioning in rural areas which gives a feeling of being rooted. Similar causal interpretations with regard to the level of expenditures for health care, although useful for those who call for money for that sector, should be made much more carefully, since assertions on such dependences are not safely confirmed.

Y_2 Mortality rate due to malignant neoplasms (per 10000 popul.)

Mortality rates due to malignant neoplasms are related with two indicators illustrating expeditures for health care. They are positively related with topical expenditures for health care, and negatively with investment expenditures for health care and social welfare proportional to the overall investment expenditures. These dependences are not easy to interpret regarding the dependences

assumed by us. It may be stated that the increase of expenditures
for health care leads to a more precise diagnosis. On the other
hand the decrease of investment expenditures leads to lower therapeutic capabilities, though it is hard to judge whether an effect
of this kind would yield immediate results as it is assumed in our
model. Further the reverse interpretation is judged likewise. We
think therefore that causal interpretation of the effect of these
two economic phenomena is highly doubtful, contrary to the interpretation of the role of the third component present in our model
- tobacco consumption - the influence of which on the mortality
rate due to neoplasms is widely confirmed.

Y_3 Infant mortality rate (per 1000 alive births)

In our model this health indicator is in negative dependence with
the expenditures for health care and hospital beds. Undoubtedly
these two phenomena may be regarded as those really affecting the
infant mortality. At the same time it is an indispensable reservation that the scope of the indicators analysed by us does not enable
us to get at the phenomena which may have much more significant influence on the infant mortality rate. We think here of the amount
of occupational activization of woman and working environment conditions with which women meet in their fertility ages.

Y_5 Incidence rate of sexually transmitted diseases (per 10000
population)

Incidences of sexually transmitted diseases, although they refer
to the somatic aspect of health are significantly related to the
social status of population and to the level of health culture of
the society. The above described break of the social net seems to
be the basic question. Our results confirm this course of reasoning.
In our model the level of incidence of sexually transmitted diseases
is positively related to the indicator of psychosomatic aspects of
health and negatively related to the number of nurses. According to
the interpretation assumed by us the nurses ratio reflects the
intensity of activities of the health care system towards the dissem-
ination of health education.

Y_6 Incidence of malignant neoplasms (per 10000 population)

According to the model, expenditures for the non-productive sphere and tobacco consumption appear to be determinants for the incidence rate of malignant neoplasms; whereas it can be hardly assumed that there are some non-accidental relationships between the first indicator (non-productive sphere) and the incidence rate. The effect of the tobacco consumption may be regarded as real.

Y_7 Natural abortion rate in proportion to the number of women aged 15 - 49

The real causes forming the level of this indicator are close, to a certain extent, to those affecting infant mortality rate. In our model we have ascertained the positive relations between the natural abortion rate and the amount of investments and the negative relation with the physicians' ratio. With necessary caution, the revealed dependences may be interpreted in terms of causal relations, especially the latter, if we take into account that the care for pregnant women is one of the best developed areas of health services in Poland. We can believe that in this case the presence of physicians in the system does not only serve for the discovery of diseases but, first of all, for real prevention and therapy. On the other hand the increase of investments leading to a rise in occupational activity, also of women, and the change of working conditions may account for the formation of conditions directly affecting this aspect of health.

Y_9 Sickness absenteeism rate due to malignant neoplasms

It may be expected that determinants of that rate are close to those which form other measures relating to malignant neoplasms. The relationships between the level of absenteeism due to neoplasms on the one hand and migration and the number of physicians on the other are confirmed in our model. The effect of the last factor was already commented. Instead, migration may be related both to sickness absenteeism as such and to the level of sickness absenteeism for a specific reason.

Y_{10} Sickness absenteeism rate due to nervous and psychiatric diseases

As has been expected the rate of one of the "nowadays diseases" shows positive relationships with the basic economic indicators: national income and the amount of investment expenditures. Too many complicated phenomena interfere with the matter to make here causal interpretation possible.

The explanation of the positive dependence between the discussed rate and the hospital beds rate is much simpler if we take into consideration that the latter also includes psychiatric beds.

Y_{11} Sickness absenteeism rate due to cardiovascular diseases

The rate of other "nowadays diseases" is affected positively - at least in our model - by the amount of the national income and the number of physicians. The remarks made earlier on difficulties in interpreting the impact of this economic variable on health still hold. The positive dependence between the rate discussed now and the physicians rate confirms the frequently formulated objections referring to the identification of incidences and the discovery of cases of certain diseases. It is indisputable that their detection is obviously related with the number of physicians. The dependences of the same kind are to be found in our alternative model in which, apart from the influence of physicians, we find a positive effect of investment expenditures on sickness absenteeism due to cardiovascular diseases. We may regard it as an evidence of "civilization impact" on the discussed health aspect.

Y_4 Incidence rate of virus hepatitis (per 10000 population)

In looking for determinants of the incidence rate of virus hepatitis, we have assumed, as a hypothesis, the principal importance of iatrogenic causes of disease. As its implication we have assumed that the higher the level of activity of the health care system is, the higher the incidence rate of virus hepatitis. Since there is no direct measure of the activity level of the health care system in our list of indicators, we have to assume that the number of physicians and the extent of absenteeism because of diseases and accidents may be treated as indirect indicators. If we accept sickness absenteeism as health indicator then the increase of health needs releases a higher activity of the health care system. Therapeutic interventions, especially if they are a consequence of accidents, can lead to iatrogenic consequences. This somewhat risky construction has not been confirmed by our results. Though the physicians ratio remains in a positive relationship with the incidence rate of virus hepatitis, the activity rate of the system adopted by us remains in a negative relationship.

5. In the passage devoted to methods, we have mentioned the use of the principle of "time lag" in looking for relationships between parameters of economic situation and health. This principle is very useful for the attempts of causal interpretation of the phenomen analysed.

   It is obvious, that a phenomenon treated as a cause should precede in time the phenomenon treated as a consequence, and the change of intensity of stimulus should precede the change of the intensity of the result.

   The data analysed by us proved to be intractable to the use of the method of this kind. The shape of our curves was such that any displacements have not increased the prediction of our models. Only in the case of the incidence rate for sexually transmitted diseases the shift in time gave a positive result. But in this case the displacement should be very big (9 years) which is very risky due to the short range of our information. What is more, with such a displacement it is difficult to speak of causal dependences and still have a full sense of responsibility. One should be fully aware that in this situation causal interpretation of the relationships, if they were to be found, has to be performed very carefully.

Conclusions

1. Summing up the results of estimation of the presented models it should be stated that these models, in respect of statistics, do not arouse greater objections. The method used seems to be sufficiently good for the estimation of regression coefficients parameters of such models. However, in two cases, at the evaluation of alternative models for Y_{11} and S_6, autocorrelation of random component occurs and therefore another method of estimation should be used here (the generalized method of the least squares). Moreover in some cases (evaluated equations for: Y_2, Y_5, Y_6, S_4 and Y_{11} and S_6) the results of the Durbin-Watson's test do not decide the problem of random components autocorrelation.

In few cases the minus marks of intercept in equations reveal an imperfect specification of variables in equations (for Y_6 and Y_{10}). However, after many attempts to estimate alternative models on the basis of our limited list of variables, it was not possible to select better estimated equations. Also coefficients R^2, which are not too high in three cases (for Y_4, Y_5 and Y_7), testify to the fact that a specification error can exist. However, all regression coefficients at selected variables are statistically significant on the level of significance = 0,05.

Only in two cases alternative equations were considered while in practice we assessed a lot of such equations. This results from the fact that at the procedure of establishing the elements of the models in such a theoretically indefinite field the method which could be mainly used was the way of "trial and error".

2. An optimistic statistical interpretation of the results obtained by us demands great precaution in their substantial interpretation. We are worried by the ease with which causality between economic status parameters, health care, and health status indicators was confirmed. The dependences determined by us were found without using the time lag method, i.e. without a shift on the time axis. The assertion that such dependences are causal type relations - which are time sequence relations - is very disturbing. We are fully aware that our attempt to interpret the statistical dependences in cause-effect terms was not always well-founded. We called for sociological or psychological assertions without any very justifiable method. The assumption that these assertions can explain but rarely predict some relationships might be hardly rejected. A further confusion is brought about by the fact that numerical data used in our analysis may only in part be regarded as fully reliable.

One of the solutions to the difficult problem of results which are extraordinarily good would be to achieve a revelation of some stability of trends reflected by our parameters.

Such a tendency is visible in our economic indicators in this time interval which has been an object of our analysis. It should be stressed that the period studied by us does not include - in the sphere of economic status - the deep depression phenomena. Extension of the analysis including the years 1955 - 1956 and 1980 - 81 would radically change the picture of situation.

According to the declared objective our paper should lead to considering the possibility of the use of causal interpretation in such a way that it would be possible to answer the practical questions put within and by social policy. We think that an analysis carried out on macro-level, for a limited period and with the use of limited data of official reporting does not give - in spite of appearances - a real answer to practical questions. Nevertheless the line of investigations is highly encouraging.

Table 1: Correlation coefficients between indicators of somatic health

		Y_1	Y_2	Y_3	Y_4	Y_5	Y_6	Y_7	Y_8	Y_9	Y_{10}	Y_{11}
Total mortality rate per 1000 population	Y_1	1,00										
Mortality rate due to malignant neoplasms per 10000 population	Y_2	0,79	1,00									
Infant mortality rate per 1000 live births occuring in the year	Y_3	-0,77	-0,99	1,00								
Incidence rate of virus hepatitis per 10000 population	Y_4	-0,46	-0,21	0,24	1,00							
Incidence rate of sexually transmitted diseases per 10000 population	Y_5	-0,32	0,04	-0,05	0,24	1,00						
Incidence rate of malignant neoplasms	Y_6	0,88	0,94	-0,95	-0,38	-0,04	1,00					
Natural abortion rate per 100 women aged 15 - 49	Y_7	-0,49	-0,81	0,77	0,21	-0,37	-0,75	1,00				
Total absenteeism rate due to diseases and accidents	Y_8	0,94	0,90	-0,89	-0,46	-0,28	0,94	-0,62	1,00			
Absenteeism rate due to malignant neoplasms	Y_9	0,85	0,95	-0,94	-0,36	-0,18	0,93	-0,70	0,95	1,00		
Absenteeism rate due to nervous and psychiatric diseases	Y_{10}	0,88	0,94	-0,94	-0,39	-0,23	0,94	-0,66	0,98	0,96	1,00	
Absenteeism rate due to cardiovascular diseases	Y_{11}	0,92	0,89	-0,89	-0,43	-0,32	0,92	-0,57	0,98	0,95	0,99	1,00

Table 2: Correlation coefficient between indicators of psycho-social aspects of health, economic indicators and indicators of health

		S_1	S_2	S_3	S_4	S_5	S_6	X_1	X_2	X_3	X_4	X_5	Z_1	Z_2	Z_3
Divorces rate per 1000 population	S_1	1,00													
Migrations	S_2	0,87	1,00												
Alcohol consumption rate per capita	S_3	0,77	0,91	1,00											
Total suicide rate	S_4	0,83	0,84	0,86	1,00										
Tobacco consumption rate per capita	S_5	0,88	0,94	0,96	0,87	1,00									
Artificial abortion rate per 100 women aged 15 - 49	S_6	-0,92	-0,90	-0,86	-0,86	-0,95	1,00								
National income per capita	X_1	0,73	0,90	0,99	0,83	0,95	-0,84	1,00							
Health expenditure as a proportion of state budget	X_2	-0,14	-0,48	-0,54	-0,35	-0,45	0,29	-0,59	1,00						
Investment expenditure per capita	X_3	0,74	0,91	0,98	0,78	0,94	-0,82	0,99	-0,59	1,00					
Investment expenditure as a proportion of state budget	X_4	-0,78	-0,80	-0,80	-0,92	-0,84	-0,80	-0,79	0,46	-0,73	1,00				
Health and social welfare as a proportion of overall investment expenditure	X_5	-0,37	-0,66	-0,68	-0,58	-0,55	0,41	-0,67	0,60	-0,66	0,56	1,00			
Physicians per 10000 popul.	Z_1	0,92	0,94	0,93	0,92	0,98	-0,95	0,92	-0,37	0,90	-0,86	-0,56	1,00		
Nurses per 10000 popul.	Z_2	0,85	0,93	0,97	0,90	0,99	-0,93	0,97	-0,48	0,95	-0,86	-0,59	0,98	1,00	
Hospital beds per 10000 popul	Z_3	0,94	0,96	0,92	0,91	0,97	-0,95	0,90	-0,35	0,90	-0,84	-0,56	0,99	0,96	1,00

Table 3: Correlation coefficients between indicators of somatic health and indicators of psycho-social aspect of health

		S_1	S_2	S_3	S_4	S_5	S_6
Total mortality rate per 1000 population	Y_1	0,70	0,65	0,85	0,92	0,80	0,91
Mortality rate due to malignant neoplasms per 10000 population	Y_2	0,93	0,90	0,93	0,88	0,91	0,94
Infant mortality rate per 100 live births occuring in the year	Y_3	-0,95	-0,92	-0,92	-0,88	-0,91	-0,94
Incidence rate of virus hepatitis per 10000 population	Y_4	-0,18	-0,16	-0,27	-0,40	-0,27	-0,40
Incidence rate of sexually transmitted diseases per 10000 population	Y_5	-0,16	0,26	-0,15	-0,32	0,13	-0,19
Incidence rate of malignant neoplasms	Y_6	0,91	0,88	0,90	0,90	0,90	-0,97
Natural abortion rate per 100 women aged 15 - 49	Y_7	-0,84	-0,83	-0,67	-0,54	-0,72	-0,68
Total absenteeism rate due to diseases and accidents	Y_8	0,80	0,75	0,91	0,96	0,85	0,97
Absenteeism rate due to malignant neoplasms	Y_9	0,86	0,79	0,96	0,92	0,86	0,96
Absenteeism rate due to nervous and psychiatric diseases	Y_{10}	0,84	0,79	0,92	0,96	0,86	0,98
Absenteeism rate due to cardiovascular diseases	Y_{11}	0,77	0,71	0,90	0,98	0,84	0,97

Table 4: Results of regression analyses for indicators of somatic health

		const	Y_8 Total absenteeism rate due to diseases and accidents	S_2 Migrations	S_3 Alcohol consumption rate (per capita)	S_4 Total suicide rate	S_5 Tobacco consumption rate per capita	X_1 National income per capita	X_2 Health expenditures as a proportion of state budget	X_3 Investment expenditures per capita	X_4 Investment expenditures as a proportion of state budget	X_5 Health and social welfare as a proportion of overall investment expenditures	Z_1 Physicians per 10.000 population	Z_2 Nurses per 10.000 population	Z_3 Hospital beds per 10.000 population	R^2	D
Total mortality rate (per 1000 population)	Y_1	9,17		0,0082					-0,271							0,90	1,45
Mortality rate due to malignant neoplasms (per 10.000 population)	Y_2	-0,98 x					0,520		0,676			-1,268				0,97	1,59
Infant mortality rate (per 1000 live births occurring in the year)	Y_3	239,6							-1,815						-3,042	0,99	2,26
Incidence rate of virus hepatitis (per 10.000 population)	Y_4	43,9	-12,56										2,57			0,64	1,70
Incidence rate of sexually transmitted diseases (per 10.000 population)	Y_5	13,84				2,394								-0,764		0,74	1,20
Incidence rate of malignant neoplasms	Y_6	2,98 x					0,713				-0,123					0,98	1,42
Natural abortion rate (per 100 women aged 15-49)	Y_7	1,26								0,011			-0,036			0,88	2,36
Absenteeism rate due to malignant neoplasms	Y_9	0,004 x		0,0001									0,004			0,98	1,57
Absenteeism rate due to nervous and psych. diseases	Y_{10}	-0,46						0,006	0,018						0,010	0,99	2,13
Absenteeism rate due to cardiovascular diseases	Y_{11}	0,036 x 0,135 x							-0,033	0,014			0,018 0,040			0,98 0,96	1,00 1,11
Total suicide rate	S_4	15,91						0,050			-0,328					0,93	1,50
Artificial abortion rate (per 100 women aged 15-19)	S_6	2,72 2,91						0,017		0,022				-0,039 -0,053		0,94 0,96	1,06 1,53

x coefficient nonsignificant at level α = 0,05

Sources of data

Rocznik Statystyczny/Statistical Year Book

1960 - tables 17/37, 9/88
1961 - tables 27/47, 28/697, 13/606, 26/46
1963 - tables 12/32, 39/59, 26/756, 30/50
1964 - tables 12/32, 39/59
1965 - tables 24/673, 6/617, 1/612, 12/31, 27/784, 32/51, 4/88
1966 - tables 40/59, 28/684, 8/750, 36/55
1967 - tables 39/73, 12/925, 30/64, 33/796
Rocznik Ochrony Zdrowia/Year Book of Health Care 1945-1967
tables 3/37, 1/6, 2/7, 20/136
1968 - tables 10/46, 39/75, 37/73, 20/764, 12/969, 33/834, 36/72
1969 - tables 10/47, 36/73, 20/753, 3/863, 32/821, 33/70
1970 - tables 11/794, 5/734, 10/439, 32/65, 30/63, 19/748, 20/749,
7/938, 39/72, 1/847, 3/849, 1/847, 11/109, 29/812, 29/62
1971 - tables 30/838
1972 - tables 6/737, 1/732, 8/42, 28/62, 26/60, 33/67, 36/70, 20/54,
1/117, 4/120, 1/841, 29/812, 25/59
1973 - tables 7/38, 36/67, 34/65, 19/709, 39/70, 32/768,
1974 - tables 9/39, 38/68, 36/66, 19/770, 4/175, 30/142, 35/65
1974 - tables 19, 11/69/Year Book of Health Care
1975 - tables 12/133, I, 8/51, 30/73, 29/72, 17/754, 33/76, 21/64,
5/101, 2/45, 24/145, 34/77
1976 - tables 4/726, 1/723, 29/77, 30/78, 13/735, 14/736, 15/737,
16/738, 32/80, 34/82, 2/767, 10/775, 1/176, 5/180,
2/767, 24/144, 33/81, 28/76
Year Book of Health Care 1976 - tables 2, 11/94
1977 - tables 21/62, 15/634, 23/64, 4/148, 1/160, 22/121
1978 - tables 10/108, 4/627, 1/624, 18/63, 19/64, 12/635, 13/636,
14/637, 15/638, 20/65, 22/67, 11/56, 2/665, 9/672,
1/46, 4/142, 1/664, 4/84, 22/120, 17/62,
1979 - tables 7/54, 19/66, 12/648, 13/649, 14/650, 15/651, 21/68,
2/678, 9/685, 1/155, 4/158, 1/677, 4/92, 22/129
1979 - tables I, 10/79 - Year Book of Health Care
1980 - tables 10/129, II, 5/668, 1/664, 7/57, 28/78, 29/79, 17/680,
19/682, 20/683, 21/684, 30/80, 32/82, 21/71, 2/709,
9/716, 1/164, 4/167, 1/708, 4/104, 3/53, 22/141, 31/81,
27/77.

NOTES:

(1) BRENNER, M.H.: Fetal, infant and maternal mortality during periods of economic instability. International Journal of Health Services 3, 2, 145-159 (1973)

BRENNER, M.H.: Health costs and benefits of economic policy. International Journal of Health Services 7, 4, 581-623 (1977)

BRENNER, M.H.: Industralization and economic growth: estimates of their effects on the health of populations. In: Assessing the Contributions of the Social Sciences to Health. (Eds.: M.H. Brenner, A. Mooney, T. Nagy). Boulder "Colorado": Westview Press (1980)

BRENNER, M.H.: Unemployment, economic growth and mortality. The Lancet, March 24, 1979, p.672 (1979)

(2) KASL, V.S.: Mortality and the business cycle: Some questions about strategies when utilizing macro-social and ecological data. American Journal of Public-Health 69, 8, 784-788 (1979)

KASL, S.V., GORE, S., COBB, S.: The experience of losing a job: Reported changes in health, symptoms and illness behaviour. Psychosomatic Medicine 37, 2, 106-122 (1975)

(3) BUNN, A.R.: Ischaemic heart disease mortality and the business cycle in Australia. American Journal of Public Health 69, 8, 772-781 (1979)

EYER, J.: Does unemployment cause the death rate peak in each business cycle? International Journal of Health Services 87, 4 (1977)

COCHRANE, A.L. et al.: Health service input and mortality in developed countries. Journal of Epidemiology and Community Health 32, 200 (1978)

PIERCE, A.: The economic cycle and social suicide rate. American Sociological Review 1967, 32, 457-62

COBB, S., KASL, S.V.: Some medical aspects of unemployment. Industr. Geront. 8, 8-15 (1972)

CATALANO, R., DOOLEY, D.: The economy as stressor: A sectoral analysis. Review of Social Economy 37, 175-187 (1979)

(4) PAWLOWSKI, T.: Concepts and methods in contemporary humanities. (in Polish) Wroclaw 9-32: Ossolineum (1977)

(5) U.S. DEPT. OF HEALTH AND SOCIAL SERVICES: Goals for the nation. p.1 (1980)

(6) WHO.: REGIONAL OFFICE FOR EUROPE: Regional strategy for attaining health for all by the year 2000. WHO: EUR/RC30/8, p.30

(7) See above, p.1

(8) WHO.: REGIONAL OFFICE FOR EUROPE: Regional health development advisory council. Report on a Meeting, Copenhagen 17. - 18.3.1980. WHO: EUR/EXM/80.2, p.2-3

(9) WHO: REGIONAL OFFICE FOR EUROPE: Measurement of levels of health. Copenhagen. WHO Regional publications European Series N. 7 (1979)

(10) MAC MAHON, B., PUGH, T.P.: Epidemiology. Polish edition, PZWL: Warszawa (1974)

BARKER, D.J.P.: Practical epidemiology. Edinburgh: Churchill Livingstone (1973)

MORRIS, J.N.: Uses of epidemiology. Edinburgh: Churchill Livingstone (1975)

(11) BENJAMIN, B.: Social and economic factors affecting mortality. The Hague, Mouton: Paris (1965)

(12) SHIGAN, E., ASPDEN, R., KITSUL, P.: Modeling health care systems. June 1979 Workshop Proceedings. International Institute for Applied Systems Analysis (IIASA), Laxenburg, Austria (1979)

(13) VENEDIKTOV, D.D.: Modeling of health care systems. In: IIASA Conference 1976, Vol. 2. Laxenburg: IIASA, Austria p. 106

(14) WHO: EVROPEJSKOIE REGIONALNOIE BIURO: Imitacionnye modeli processov upravlenia zdravoochraneniem, Otčet o soveščanii Rabočej gruppy VOZ. WHO: Kopenhagen (1980)

(15) BRENNER, M.H.: Mortality and the national economy. The Lancet, 15.9.1979, 568-572 (1979)

UNEMPLOYMENT, NUTRITION AND INFANT MORTALITY IN BRITAIN
1920 - 1950

Jay M. Winter

Pembroke College, Cambridge
Great Britain

The paths of labour historians and demographic historians have crossed all too rarely in Britain. Part of the cause of separate but equal development is a current of mutual suspicion, largely based on misapprehensions, which should have been swept away long ago. Among some labour historians there is a profound distrust of quantification, either as the art of proving laboriously what we already know, or as a cult replete with mysteries into which all but initiates enter at their peril. Among demographic historians, the explicit political commitments of some historians of labour seem to violate canons of scholarly objectivity, as if population questions and policies have had no ideological content.

The present plea for colloboration is based on the view that it is both profitable and necessary. Scholars in the fields of labour history and demographic history have distinctive contributions to make on many subjects of mutual interest. Among them is the history of the health of the working population. Demographic historians can learn much from studies of class structure about the changing meaning and complexity of the social and economic variables which they relate to vital statistics by means of sophisticated statistical analysis. Labour historians can learn much from demographic analysis about the costs of social inequality and the degree to which working people have managed to cope successfully with chronic deprivation and economic insecurity.

Scholars of both disciplines can also help in different ways to unravel the difficult problem of what is the appropriate time scale on which to analyse the relation between trends in public health and variations in levels of employment or income. In some quarters, a short-term perspective is adopted 'faute de mieux', and movements in vital statistics are reduced to reflex reactions to changes in economic variables. In these cases a joint effort is necessary in order to bring current historical and epidemiological research to bear on problems of public health in the past. Only then will it be possible both to relate short-term developments to long-term trends and to transform abstract economic and social categories into descriptions of real and at times contradictory social situations.

A case in point is the relation between unemployment and mortality rates. In the American context, one student of demographic trends has argued recently that unemployment was a killer. (1) The victims were not workers, but rather their infants, whose survival chances, it is claimed, were significantly reduced immediately after surges in unemployment in the United States in this century. Partly by adversely affecting the physical or emotional health of the mother, partly by reducing expenditure on public health care and partly by diminishing the quantity and quality of the food intake of infants, economic slumps quickly took their toll of the lives of the most vulnerable sections of the population.

In the light of recent employment trends in Britain, this subject has more than historical significance. (2) No one denies that deprivation has made the struggle to improve public health much more difficult in this century, but few have succeeded in untangling the complex web of relations between economic fluctuations and infant mortality. In order to do so, we must go beyond the short-term perspective of studies such as that cited above. One of the objectives of this essay is to show why this is necessary, with reference to the experience of Britain in the years 1920-50.

This period is an appropriate one about which to pose the methodological and substantive problems related to the question of the effects of employment levels on infant survival chances since between 1921 and 1948, statistics which accurately reflect fluctuations in levels of unemployment among workers were collected under the workings of the National Insurance Act. Between 1911 and 1921, only workers in certain 'precarious' trades were covered by the insurance scheme, and for the period before 1911, the historian must deal with statistics drawn from trade union records, the representative nature of which is highly doubtful. After 1948, virtually the whole population whether in the labour force or not, came under the protection of the Act. Since accurate unemployment statistics are essential to this study, it is necessary to restrict it to the three decades after the end of the First World War.

There are other reasons why this period has been chosen as a test case. The contrast between mass unemployment in the interwar years and 'full employment' in the periods during and after the Second World War is a commonplace of economic and social history. (3) It is well known too, that a major redistribution of income levels took place in the period 1938-48, thereby significantly reducing income inequality in this country. (4) By focusing on the second quarter of this century, it is possible to see in what ways a major break in the pattern of unemployment and income distribution affected infant health.

The conclusion that will be drawn is that unemployment was not the decisive cause of fluctuations in infant mortality rates during this period. It will be shown that while short-term changes are important, we must look both before and after this period to appreciate the full demographic meaning of economic instability. On the one hand, we must seek in much earlier developments the primary source of movements in infant mortality rates in these years. By doing this, it is possible to see how the slow but steady progress of sanitation and nutrition since the 1850s is reflected in the demographic experience of later generations. The shadow effect of the rise in working-class living standards over the past century is at once more subtle, more significant and more stubbornly irreversible than many students of the period have acknowledged. These gains have left (and still leave) a legacy that even foolish economic policies or politically imposed impoverishment cannot obliterate completely. It is in this context that we must place the downward trend of infant mortality in the period 1920-50. On the other hand, we can find evidence of the deleterious effects of the Depression of the interwar years and the beneficial effects of economic conditions in the 1940s in certain aspects of infant mortality trends in the years since 1950. The development of a long-term perspective is, therefore, the key to an understanding of one important part of the history of public health in Britain over the last one hundred years.

What I propose to do in this essay is to describe first the character and components of infant mortality in the period under review. Secondly, I shall examine the statistical evidence to show that in the British case, it is a vast over-simplification of the interaction of economic and demographic behaviour to argue with M.H. Brenner that there is a demonstrable, direct, short-term relation between 'national economic changes and infant mortality under one year in each of the major age categories.' (5) Thirdly, I shall discuss the ways in which the upheavals of the Second World War affected infant mortality rates in England and Wales. Finally, I shall try to relate the arguments about short-term and long-term changes to an interpretation of aspects of the demographic and social history of Britain.

1. The course of infant mortality decline in Britain, 1921-48

During the period 1921-48, infant mortality rates in England and Wales declined by more than 60 per cent, from 83 to 33 deaths per 1.000 live births. A decline of similar magnitude was registered in Scotland. This constituted a continuation of the trend towards increasing infant survival rates which began at the turn of the century. Similar improvements were made in Europe during this period, as figure 1 illustrates. While experiencing significantly lower infant mortality rates than Scotland and France, England and Wales lagged behind the Netherlands and Switzerland in terms of infant survival chances throughout most of the period.

Three aspects of the trend are clear. First, between 1929 and 1948, there seems to have been a periodicity of two to four years in the appearance of peaks of mortality. Increases in infant mortality punctuated the trend of economic decline in a number of European countries in 1929, 1932, 1935-36, 1940-41, 1944-45 and 1947. Some of the fluctuation in infant mortality in this period may be a function of the virulence or periodicity of viral and bacterial infections. (6) During the Second World War, peaks of infant mortality such as those in the Netherlands in 1945 and in France in both 1940 and 1945, were obviously attributable to war conditions. The fact that increases were registered in the war years by countries occupied (France and Holland), unoccupied but combatant (Britain) and neutral (Switzerland and Ireland) suggests that part of the upward disturbance in infant mortality rates between 1939 and 1945 probably would have occurred even had war been avoided. There is an epidemiological component of the history of infant mortality which cannot be ignored.

Secondly, as is shown in figure 2, the upward surge in infant mortality in 1940-41 in England and Wales is shown in all categories of births with the exception of illegitimate births. The steady decline in illegitimate infant mortality rates after 1939 suggests in part that the maternity services reached many unmarried mothers and thereby reduced the greater risks that their infants faced in the first year of life. In addition, the proportion of married women among all women who gave birth to illegitimate children rose to about one-third of the total. Herein may be one reason for the wartime continuation of the tendency for a narrowing of the gap between legitimate and illegitimate infant mortality rates.

Thirdly, it is possible to compare the contribution of different periods within the first year of life to the overall trend of decline. A glance at figure 3 will suffice to show that mortality rates under

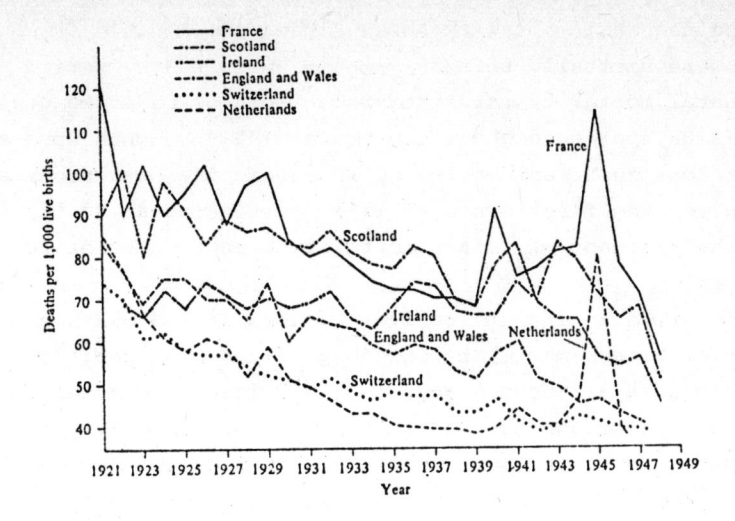

Fig. 1: Infant mortality rates in selected European nations, 1921-48

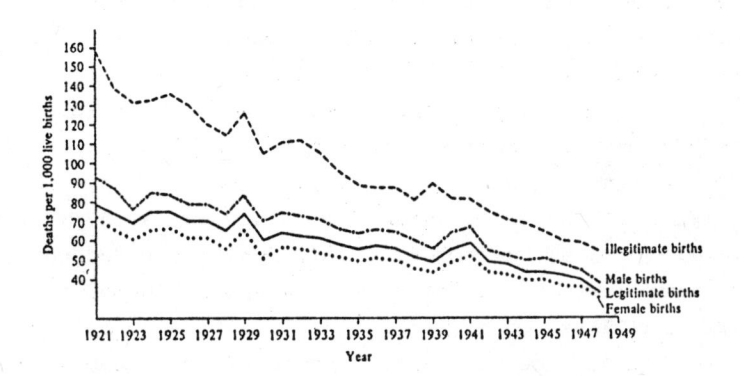

Fig. 2: Infant mortality rates for legitimate, illegitimate, female and male births in England and Wales, 1921-48

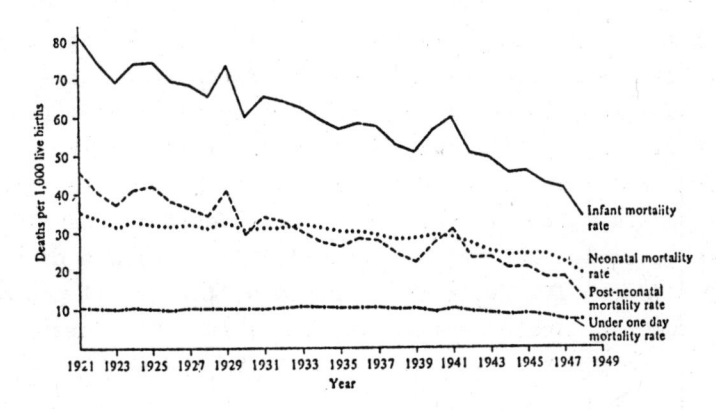

Fig. 3: Infant mortality rates at different periods of the first year of life in England and Wales, 1921-48

one day and neonatal mortality rates (under one month) for England
and Wales were virtually static throughout most of the period under review. Neonatal mortality rates started a more precipitate decline in
the late 1940s, but throughout the period 1921-48, much more signigfi-
cant reductions in infant mortality appear in the post neonatal period,
that is, after the first month of life. Post-neonatal mortality trends
governed the movement of infant mortality trends, a point to which we
shall return.

The deterioration in infant survival chances in 1941-42 was primarily
a function of higher mortality in the post-neonatal period, during
which most babies are weaned and, in time, lose the protection of their
mothers' antibodies against infectious disease. In contrast, gains in
survival rates for infants in the second half of the Second World War
were registered at both the early and the later stages of the first
year of life. The point is supported by data presented in table 1,
which describe wartime declines in both the developmental and wasting
diseases, which primarily affect neonatal mortality rates, and infectious diseases, which primarily affect post-neonatal mortality rates.
It is equally striking that diarrhoea and enteritis, historically the
great scourge of infant life among malnourished populations, did not
contribute to either the increase in infant mortality rates in 1940-41
or their decline in the later years of the war.

An overall trend of declining infant mortality rates in Britain was
interrupted, therefore, but not reversed, during the Second World War.
The same is true for maternal mortality rates, the decline in which
began in the mid-1930s. Chemotherapy was not the sole cause of this
important development, but the introduction of sulphonamide drugs in
the 1930s enabled doctors to control puerperal sepsis, the greatest
single cause of maternal deaths. (7)

The war period was a turning-point, though, in the trend of still
births. Reliable statistics are available only since the late 1920s,
when the still-birth rate for England and Wales stood at 40 per 1.000
total births. Virtually no change occurred in the decade before the
outbreak of war, but, as we can see in table 2, a decline of approximately 30 per cent took place throughout England and Wales between
1938 and 1946. The greatest gains were registered in the mining regions
of South Wales (Wales II) and in the industrial regions of Lancashire
and Cheshire (North IV), with other regions, more rural and agricultural in character (South West), not far behind. Of course, massive
internal migration makes regional comparisons between pre-war and

Table 1.   Infant Mortality Rates from Certain Causes, England and Wales, 1937-1946 (Deaths per 1,000 Live Births)

	1937	1938	1939	1940	1941	1942	1943	1944	1945
All Causes	57.68	52.81	50.57	56.77	60.04	50.62	49.12	45.44	46.00
1. Infectious Diseases Excluding Tuberculosis	3.23	2.43	2.28	2.81	4.24	2.09	2.60	1.98	1.81
2. Tuberculosis	0.63	0.60	0.51	0.60	0.67	0.54	0.51	0.44	0.42
3. Diarrhoea and Enteritis	5.30	5.07	4.31	4.44	4.82	5.17	4.94	4.84	5.12
4. Developmental and Wasting Disease	26.91	24.94	24.76	25.41	25.56	23.79	21.69	20.40	20.33
5. Other Causes	21.61	19.77	18.70	23.50	24.75	19.03	19.38	17.78	18.32

Table 2. Still-birth rates, England and Wales, 1938-46, by region (deaths per 1,000 total births)

	1938	1939	1940	1941	1942	1943	1944	1945	1946
England and Wales	38	38	36	35	33	30	28	28	27
South East	32	31	30	30	29	27	25	24	24
Greater London	31	31	29	30	29	26	24	24	24
Rest of South East	34	33	31	29	28	27	25	25	25
North	42	42	40	39	37	33	30	30	30
North I	39	40	40	36	37	32	30	31	31
North II	37	39	36	39	35	30	29	30	29
North III	41	42	39	38	36	32	30	30	29
North IV	46	44	41	40	38	34	31	30	31
Midland	38	38	36	34	33	30	26	27	26
Midlands I	37	38	36	34	33	30	26	27	26
Midlands II	39	38	36	33	33	31	26	28	25
East	37	36	34	34	32	29	26	28	27
South West	39	37	36	32	32	30	27	26	26
Wales	51	49	47	43	40	36	34	34	33
Wales I	51	49	47	44	39	36	34	35	33
Wales II	48	47	47	39	41	35	33	32	33
County Boroughs	40	40	38	36	34	31	29	29	29
Other urban districts	41	40	38	36	34	32	28	29	28
Rural districts	38	37	37	34	32	30	27	28	26

Regions

South East
Bedfordshire
Berkshire
Buckinghamshire
Essex
Hertfordshire
Kent
London
Middlesex
Oxfordshire
Southampton
Surrey
Sussex
Isle of Wight

North I
Durham
Northumberland

North II
Cumberland
Westmoreland
Yorkshire-
  East Riding

Yorkshire-
  North Riding

North III
Yorkshire-
  West Riding
Yorkshire-
  County
  Boroughs

North IV
Cheshire
Lancashire

Midlands I
Gloucestershire
Herefordshire
Shropshire
Staffordshire
Warwickshire
Worcestershire

Midlands II
Derbyshire
Lincolnshire,
  parts of
Northamptonshire
Nottinghamshire
Peterborough,
  Soke of

South West
Cornwall
Devon
Somerset
Wiltshire

East
Cambridgeshire
Ely, Isle of
Huntingdonshire
Lincolnshire,
  parts of
Norfolk
Rutlandshire
Suffolk

Wales I
Breckonshire
Carmarthenshire
Glamorganshire
Monmounthshire

Wales II
Anglesey
Caernarvonshire
Cardiganshire
Denbighshire
Flintshire
Merionethshire
Montgomeryshire
Pembrokeshire
Radnorshire

post-war populations highly suspect. It is best, therefore, to interpret the decline in still-birth rates in this period as a reflection of a process which affected the population in Britain as a whole. That process, it will be argued below, was set in motion long before the outbreak of the Second World War. Much smaller gains were made, both relatively and absolutely, in infant survival chances during the war against Hitler, than during the First World War a generation earlier (8). It was perhaps easier to effect a reduction in the infant mortality rate when it stood at about 100 per 1.000 live births in 1914, than when it was about 50 per 1.000 live births in 1939. But the greater impact of the earlier conflict must be understood in the context of pre-war social conditions which were significantly worse than those of the interwar years. Our interpretation of the stability of mortality trends in the period 1921-48 rests on the assumption that they were determined largely by prior changes in the standard of living in the British working class.

In order to complete the general demographic picture, it is necessary to examine the possibility that movements in the birth rate influenced the course of the decline in infant mortality. By the 1920s, resort to contraception was, if not universal, extremely widespread in British society. The decline in fertility, dating from the 1870s, enabled working-class parents to provide more food and greater attention to each child in a smaller completed family. In the interwar years, however, the long-term trend was either interrupted or broken, a distinction which depends upon an interpretation of demographic trends today. There is no argument, though, that the birth-rate moved downward in the first half of our period (1921-34) and upward in the second half (1935-48). Since the infant mortality rates declined both during the upswings and the downswings of the birth-rate, and since changes in maternal age and parity in this period were dismissed long ago as decisive factors in the downward mortality trend, (9) we can conclude that purely demographic changes were not directly responsible for the gains made in infant survival chances during the period under review.

2. Unemployment and infant mortality

A) Time-series analysis

With this set of descriptive statistics in mind, let us consider the problem of the nature of the relation between unemployment and infant mortality during this period. Professor Brenner's case is that standard statistical methods can establish both the existence and nature of a strong correlation between movements in employment levels and movements in infant mortality rates. His approach is fairly simple. In order to make the unemployment rate consistent with other major but positive economic indicators, he used what he called an 'inverted' unemployment rate, namely 100 minus the percentage of the labour force unemployed. This was deemed to be the independent variable, the trend of which he determined. With the trend line equation in hand, he then calculated annual deviations from the trend. When a positive deviation was recorded, it indicated better than average employment conditions. Conversely, a negative deviation from the trend indicated worse than average employment conditions. Using US data for the period 1915-67, the bad years of the 1930s and the good years of the 1940s stand out clearly (figure 4). Against this set of deviations from the trend of employment, some of which were smoothed out by the use of moving averages, Brenner plotted deviations from the trends of under one day, post-neonatal and infant mortality rates. A positive deviation from these trends meant higher than average infant mortality; a negative deviation, lower than average infant mortality. What Brenner was after was a sort of 'double helix', confirming his hypothesis that employment levels and infant mortality rates were related in a statistically significant way. His primary conclusion was that when unemployment rose, mortality in the first day of life rose one year later, and post-neonatal mortality and infant mortality as a whole rose three to five years later.

There are theoretical objections to the method Brenner used to generate his evidence of the supposed inverse relation between employment and infant mortality, and I shall discuss these difficulties below. It seems reasonable, though, to try to test Brenner's hypothesis in an indirect way, by repeating the exercise for data on unemployment and infant mortality at various stages of the first year of life in Britain in the period 1921-49.

The results using British data are strikingly different from those reported by Brenner in his examination of the American case. On the one hand, his hypothesis seems to be confirmed in the case of early infant mortality. Figure 5 displays the 'double helix' predicted by Brenner in the case of day-one mortality in England

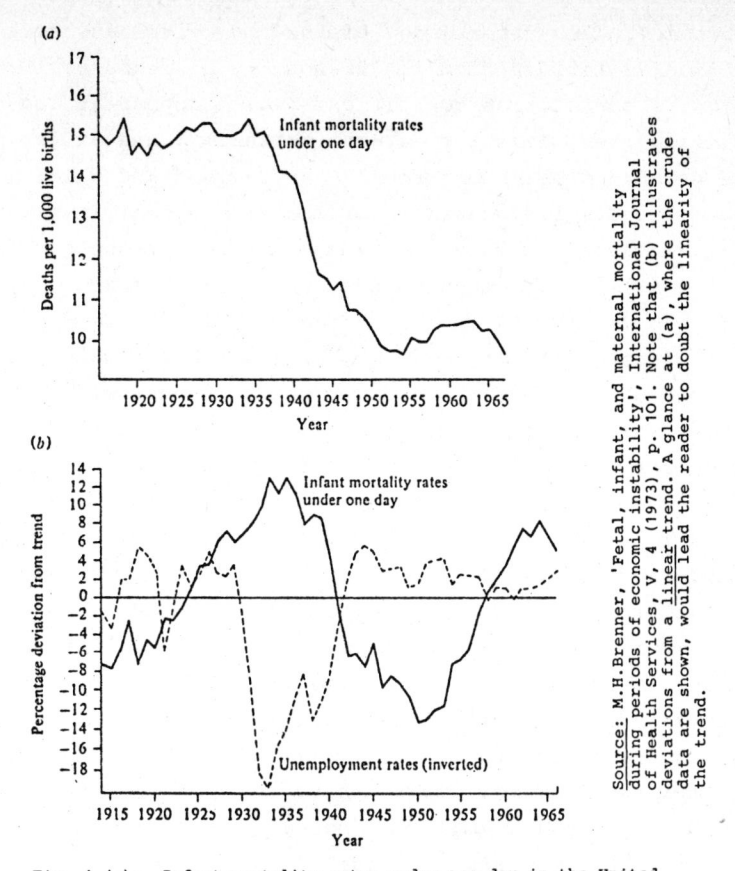

Fig. 4 (a): Infant mortality rates under one day in the United States, 1915-67.
(b): Percentage deviations from the trends of under one day mortality rates and unemployment rates (inverted), 1915-67 (relation shown at one-year lag)

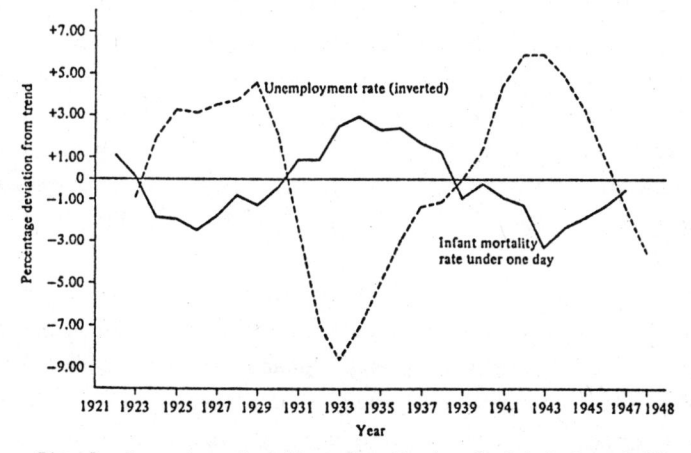

Source: M.H. Brenner, 'Fetal, infant, and maternal mortality during periods of economic instability', International Journal of Health Services, V, 4 (1973), p. 101. Note that (b) illustrates deviations from a linear trend. A glance at (a), where the crude data are shown, would lead the reader to doubt the linearity of the trend.

Fig. 5: Percentage deviations from the trend of infant mortality rates during the first day of life and from the trend of unemployment rates (inverted) in England and Wales, 1921-48 (unemployment rates moved forward by one year, three-year averages).

and Wales. The mirror image of the two curves describing percentage deviations from the trends may be measured in terms of negative correlation coefficients which appear at lags of zero, one, and four years for day-one mortality, and at lags of zero and one year for week-one mortality in England and Wales (appendices 1 and 2). Similar negative correlations appear in the case of early infant mortality in Scotland at lags of one and four years. On the other hand, though, Brenner's findings are not replicated at later periods of the first year of life. Indeed, as in the case of total infant mortality in England and Wales, the numerous positive correlations imply that when unemployment rose, infant mortality actually fell, which is completely at variance with Brenner's argument. The weight of the statistical evidence concerning Britain, therefore, is against the contention that movements in infant mortality 'respond' to movements in unemployment.

I shall argue below that the positive findings in support of Brenner's hypothesis are probably statistical aberrations. It is necessary, though, to consider the possibility that early infant mortality is a special case. Time-series analysis seems to show two contradictory things:

1) when unemployment rates dipped below the trend line for the period 1921-49, first-week mortality rates either rose to levels well above the trend or failed to fall with it;

2) no such relation existed at later stages of the first year of life. It is extremely difficult to accept at face value this apparent indication of a correlation between unemployment and early infant mortality, since there is no evidence that unemployment resulted in deprivation which affected new-born babies in the first seven days of life but not thereafter. It could be argued that unemployment interfered indirectly with the access which women had to hospitalization or professional care at home immediately after childbirth, but this argument is unconvincing for several reasons. First, the proportion of all deliveries undertaken in hospitals was rising throughout this period. Secondly, even before the outbreak of war in 1939, major improvements had taken place in provision for antenatal and postnatal care in maternal and child welfare centres. Both developments helped to protect the maternal population against the worst effects of the Depression. The exception was in

South Wales, where maternal morbidity and mortality rates rose in the aftermath of increases in unemployment. Fortunately, the state of health of women in childbirth in the mining communities of South Wales was not representative of that of British women as a whole. When the decline in maternal mortality rates for Britain as a whole did come in 1936, it was not as a result of declining unemployment rates or the alleviation of the fear of unemployment. No one would deny that joblessness created stress among working women and the wives of working men, but the evidence that such anxiety affected pregnancy or its outcome is too weak to be conclusive.

Other doubts must be raised about accepting the contention that unemployment affected early but not late infant mortality rates. The most rigorous examination of the effect of unemployment on aspects of the mortality experience of the British population is the analysis of rheumatic heart disease among children in the period 1927-38 by Morris and Titmuss. They demonstrate conclusively that an increase in unemployment led to an increase in juvenile deaths due to rheumatic heart disease. A time lag of three years separated the two trends and represented the latent period of the disease. (10) Its toll was undoubtedly a reflection of malnutrition and squalor, conditions which also affect infant survival chances as a whole, and in particular those during the later months of the first year of life. If corroboration for the findings of Titmuss and Morris are to be sought in application of Brenner's method to British data, then it is to the post-neonatal period that we must direct special attention. And it is precisely at this later stage of infant mortality that Brenner's hypothesis is refuted by the data.

Another line of reasoning about the relation between unemployment and infant mortality is that a decline in protein intake during pregnancy increased early infant mortality due to the congenital disease and deformity. There is some confirmation for this argument in the fact that the infant mortality rate due to spina bifida and anencephalus increased in the early 1930s. This rise continued, however, in the later 1930s when unemployment rates dropped, and during the Second World War when unemployment reached negligible levels. (11) It is puzzling, though, that infant mortality after the first week of life does not register evidence of diminished resistance to disease through maternal protein deficiency.

A further problem is that it is very difficult to reach firm conclusions about nutritional levels in general or those of the unemployed in particular for this period. Lord Boyd Orr's work suggests that aggregate protein intake was constant over the period 1924-34, but that in the same decade, consumption of animal fat, fruits and vegetables increased significantly. During the Second World War, it was precisely these foodstuffs that were in very short supply. (12) A link between protein intake and early infant mortality is therefore plausible but unsubstantiated for the period under review. The shadow effect of such food deprivation after the Second World War is a point to which we shall return below.

Another look at figure 3 will suffice to show a further, more technical, reason for doubting Brenner's hypothesis. Statistically significant correlations between deviations from the trends of unemployment and infant mortality were found for the case of mortality in the first week of life, that is, in a time series which shows little or no absolute movement over three decades. The method of fitting a trend line to such data may exaggerate tiny changes and make them appear to be of equal significance to much greater movements around different trend lines. Brenner's use of a 'linear' trend line in the case of day-one mortality is highly debatable, to say the least, (13) and it is no accident, therefore, that the relation between post-neonatal mortality and unemployment was found to be non-existent, while such a relation seemed to be proved in the case of early infant mortality. The method itself may produce such anomalies. Indeed, some statisticians raise objections to the way in which trend lines are 'fitted' to data, regardless of their character. As a 'reductio ad absurdum', it can be shown, using this approach, that sunspot eruptions cause business cycles. For this reason, alternative techniques of time-series analysis have been devised. Among them is a sophisticated procedure known as the 'Box Jenkins' method. Through the integration of an autoregressive and moving average model, the Box-Jenkins approach solves problems built into more traditional modes of detrending series. It is also a powerful tool in the analysis of the structure of time series and of any lagged relation between serially correlated variables, which is precisely what we need. (14) Using this method, I was unable to identify any correlation between unemployment rates and infant mortality rates at any lag from one to ten years. (15)

B) Class differentials in infant mortality rates

In other ways too, we can show that it is necessary to view the relation between unemployment and infant mortality in a manner more complex than that suggested by Professor Brenner. Let us examine evidence related to the infant mortality experience of different social classes, regions, and urban administrative areas.

The shift from high to low unemployment in the 1930s and 1940s seems to have left undiminished class differentials in infant mortality. Evidence on this point has been available since the 1920s, when Registrars-General started regularly to use a five-tiered taxonomy of social classes to measure in a very rough way the demographic disadvantage of being born into a working man's family. Not too much should be made of such comparisons, which rely upon an inadequate definition of social class in terms of male occupation. Still, we can learn something from them. As it is shown in table 3, in 1911 the mortality rate of infants born to the families of unskilled workers was double that of infants born to professional men's families. Between 1911 and 1939 the aggregate infant mortality rate for England and Wales dropped from 130 to 51 deaths per 1.000 live births. Yet over the same period, the advantage of Class I over Class V babies was not only maintained, but actually increased. This was only marginally true in the first month of life. At ages between six and twelve months though, when infectious diseases predominate, the advantage in survival chances which infants of well-to-do families had over those of poorer families increased substantially in the period between 1911 and 1931-32.

Assuming for a moment the very unlikely fact of low inter-class mobility, it is possible to compare only very imperfectly trends in demographic inequality in the pre-war decade and in the years between 1939 and 1951. Again we see that shifts in levels of unemployment were not decisive determinants in shifts in relative levels of infant mortality. In the 1930s, the gap between Class V and Class I narrowed both at ages six to twelve months and in terms of infant mortality rates as a whole. By 1951, the elimination of mass unemployment ought to have had some differential effect on the relative position of families of unskilled workers, if the Brenner hypothesis is valid. The evidence, however, points the other way.

Table 3. Infant mortality rates of legitimate children, England and Wales, 1911, 1920-22, 1930-32, 1939 and 1951 (deaths per 1,000 live births), with respect to excess mortality in Social Class V compared to Social Class I

	1911	1921-23	1930-32	1939	1951
Neonatal Mortality					
Class V	42.5	36.9	32.5	30.1	22.8
Class I	30.2	23.4	21.7	18.9	14.0
Excess	12.3	13.5	10.8	11.2	8.8
% Excess	40.7	57.7	49.7	59.3	62.9
Post-neonatal Mortality					
Class V	110.0	60.1	44.5	30.0	18.0
Class I	46.2	15.0	11.0	8.0	4.7
Excess	63.8	45.1	33.5	22.0	13.3
% Excess	138.1	300.1	304.5	275.0	283.0
Mortality at 6-12 months					
Class V	50.0	24.6	19.4	10.4	—
Class I	18.3	5.8	3.6	2.3	—
Excess	31.7	18.8	15.8	8.1	—
% Excess	173.2	324.1	438.9	352.2	—
Infant Mortality					
Class V	152.5	97.0	77.0	60.1	40.8
Class I	76.4	38.4	32.7	26.9	18.7
Excess	76.1	58.6	44.3	33.2	22.1
% Excess	99.6	152.6	135.5	123.4	118.2

Sources: R. Titmuss, Birth, Poverty and Wealth (1943), pp.44-5.
Registrar-General's Decennial Supplement. England and Wales 1931. Part IIB. Occupational Fertility.1931 and 1939, Table Q1, p.86.
Registrar-General's Decennial Supplement. England and Wales 1951. Part II, vol. 2, Table 14A, Occupational Mortality.

The excess of Class V infant mortality rates over those of Class I in 1951 and 1939 was virtually the same.

It is a commonplace of the history of the interwar years that the slump completely bypassed large parts of the south and east of England. It did not require Orwell's journey to Wigan pier to make known the fact of wide regional and industrial variations in economic hardship. Among the worst-hit populations were those who lived in the 'Special Areas' of England, encompassing the counties of Durham, Cumberland and Northumberland, and the 'Special Areas' of Wales, that is, Glamorgan, Brecknock, Pembroke and Monmouth. In each of these counties, unemployment rates in the early 1930s reached between 30 per cent and 40 per cent, or double the national average. In parts of these areas, unemployment rates of 70 per cent to 80 per cent were not unknown. What does the experience of infant mortality in these regions during the age of mass unemployment in the 1930s and in the period of 'full employment' in the 1940s contribute to the debate over Brenner's hypothesis?

The first point to be made is that these regions are highly heterogeneous, and that, therefore, we should expect wide fluctuations in their demographic behaviour. Still, it is no comfort to supporters of Brenner's case that improvements were registered in Northumberland in the early 1930s, in Glamorgan in the mid-1930s, and in Durham in the late 1930s, despite the persistence of very high unemployment rates compared to the nation as a whole throughout the pre-war decade. It is even more surprising that in the years 1945-49, when the Attlee government made certain that there would be no immediate return to the age of mass unemployment, there occurred in Glamorgan and Durham a slow-down in the rate of decline of infant mortality. Data on county boroughs in these regions show the same pattern of irregularity in the relation between unemployment and infant mortality.

Statistics relating to areas outside those worst hit by unemployment also show a persistent trend for the better during the 'bad' 1930s and the 'better' 1940s. If anything, there are indications that the difference between the national rate of infant mortality and that of industrial regions in the post-war period was actually greater than in the pre-war period. For instance, infant mortality rates in Lancashire and Cheshire in 1937 were 21 per cent above the national average. Ten years later, the gap had grown to 32 per cent.

The greatest gains in infant survival chances were registered in London and Southeast, that is to say, in those areas which were not afflicted by mass unemployment in the 1930s.

C) Variance in infant mortality rates in urban administrative areas

Finally, let us compare the trend of infant mortality in smaller administrative areas. Brenner's hypothesis suggests that the pace of infant mortality decline was greater in areas of low unemployment such as Oxford and Eastbourne than in high unemployment areas such as Wigan or Sunderland. If this assumption were true, it would mean that the variance among the mortality rates of all county boroughs would increase when unemployment hit some harder than others. The statistical variance among all county boroughs of England and Wales and among all metropolitan boroughs of London in the period 1920-50 is, though, astonishingly uniform. Whatever their experience of unemployment, virtually all urban areas went through the process of infant mortality decline together, as it were. (16) Here again it appears that demographic trends cannot be reduced to reflections of the workings of the labour market.

3. Infant mortality during the Second World War

The decline in infant mortality in England and Wales was unshaken by the slump. It is hardly surprising that there was a further drop in the later 1930s: partly because of a brightening economic climate and partly because of the introduction of the early sulphonamide drugs. As the late Richard Titmuss showed, these gains were not only maintained but in some respects amplified during the Second World War. (17) In this context the importance of short-term social and economic changes for improvements in public health can be seen in sharp relief.

It was inevitable that an increase in civilian mortality rates would occur in the aftermath of aerial bombardment. To avoid such casualties over one million Londoners and other city dwellers were evacuated as the war began. When the anticipated Blitz did not materialize, there was a drift back to the cities. This trend was reversed, though, when

bombing began in earnest in late 1940. On balance, migration took out of the line of fire, and probably saved the lives of a significant number of mothers and infants. In March 1942, when the worst of the first phase of the Blitz was over, more than 600.000 people were still billeted in government reception areas. (18) Such policies helped to ensure that operations of war did not significantly add to infant mortality rates in the period 1940-42, as is shown in table 4.
The dislocation, anxiety and hardship caused by evacuation and relocation of bombed-out families apparently did not endanger the health of pregnant women or their children in early infancy. Infant mortality rates due to prematurity and to birth injuries declined slightly in 1940-41 compared to those of the immediate pre-war period. A widespread outbreak of German measles in 1940-41 was probably the source of a small, but real increase in the rate of death due to congenital abnormalities in 1941-42. The slight decline registered in 1940-41 in neonatal mortality rates as a whole, though, further supports the view that the disruption of war did not undermine the progress made in the pre-war period in terms of the survival chances of mothers or their infants in the early period of the first year of life.
It is rather in the context of post-neonatal mortality that we can find evidence of the deleterious consequences of the upheaval of the first three years of the war. Migration and overcrowding in relocation areas helped to spread viral and bacterial infections. Less parental supervision and more exposed gas pipes and electric leads were responsible for an increase in fatal household accidents and in 'overlying' or asphyxiation of infants. At the same time, a sharp fall in food supplies, particularly in meat, fats, sugar and fruits, added to increased stress and overwork among women, reduced resistance to infection among mothers and infants. If we recall that rehousing of bombed-out families often took place in inadequate dwellings and that the winters of 1939-40 and 1940-41 were unusually cold, it should come as no surprise that infant mortality due to bronchitis and pneumonia, as well as to other bacterial and viral diseases, increased sharply at this time. (19)

Table 4. Infant mortality rates by cause and sex, 1940-45
         (deaths per 1,000 live births)

| | 1940 - 42 | | 1943 - 45 | |
Cause	Male	Female	Male	Female
Whooping cough	1.05	1.24	0.75	0.89
Tuberculous diseases	0.64	0.54	0.49	0.42
Measles	0.42	0.37	0.28	0.29
Convulsions	1.41	0.94	0.77	0.51
Bronchitis and pneumonia	13.23	10.18	10.35	8.22
Entiritis and diarrhoea	5.60	3.98	5.71	4.16
Congenital malformations	6.97	6.14	6.01	5.31
Premature birth	16.07	12.38	12.93	10.73
Injury at birth	3.13	2.07	2.96	1.91
Asphyxia, atelectasis	2.39	1.88	2.50	1.83
Haemolytic diseases	0.68	0.44	0.80	0.49
Operations of war	0.25	0.28	0.07	0.08
Other violence	1.52	1.28	1.46	1.23
Other and ill-defined causes	9.22	6.63	7.05	5.06
All causes	62.61	48.35	52.13	41.13

Source: Registrar-General's Statistical Review of England and
          Wales for the Six Years 1940-45, vol. 1, Medical, p. 50

The evidence in table 4 confirms Titmuss' view that it is essential to divide the demographic history of the Second World War into two periods, 1939-42 and 1943-45. The first period is one of marked deterioration in infant survival chances; the second, of striking and substantial gains in infant survival rates. The causes of the transition from phase one to phase two lie in part in the vagaries of enemy action. Of perhaps greater importance, though, is that by 1941, the British population had been insulated from some of the worst features of this country's economic frailty by specific policy decisions.

It was a central tenet of the economic strategy of Churchill's Coalition that the cost of the war should not be placed on the shoulders of those least able to bear it. Consequently, increases in wages were not passed on to consumers but were covered by subsidies. These kept down the cost of the relevant commodities and of other goods, the prices of which were unaffected by rising wage bills. It took time, though, for the mechanism of price controls to operate effectively. Hence only in late 1942 did the index of weekly wage rates finally catch up with and surpass the cost of living index. Because of overtime and piecework, as well as separation allowances for wives

of servicemen, family incomes may have reached the price level even
earlier. At the same time, a more progressive tax structure helped
to redistribute income away from salaries, rents, interest and profits,
that is, middle-class incomes, and towards wages. (20) The period of
undeniably rising real incomes in 1943-45 coincides, therefore, with
the period of steeply declining rates of infant mortality.

Effective food rationing, the introduction of provision of free milk
under the National Milk Scheme, strict limitations on the production
and distribution of alcoholic beverages and rent control helped to
stabilize the family economy of the working class more than that of
the middle class. This was largely because manual workers' families
spent a much greater proportion of their incomes on food, drink and
rent than did families of non-manual workers or professional people.
A rise in the price of luxury items, or in the costs of motoring,
travel and services significantly affected the cost of living of the
middle class. Such relatively minor deprivation, annoying though it
may have been, in effect paid for the improvement in working-class incomes and indirectly in working-class nutritional levels during the
war.

Still, the per capita consumption of food dropped by 18 per cent in
the difficult years of 1938-41 and was 10 per cent below the pre-war
level three years later. Consumption of milk, poultry, eggs, meat and
fish was substantially reduced. The nutritional effect of the inevitable shortage of animal protein and fats in the nation's diet was
balanced in part by an increase on consumption of vitamins and minerals
due to the greater prominence of vegetables in the diet. Such adjustments meant that there was only a 2 per cent drop in the daily per
capita calorific intake over the decade 1934-44. This relatively minor
squeeze in food consumption would have been much worse, though, had
not home farmers succeeded in raising agricultural output which, together with lend-lease aid, kept food supplies at a safe level throughout the war. Similar developments had occurred in muted form in the
1914-18 war, but a generation later, agricultural and food policy was
more effectively planned and carried out. (21)

A similar parallel may be found between the two world wars in terms of
a growing commitment by the state to defend the health of mothers and
children as casualty lists lengthened. The fact that until D-Day in
1944 more civilians than soldiers died from enemy action no doubt
helped to bring civilian needs to the fore. The demands of the war
economy also made the extension of provision for mothers and infants

into an act of national importance. Factory crèches, nurseries and
child and maternal welfare centres were built at an unprecedented
rate during the war. In addition, women's attitudes changed.
By 1943, and for the first time, a majority of pregnant women attended
antenatal-care centres early in their pregnancy. By the end of the war,
it had become much easier for doctors, nurses and midwives to identify
problem cases, to remedy deficiencies in nutrition during pregnancy
and to ensure effective care during and after labour. By 1945, over
70 per cent of the infants born in the previous year were brought to
infant welfare centres. (22) Between 1939 and 1945, therefore, the
pre-war patchwork of voluntary and local authority-sponsored institutions began to take on the unified form in which the maternity
service exists today, and more women began to see it as a right rather
than as a privilege.

It is more difficult to locate the impact of wartime medical provision
on the deterioration in infant survival chances in 1940-42 or in the
pattern of improvement in 1943-45. As in the First World War, civilians
had a much diminished chance of seeing a doctor in wartime due to
military mobilization. (23) Titmuss estimated that fully one-third of
general practitioners were called up and that of the remainder, a substantial number were old-age pensioners. The scarcity of medical
attention was particularly marked in rural areas. (24) Some of the
gap was filled by the patent medicine industry and the corner chemist,
but more seriously ill people were indoubtedly disadvantaged during
the war. When tuberculous people were sent home early in the war to
make room in sanatoria for the wave of bombing casualties which never
came, that disease was bound to spread. The data in table 1 show that,
fortunately, infants in Britain did not suffer from this recrudescence
of the 'White Plague'.

It is possible, though, that wartime medical developments helped to
control the spread of disease. Advances in chemotherapy and in the
efficient operation of the blood transfusion service, which were of
direct use in dealing with war casualties, may have helped civilians
as well. It is likely, however, that the militara had first access to
the limited supplies of penicillin and other drugs, and that it was
only long after 1945 that the civilian population enjoyed the full
fruits of the pre-war chemotherapeutic breakthrough. Medical intervention was, therefore, less important than economic and social policy
in curbing the hardships of the early part of the war and in ensuring
that Britain's military effort did not undermine the health and survival chances of mothers and infants.

4. Conclusions and implications

This examination of a chapter of the demographic history of England and Wales has tried to establish that the relation between economic change and demographic change is anything but a simple one of short-term cause and effect. It is profoundly misleading to treat unemployment as an independent variable and infant mortality as a dependent variable, in the way Brenner has done. To make sense of the immediate consequences of unemployment, it must be seen as a part of a network of economic relations, support systems and social attitudes that are deeply embedded in the class structure. The worst way to approach the problem of unemployment is to reify it. In addition, Brennner's analysis assumes that unemployment is one phenomenon, when, of course, it is many. We need to know much more about the way in which unemployed people and their families cope with undoubted difficulties of joblessness. To assume that men and women who lose their jobs will by definition be unable to support their families or to keep their children alive is unwarranted and demonstrably untrue.

In the period under review, one reason why infant mortality rates did not follow in the immediate wake of movements in unemployment rates is that unemployment insurance, however miserly and demeaning in its application, and council housing, however drab and dispiriting in its appearance, provided a buffer for the unemployed which helped to separate deprivation from destitution. (25) Perhaps these forms of state support distinguish the British and American cases, and provide the basis for a comparative study of the impact of economic crises on different populations.

On another level, though, the lack of symmetry between economic change and demographic development suggests that it is necessary to use different time perspectives in analysing these discrete phenomena. Even in the twentieth century, demographic history may require a touch of what French historians call the style of 'la longue durée'. In other words, we shall not be able to appreciate the demographic costs of a depression or a war by concentrating solely on the events themselves.

Some immediate repercussions of either political or economic upheavals can, of course, be seen. It is clear that the combination of aerial bombardment in the first part of the Second World War and delays in the emergence of an efficient war economy contributed to the increase in infant mortality in 1940-41. Abundant evidence exists too about the beneficial effects of rising real wages and extended social provision for the health of mothers and infants in the latter part of the war. It is necessary, however, to take a longer-term view in order to place both the pre-war and war-related events in their appropriate context.

If there is any single change which ought to govern comparisons of the social history of the late nineteenth century with that of the twentieth century, it is the eradication of much of the appalling poverty which was endemic in Victorian cities and in large parts of the Victorian countryside. Alterations in the labour market and the growth of state and local authority provision were in part responsible for these developments. Consequently, communities where unemployment was high in the interwar years did not bear the worst features of nineteenth-century capitalism, and it would be foolish to look for demographic evidence that it did so. Similarly, the deprivation occasioned by Hitler's war did not alter in any lasting way the pre-war pattern of improvement in social conditions and in public health.

The demographic experience of this turbulent century can be understood fully, therefore, only by adopting a long-term view. The case of the Netherlands during the Second World War may help to clarify this point. In 1944-45, there occurred in Holland a man-made famine imposed by the Nazis on Dutch city dwellers in the aftermath of a railway strike intended to spark off an insurrection or at least to interfere with German troop movements after the Normandy landings. Unfortunately for the Dutch, the Allies finally arrived only in the last days of the war, by which time nutritional levels had been reduced below subsistence. The consequence was a severe short-term demographic crisis. Mortality rates soared, and the birth weight of new-born babies conceived in this period diminished significantly. (26) But the crisis struck a population whose nutritional standards had been rising over several generations. Once normal conditions had been restored, the trend of infant mortality continued on its downward path. Twenty years later, indeed, the newborn babies of the 'hunger winter' were found to be virtually indistinguishable in physical and mental characteristics from people born either slightly earlier or slightly later. At least on one level, the physical scars of war healed almost without trace. (27)

Nothing even remotely like the 'hunger winter' of 1944-45 occurred in Britain during the Second World War. It is true, nonetheless, that the capacity of the civilian populations of both Britain and Holland to adjust to the shortages, deprivations and unjustices of war was a reflection more of the trend of nutritional and sanitary improvement over the generations preceding the 1939-45 conflict than of any particular aspect of the war itself.

The trend towards better nutrition was initiated by the sustained rise in real wages during the third quarter of the nineteenth century. Working-class children born in the 1850s and 1860s were the first to receive unambiguously some of the fruits of economic growth. As they grew into adolescence and early adulthood, their death rates began to decline. The same generation married in the 1880s and 1890s and were more likely by the turn of the century to give birth to infants with an improved chance of surviving the first year of life. Improvements in parental, and in particular in maternal health, were, therefore, prerequisites of improvements in infant health. After 1900, the secular improvement in standards of living and nutrition continued and was reflected both in increasing life-expectancy for adults and in significant increases in the age-specific height and weight of schoolchildren. (28)

Better nutrition meant increased resistance to viral and bacterial infection. In addition, sanitary and medical intervention helped to reduce exposure to disease. After 1936, advances in chemotherapy enabled doctors to control many previously lethal diseases. Before this period, though, the enhancement of recovery rates from endemic infant diseases such as diorrhoea and measles was a result of improved nutrition, both among pregnant women and among their children. Unfortunately, we do not have relevant morbidity and case-fatality rates to prove this argument beyond question. The overwhelming evidence from studies of the synergistic relation between nutrition and infectious disease (29) leaves little doubt, though, a sustained decline in infant mortality rates such as Britain experienced before the 1930s was impossible without major improvements in the quantity and quality of the per capita food intake.

The way in which a female child is fed is likely, a generation later, to affect her ability to conceive, to carry a pregnancy to full term and to give birth to a baby healthy enough to survive the first year of life. By examining this cohort effect it is possible to see, finally that the shadow of chronic deprivation is just as important as the shadow of nutritional improvements. In a series of remarkable studies, Sir Dugald Baird and his colleagues at Aberdeen have shown conclusively that the quality of a mother's environment before and soon after _her_ birth influences her reproductive efficiency and the survival chances of her children a generation later, and even those of her children's children two generations later. For instance, there was a rise in the perinatal mortality rate due to low birth weight in Aberdeen 1968-72. Particularly affected were the 15-19 and 20-24 cohorts who had been born in 1949-57 and 1944-52, when the indicence of low birth weight was also high. <u>Their</u> mothers had been born between 1928 and 1932, during the worst years of depression. (30) Similarly, in Scotland as a whole, there was an increase in the perinatal mortality rates due to central nervous system malformations among three cohorts of babies: those born in the early 1930s, those born in the 1950s and those born in 1971 - 72. (31) Here is evidence of the human costs of the depression, which Brenner's short-term approach could not detect.

Similarly, Baird has shown that the full effects of wartime food policies can only be seen after one generation. As we have noted, the still-birth rate fell substantially between 1940 and 1947. Among deliveries in Aberdeen, it dropped sharply as well after 1963 for women in the 20-24 age group, after 1967 for women in the 25-29 age group and after 1972 for women in the 30-34 age group. In other words, it is in the 1970s that we can see the beneficial outcome of giving priority in food allocation to pregnant women and children in the 1940s. We can understand, therefore, why girls born in the mid-1940s had a greater reproductive efficiency in the period 1974-79, when there occurred a 38 per cent drop in the perinatal mortality rate. (32) A recognition of such cohort effects is thus essential to an interpretation of the relation between economic and demographic change. (33)

There is, in sum, a momentum in Britain's demographic history which is the product of slow but cumulative changes in the adequacy of the diet of the working population. The record is certainly not one of uniform and unbroken improvement. On balance, though, it is only by recognizing the significance of the long-term legacy of better nutrition that we will understand why the process of infant mortality decline survived intact the economic dislocation of both the slump and the Second World War.

Appendix 1. Estimates of trends in unemployment rates (inverted) and in infant mortality rates at some sub-periods of the first year of life in Britain, 1921-49

Infant mortality rates	Equations used to detrend rates	R^2
England and Wales 1921-48		
Day 0-1	$y = -0.01905912x + 0.0000424 8094x^3 - 0.000000000545 0923x^6 + 10.38337$	0.91
Days 1-7	$y = +0.157189x - 0.0000014 67553x^4 - 8.115394$	0.91
Days 7-28	$y = -0.248112x + 0.00000000 2723914x^5 + 17.14570$	0.90
Days 0-28	$y = +0.06122582x - 0.0000002 617767x^4 - 32.32186$	0.94
Months 1-12	$y = -0.9836474x + 0.00000002 039225x^4 + 63.58606$	0.89
Year 0-1	$y = -0.9198079x - 0.00000024 21507x^4 + 95.84295$	0.92
Scotland 1922-49		
Days 0-7	$y = -0.03957798x + 0.0001447 995x^3 - 0.0000000001472 9946x^4 + 22.85896$	0.84
Days 0-28	$y = -1.470707x + 0.0007926205x^3 - 0.00000000448 8805x^6$	0.90
Months 1-12	$y = -2.120373x - 0.000624 2913x^3 - 0.0000000034 72773x^6 + 96.37800$	0.86
Year 0-1	$y = -3.605271x + 0.00143 8913x^3 - 0.0000000080 67815x^6 + 158.4418$	0.89
Unemployment (inverted) in United Kingdom		
	$y = -0.5059029x + 0.000005 95640x^4 + 96.24721$	0.63

x = year
y = infant mortality rate or unemployment rate (inverted)

Appendix 2. Correlation coefficients between percentage deviations from trend of unemployment rates (inverted) and trends of infant mortality rates at sub-periods of the first year of life in Britain, 1921-49

Rate	No lag		1-year lag		4-year lag	
	No average	3-year average	No average	3-year average	No average	3-year average
England and Wales 1921-48						
Day 0-1	-0.4077[a]	-0.7058[a]	-0.5788[a]	-0.8798[a]	-0.1442[a]	-0.5235[a]
Days 1-7	-0.3257[a]	-0.4467[a]	-0.4413[a]	-0.5170[a]	-0.0437[a]	-0.0220
Days 7-28	+0.2749[a]	+0.2940[a]	+0.2556[a]	+0.3288[a]	+0.1241[a]	+0.3993[a]
Days 0-28	+0.0294	-0.0549	-0.0896[a]	-0.2035[a]	+0.0110	-0.0549
Months 1-12	+0.0401[a]	+0.6296[a]	+0.3940[a]	+0.6201[a]	+0.0883[a]	+0.1634[a]
Year 0-1	+0.3396[a]	+0.5604[a]	+0.3052[a]	+0.4928[a]	+0.0787[a]	+0.1434[a]
Scotland 1922-49						
Days 0-7	-0.0185	-0.0003	-0.2577[a]	-0.2694[a]	-0.1374	-0.3286[a]
Days 0-28	+0.1237[a]	+0.1944[a]	-0.0971[a]	-0.1011[a]	-0.2655[a]	-0.4914[a]
Months 1-12	+0.0941[a]	+0.1190[a]	+0.1242[a]	+0.2052[a]	+0.1424[a]	+0.2331[a]
Year 0-1	+0.0926[a]	+0.1524[a]	+0.0686[a]	+0.1114[a]	+0.0284[a]	-0.0116[a]

[a] Significant at the 5% level.

The Durbin–Watson test showed positive serial correlation only in the case of the trend of unemployment rates. Since none of the time series of infant mortality rates displayed evidence of autocorrelation, it is possible to accept the significance of the correlation coefficients shown above.

REFERENCES:

For advice on this paper, thanks are due to Sir Dugald Baird, Volker Berghahn, Peter Clarke, Jo Garcia, Ann Oakley, Jim Oeppen and Henry Pelling.

(1) BRENNER, M.H.: Fetal, infant, and maternal mortality during periods of economic instability. International Journal of Health Services III, 155 (1973)

(2) See the citation of Brenner's work in the recent report of a working party ot the DEPARTMENT OF HEALTH AND SOCIAL SECURITY: Inequalities in Health (1980)

(3) MATTHEWS, R.C.O.: Why has Britain had full employment since the war? Economic Journal LXXVIII, 555-69 (1968)

(4) SEERS, D.: The levelling of incomes since 1938. (1950)

(5) BRENNER, M.H.: Economic instability. 153

(6) BEVERIDE, W.I.B.: Influenza (1977)

(7) MC KEOWN, T.: The modern rise of population. (1976)
The advice of Ann Oakley was particularly helpful on this point.

(8) WINTER, J.M.: The impact of the first world war on civilian health in Britain. Economic History Review, 2nd ser., XXX, 487-508 (1977)

(9) HEADY, J.A., STEVENS, C.F., DALY, C., MORRIS, J.N.: Social and biological factors in infant mortality. IV. The independent effects of social class, region, the mother's age, and her parity. Lancet, 5 March 1955

(10) MORRIS, J.N., TITMUSS, R.N.: Health and social change: I. - the recent history of rheumatic heart disease. Medical Officer, 26. Aug.; 2., 9. Sept. 1944

(11) ROGERS, S.C., WEATHERALL, J.A.C.: Anencephalus, Spina Bifida and Congenital Hydrocephalus. England and Wales 1964-1972. Office of Population Census and Surveys. Studies in Medical and Population Subjects 32 (1976)

(12) BOYD ORR, J.: Food, health and income 24-5 (1937)
The impact of the war on civilian consumption in the United Kingdom, the United States, and Canada. 26-31 (1945)

(13) This point has already been made with reference to Brenner's work. See
KASL, S.V.: Mortality and the business cycle. Some questions about research strategies when utilizing macro-social and ecological data. American Journal of Public Health LXIX, 784-8 (1979)
and the same author's comment. In: Stress and Mental Disorder (J.E. Barrett et al). New York 217-18 (1979)

(14) ANDERSON, O.D.: Time Series Analysis and Forecasting. The Box-Jenkins Approach (1975)
Thanks are due to Jim OEPPEN of the SSRC Cambridge Group for the History of Population and Social Structure for statistical help on this and other points.

(15)   Firm conclusions cannot be drawn, though, since the Box-Jenkins approach requires a time series of at least fifty years. Pre-1920 measurements of unemployment rates are thereby introduced, which vitiates comparisons.

(16)   A full report of the findings of the analysis of variance will be published by Dr. Brian BENSON and the author

(17)   TITMUSS, R.N.: Problems of social policy, ch. 25 (1950)

(18)   On the state of the public during six years of war p.42 (1946)

(19)   PARSONS, Sir L.: The war in Britain. An experiment in social pediatrics. Birmingham Medical Review xv, 3, 125-38, (1947).
I am grateful to Dr. Robert DARE for having drawn my attention to this article.

(20)   SEERS, D.: The levelling of incomes. chaps. 1-2 (1950)

(21)   OLSON, M.: The economics of the wartime shortage. Durham, North Carolina, USA (1960)

(22)   ROYAL COLLEGE OF OBSTETRICIANS AND GYNAECOLOGISTS: Maternity in Great Britain (1948)

(23)   WINTER, J.M.: Military fitness and public health in Britain during the first world war. Journal of Contemporary History XV, 211-44 (1980)

(24)   TITMUSS, R.N.: Problems of social policy. 530 (1950)

(25)   This help could backfire if council housing rents were too high. See:
M'GONIGLE, G.C.M.: Poverty, nutrition, and public health. Proceedings of the Royal Society of Medicine XXVI, I, 677-87 (1933)

(26)   SMITH, C.A.: Effects of wartime starvation in Holland on pregnancy and its Products. American Journal of Obstetrics and Gynecology LIII, 599-608 (1974)

(27)   STEIN, Z., SUSSER, M., SAENGER, G., MOROLLA, F.: Famine and human development. The Dutch hunger winter of 1944-45. Oxford (1975)
The only exception, which is interesting for our purposes, is a disproportionately high incidence of central nervous system disorders detected during medical examination of recruits who were born during the 'hunger winter'

(28)   WEIR, J.B.de V.: The assessment of the growth of schoolchildren with special reference to secular changes. British Journal of Nutrition XI, 19-33 (1952)

(29)   SCRIMSHAW, N., TAYLOR, C., GORDON, J.: Interactions of nutrition and infection. New York (1968)

(30)   BAIRD, D.: The Epidemiology of low birth weight: Changes in incidence in Aberdeen 1948-72. Journal of Biosocial Science VI, 323-41 (1974)
BAIRD, D.: The interplay of changes in society, reproductive habits, and obstetric practice in Scotland between 1922 and 1972. British Journal of Preventive and Social Medicine XXIX, 135-46 (1975)

(31) BAIRD, D.: Epidemiology of congenital malformations of the central nervous system in (a) Aberdeen and (b) Scotland. Journal of Biosocial Science VI, 113-37 (1974)
BAIRD, D.: The changing pattern of human reproduction in Scotland 1928-72. Journal of Biosocial Science VII, 77-97 (1975)

(32) BAIRD, D.: Environment and reproduction. British Journal of Obstetrics and Gynaecology LXXXVIII, 1057-67 (1980)

(33) On cohort effects, the literature is enormous. See W.O. KERMACK, A.G. MC KENDRICK and P.L. MC KINLAY. 'Death-rates in Great Britain and Sweden. Some General Regularities and their Significance', Lancet, 31 March 1934; J.N. MORRIS and J.A. HEADY, 'Social and Biological Factors in Infant Mortality. V. Mortality in Relation to the Father's Occupation', Lancet, 12 March 1955. On the specific subject of this essay, see TITMUSS, Problems of Social Policy, p.538: 'But just as the advances of one generation may show their full effects through the lives of succeeding generations so, too, may the retreats'.

INVOLUNTARY UNEMPLOYMENT AND HEALTH STATUS:
A REGIONAL CASE STUDY UTILISING SOCIOLOGICAL AND
MICRO-EPIDEMIOLOGICAL PERSPECTIVES

Malcolm Colledge
Michael Kingham

School of Behavioural Science
Newcastle upon Tyne Polytechnic
Great Britain

The sharp rise in unemployment levels to the late seventies reaching a benchmark of three million in 1982 has made unemployment the major socio-political and economic issue of the decade. Also, the forecast that levels of unemployment will remain high for some time has resulted in a change of emphasis in the debate about the effects of redundancy and loss of work. Discussion in recent years of unemployment and the unemployed has mainly concentrated on demographic and labour market predictions, ignoring with a few notable exception (Jahoda et al.1933, Hill et al.1973, Townsend 1979) unemployment in its wider social context. Recently, however, the increasing concern with the social context has been apparent in the debates of academies and policy markers.

Sinfield (1981) draws attention to the need to examine unemployment in the context of a work orientated society where employment for the majority provides the main access to reward, status and security. When we look at the social meaning of job loss and its effects on the individual and family life, the effects of poverty and deprivation can be readily identified. One aspect that has been raised, and is less easy to document, is the effect of unemployment on the health of an individual and the family. Recently, the statistical analysis of Brenner (1973, 1977, 1979) has drawn attention not only to the social problems resulting from unemployment but also that there is evidence to suggest a relationship between mortality rates and cycles of economic activity.

The recent work of Fagin (1981), Colledge (1981), and Popay (1981) has added to the evidence, suggesting a link between unemployment and health status. Although this evidence is open to criticism, it has stimulated the need for further research to evaluate the possible link between ill health and high levels of unemployment.

This article is an attempt to overview some of the literature to date, showing a relationship between unemployment as a stress factor, and its possible effects on large sectors of the population, who are already vulnerable because of their class position.

Social class and unemployment are related. The lower down the social scale the worker the greater are the chances of becoming unemployed. Also the difference between skilled and unskilled workers is quite dramatic, both in terms of the frequency and chances of becoming unemployed (see Table 1). Not only is the burden of unemployment shouldered on a class basis, but also the mortality of working men shows a positive deterioration from social class I to V (see Table 2). To add to this burden, where high regional pockets of unemployment are observed this can be matched with high levels of mortality. For example, the general death rate in 1972 for workers in East Anglia, Oxford and Wessex was 13% below average, whereas in Liverpool and Newcastle upon Tyne it was 12% above the England and Wales average. Therefore one of the most consistent findings is an inverse relationship between socio-economic status and mortality placing the burden squarely on the shoulders of socio-economic groups IV and V who are also the most vulnerable to unemployment. At this level what unemployment and mortality have in common is that they seem to be shared on an unequal basis (Colledge 1982).

The social meaning of work, a key variable?

Given the above discussion what is the evidence to suggest that unemployment as a factor can make a direct impact on health? After all it could be said that it is just another stress that certain groups have to face in their life chances because of their position in the socio-economic structure, and should therefore be given no more status than bereavement, or the effects of work on health.

For the authors the key lies in an understanding of the social meaning of work and unemployment.

To be able to understand the social meaning of unemployment, not only do we need to know the characteristics of the unemployed, but also what the general idea of unemployment means. The term is full of ambiguity and can mean different things to the individual. It can mean "being without a job", but it can also refer to a state of leisure. According to Garraty (1980) the English word "unemployment" did not come into general use until the latter part of the 19th century: prior to that, circumlocutions such as "want of employment" and "involuntary idleness" were used.

The development of the use of the word "unemployment" suggests a social dimension, which can be characterised as a relationship to production. You really cannot be unemployed unless you have to sell your labour in the market place. An artist or a writer may find it difficult to earn a decent living but technically they are never unable to work. Therefore only those who work for a wage or salary can become unemployed. In the context of this paper unemployment is taken to mean "involuntary unemployment", which means the inability of the individual to sell their labour in the market. It is necessary to categorise job loss in this way because some people may find unemployment a pleasant experience (the older worker near retirement for instance).

In the article we are principally concerned with those for whom work is a major part of their status and financial security. For this group of workers unemployment or the threat of unemployment is an assault on their social identity and wellbeing. The total lack of control felt by the worker over the situation, their inability to sell their labour and worth to capital, plus a deeply ingrained work ethic could be the key variable determining the health of the unemployed, lending weight to the evidence at a macro and micro level of analysis.

Historical Dimension

The idea that there could be a link between the business cycle and health indicators is not new. Durkheim in 1897 discussed the incidence of suicide in relation to peaks and falls of economic activity. Studies during the great depression looked at the impact of economic decline on psychological wellbeing (Komora and Clark 1955), and psychiatric hospital admissions. Morris and Titmuss as early as 1944 used multivariable methods to examine the relationship between unemployment rates and rates of heart disease mortality in young people aged 5 - 24 years during the depression of the thirties showing a 2 - 4 year lag period. The interesting point to note is that Morris and Timusses figures are identical to those reported by Brenner in the USA in all major categories of heart disease for all ages.

Jahoda and Lasarzfeld's classic study of the thirties "Marienthal" examining the impact of unemployment on family life during the Great Depression, noted how a lowering of living standards was central to mental and physical deterioration in the villagers.

This historical tradition has, however, looked at the effects of unemployment on health marginally rather than directly, with the exception of Titmuss and Morris. That is not to say that the effects of unemployment on health were not debated during the thirties, but that is an issue beyond the scope of this article.

During the recession the main impetus to discussion and research has been through the work of Harvey Brenner. The publication of his findings has led to the medical profession debating the issue in the Lancet, demonstrating the need for doctors and researchers to reassess this issue. Peter Draper and his colleagues at the Unit for the Study of Health Policy at Guys medical school have in their work highlighted the importance of Brenner's analysis against a tide of medical scepticism, by drawing attention to the research evidence that adds weight to Brenner's arguments.

Macro analysis: the evidence

Brenner's basic hypothesis is that pathological reactions follow increased unemployment, and these reactions will be dispersed over time so that there will probably be a time lag between the stress of being unemployed and the onset of illness. Examining unemployment in the USA, Brenner claims that a 1% increase in unemployment in the USA over a period of six years has been associated with a 2% increase in deaths. This correlation is supported by the following arguments. Namely that changes in mortality and indicators of morbidity will be dispersed over time, creating a time lag between the periods of unemployment and the onset of illness, which is reflected in the changing patterns of mortality e.g. cardiovascular disease, cirrhosis of the liver. Other indicators such as the suicide rate, homicide rate and admissions to psychiatric hospitals follow a similar trend (see Table 3).

"Instabilities in the national economy have been the single most important source of fluctuation in mental hospital admissions"
(Brenner H., Mental Illness and the Economy, 1973)

Also it should be noted the increase in admissions is not among those with a history of mental disorder but rather newly diagnosed cases.

Other research at this level, has generally confirmed Brenners findings. Graham Stokes at Birmingham University used similar methods to Brenner, to trace the relationship between unemployment levels and mental hospital admissions in Britain 1952 to 1976. Not only did he find similar results but also concluded that women show a greater sensitivity to economic change and the most vulnerable groups are women between the ages 20 - 24 and men between the ages 35 - 44. In Australia Bunn using a similar methodology shows a relationship between annual changes in Ischaemic heart diseases, infant mortality and suicide. Bunn also found that a change in prescribing practice followed eighteen months after a peak in the unemployment rate, this he saw as an indicator of "National stress". A report commissioned by North Tyneside Community Health Council found that in the first quarter of 1980 psychiatric hospital admissions were up by 30% with a greater demand for outpatient appointments. This occurred during a steeply rising period of unemployment (see Fig.1). It also documents mortality rates from Bronchitis and heart disease twice as high as the national average in areas of long term unemployment.

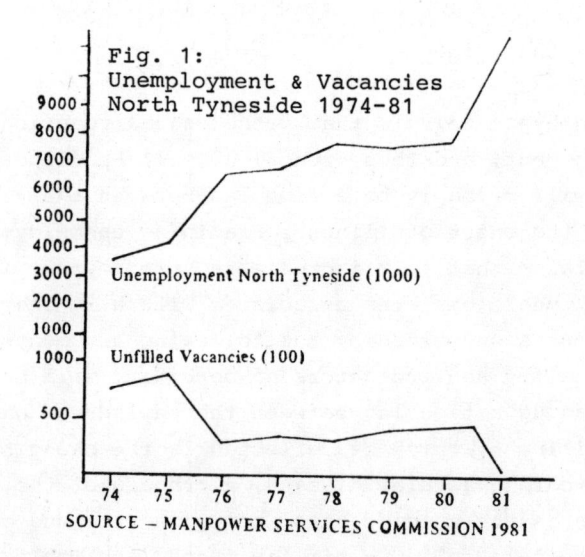

Fig. 1: Unemployment & Vacancies North Tyneside 1974-81

SOURCE – MANPOWER SERVICES COMMISSION 1981

It is important to note that Brenner's work and similar research is looking at the overall impact of unemployment and mortality on the whole community and not just the individual. Taken at this level of analysis it is easier to accept these results than if an attempt were made to make a causal connection between a group of unemployed individuals and mortality. However even though we must treat the results of Brenner and others with some caution, recent evidence from the British Regional Heart Study showed a link between unemployment and heart disease, obstructive lung disease, and bronchitis. The data was collected before unemployment dramatically rose and did not include those hard hit in the inner city areas. Separating out those who were out of work because they were ill, Cook and his colleagues showed that 18% of those interviewed who were fit when they lost their jobs subsequently suffered from ischaemic heart disease compared with 9% of those in work. Also 26% unemployed had obstructive lung disease compared with 15% of the workers in the study. There was a similar ratio in the case of chronic bronchitis. Taking adjustments for region, social class and smoking habits the rate of heart disease was still seen to be significantly higher than for those in work. Against the background of these findings we return to Brenner and explore his analysis of the situation in the United Kingdom, this will give a general understanding of the likely affect of this recession on the health of the population and future health care demands.

Looking at the experience of England and Wales 1936-1976 Brenner notes that the long term upward trend in real per capita income is associated with better health, but that recessions followed by periods of rapid economic growth can be stressful to certain sections of the working population i.e. the less skilled, who are the first to lose their jobs and the last to get work when the recession ends. Brenner claims that his work in Liverpool indicated that each 1% increase in unemployment in the period 1970-1975 was accompanied by an additional 230 deaths over and above those forecast for the 45+ age group. Brenner suggests that economic instability and insecurity increase the likelihood of immoderate and instable life habits. Tie this to the downward mobility and other stresses, the likelihood of increased mortality and other social indicators is self-evident. Recently Brenner has looked at the United Kingdom in greater detail and included Scotland in his analysis noting that the effect of unemployment on mortality occurs sooner than in the rest of the UK, six year lag compared with ten. At the same time Scotland tends to show a more severe health response to the effects of economic recovery after the recession. This may be due to the actuality of harsher and longer recessional periods in Scotland. This thesis could also in our opinion apply to parts of Wales, the North East and areas like Liverpool, who share with Scotland a long history of chronic unemployment and industrial decline. North Tyneside is a classical example as one of the ten areas - special areas designated by the "Black

Report".

The Metropolitan Borough of North Tyneside was created in the 1974 reorganisation of Local Government. Situated in the Northern Region it lies on the northern side of the River Tyne and is bounded by the North Sea to the east. To the north it reaches the boundary of Northumberland and on the west side lies the city of Newcastle upon Tyne.
The reorganisation brought together areas with different characteristics. Along the coast there are the resorts of Whitley Bay and Tynemouth, residential areas providing housing for people who commute to work in Newcastle. These contrast with the shipbuilding and repair industry communities that lie along the Tyne predominantly in Wallsend. The administrative centre of the Borough is North Shields, historically dependent on marine industries, but now with employment in retail and administrative services. Moving inland, to the north west, are the large housing estates of Longbenton and Killingworth Township, originally developed as important overspill areas for the former Newcastle upon Tyne Council.

Whilst North Tyneside shares the major socio-economic characteristics of the Northern Region there are variations in local employment structures which are unique to the Borough. The recruitment for work is complex, and even developments in light and service industries in North Tyneside have had less impact on local employment levels than have been expected. The catchment area for professional and managerial jobs is not only regional but national.

The pattern of industrial structure and employment in North Tyneside is broadly similar to that of the Northern Region as a whole (see Table 4) with the main emphasis on manufacturing and service industries.

However as the authors of The Jobless (1980) report point out their presentation conceals variations in local employment structures. In the case of North Tyneside it can be seen that Whitley Bay has a concentration of jobs in the service sector, whereas in Wallsend the main sector is manufacturing. North Shields, as the administrative centre, shows an emphasis on both professions and services, but retains its traditional manufacturing role. However there is much more light industry compared with the heavy engineering in Wallsend. West Moor shows a diverse spread of employment.

Unemployment in North Tyneside

Historically as with the Northern Region, North Tyneside has had above-average unemployment rates. Variations in the employment situation since 1974 have followed national trends, including the sharp deterioration during 1980.

As with the differences in the institutional structure of the sub areas so is the burden of unemployment. North Shields and Wallsend carry the major burden, with unemployment doubling in the last five years. All four Employment Offices have shown a general decline in vacancies notified and the concern with the general labourer as outlined by Pimlott (1981), is borne out in North Tyneside especially in Wallsend, North Shields and West Moor (see Table 5).

When we look at Wallsend and North Shields (which accounted for two out of every three jobs in North Tyneside in 1976) the picture of a declining industrial base becomes apparent. According to North Tyneside Trades Council (1979) overall employment in Wallsend declined by 25% over the period 1959-1976. Losses occurred in the primary and manufacturing sectors. In the same period manufacturing jobs fell by 36% leading to a fall in the proportion of all jobs in that sector from 71% to 61%. In numerical terms this represents the loss of about 7,000 jobs. A similar chronic situation exists in North Shields.

Studies conducted by North Tyneside C.D.P. between 1972 and 1977 culminated in a series of publications which present a comprehensive socio-economic, historical and contemporary analysis of North Shields.

Also Sinfield in the sixties interviewing men out of work, talks about his experiences in North Shields and how the town seemed typical of the region, but had less long term unemployment. So he planned his questions to deal with families coping with the crisis of sudden unemployment.

> "My mistake became evident very quickly. Very few of the 92 unemployed men I spoke to had not been out of work before. More than one quarter of the previous five years had been totally unproductive for this sample of unemployed men - an average of one year and five months had been spent 'signing on the dole'. The information given by the men was confirmed by data from the Employment Exchange". (Sinfield 1981)

In 1975-76 a second sample of unemployed was drawn by the C.D.P. project in the same way as the Sinfield study. The evidence suggests that North Shields has been severely affected by the deterioration in the economy in the intervening twelve years. More than 1 in 3 of the second sample has been either mainly or wholly out of work for three years in contrast to Sinfield's finding in 1963-64 which reported one in ten of those interviewed. These figures indicate that long term unemployment has increased in North Shields. What was shown for the majority of workers was "work but not security", going through periods of unemployment was the norm. Table 6 compares the length of unemployment for 92 men aged 18 and over in the sample, and the authors note that the men interviewed had been unemployed on average for sixteen months.

They also reported the relationships between the age of the unemployed, family type, industrial sector and skill level.

In North Tyneside there is evidence to suggest that where the employment is concentrated so is social disadvantage. The North Tyneside Metropolitan Borough Council's first Inner Areas Programme identified nine areas for which special Government funding was recommended, and which should be given special preference by the Borough. Eight of the nine areas are in North Shields and Wallsend, in the town centres, and also along the riverside and the Meadowell Estate. Outside the inner town area the other special area is in the Longbenton Council Estate. These nine areas only show the worst of the deprivations and concentrations of bad housing and poor environmental conditions. It should be noted that these areas are selected by political processes and there are other areas suffering social deprivation. As the Jobless (1980) report notes, the severity of the North Tyneside problem is highlighted by the fact that these nine areas cover almost one in four of the 200,000 population.

Against this background of industrial decline if we look at the health profile of North Tyneside we find that in the periods 1975-1979 the perinatal mortality rate was high causing concern locally and nationally.

The Strategic Plan for North Tyneside Area Health Authority 1979-1988 draws attention to a letter from the Secretary of State of 9th August 1978 identifying North Tyneside as an area where high infant and perinatal mortality rates persist. The situation was also highlighted by the Black Report 1980 and reinforced the need for special provision. In 1978 a Working Party of local Health Services staff examined arrangements for ante-natal care and studied individual records of all deaths during pregnancy to identify cause of death, geographical location, social class and legitimacy.

The following features were identified:

(a) The North Tyneside area has the highest Standardised Mortality Ratio in the Northern Region (1974-1976), this being 118.

(b) The area has only reached 89% of its target allocation under the R.A.W.P. formula and is the second furthest away from the target in the region.

(c) The area has a high illegitimacy rate - 12% as compared with a regional and national level of 9.6% and 9% respectively.

(d) The socio-economic structure of the North Tyneside population leans heavily towards Social Class V - 10.7% of economically active males compared with 8.7% in the Region and 6.6% Nationally (source 1971 Census). In 1976 the National Perinatal Mortality Rate for Social Class V was 24.9% per 1000 births; over five deaths per thousand higher than for Social Class IV.

If we examine the general death rate for the Northern region North Tyneside 1975-1979 comes second for all causes and first for neoplasms.

Table 8 gives a detailed profile for mortality in North Tyneside 1975-1979 contrasted with the Northern Region. Generally, the health profile is not a good one but the figures are difficult to interpret <u>and make sense</u> of because of the differences in the various parts of North Tyneside. Just as the unemployment characteristics are different so indeed is the mortality profile.

Small area analysis by Maclean reveals that relationships can be drawn between unemployment, social class and health in North Tyneside. Standardised mortality ratios for bronchitis and emphysema 1975-1978 were concentrated in the areas of North Shields and Wallsend reflecting the environmental and industrial history of these areas together with other social class variables such as cigarette smoking. In examining the data we must bear in mind the long term effects of these diseases and that the stress of unemployment may exacerbate their effect. Corresponding data for two other major indicators, namely, ischaemic heart disease and cancer of the lung followed a similar pattern.

Areas in the United Kingdom like North Tyneside reinforce the overall findings of Brenner outlined so far and also general factors that emerge from his recent analysis. First, the over 40 male unemployment ratio is significantly related to total cirrhosis and cardio vascular mortality for England and Wales. Secondly that the 20-40 year old female unemployment ratio is significantly related to infant mortality without any time lag. Brenner's study for the US Department of Labor Manpower Administration 1972 also demonstrated an inverse relationship between National economic change and Infant mortality. The longer the change in the economic indicators the stronger the relationship.

Third recessional decline in the United Kingdom in average weekly hours worked in manufacturing industry show strong relations to increased mortality as do short term losses in income. Also the total unemployment rate as well as high unemployment among certain groups correlates significantly with increased mortality for different causes.

The findings suggest the implications of the recession for health go far beyond unemployment alone. The very threat of economic loss or breakdown of social networks could increase the risk to workers who do not experience unemployment.

Criticism of Brenner comes initially from Eyer and more recently from Gravelle and Stern et al. For Eyer, although he acknowledges the stress of unemployment, questions Brenner's interpretation by suggesting that economic growth is harmful to health and the death rate falls during periods of unemployment. Eyer then goes on to look at the evidence of time lag and suggests that stress associated with work and social relations in the class struggle are more important. To give strength to his arguments Eyer draws on the work of Kasl and Cobb, who followed a group of workers threatened with plant closure demonstrating changes in blood pressure, uric acid and cholesterol levels. The change in blood pressure occurred in anticipation of closure and for Eyer suggest that the factors which anticipate unemployment effect mortality rather than lagging behind it. This leads Eyer to the conclusion that the lag in stress appearing during unemployment is short and does not account for a large variation in the death rate. By Eyer's calculations unemployment change accounts for only a 1% change in the death rate as opposed to the claims made by Brenner. The more likely factor, as mentioned earlier is the "alienation" in the majority of the population in the work process and the relationship to production.

What Eyer fails to take into account is that Kasl and Cobbs work also supports Brenner's thesis in that elevated blood pressure could be seen as precipitative of heart disease if it persisted for any lenght of time and therefore account for the time lag between the recession and the onset of illness.

The central critiscism emerging from the work of Gravelle and Stern is that it is difficult to show how unemployment as a factor can be separated from poverty, bad housing, inadequate diet, etc. Also Gravelle tested Brenner's 1936-1976 model and reported that its performance in presenting accurate results was not impressive. The question of drop in personal income as the main indicators is refuted in that in 1930 and 1970 high unemployment was associated with high disposable income. Also the criticisms of Gravelle and Stern concentrate on statistical methods and the appropriate formula for time series, which in the authors' opinion detract from the real issue. However Gravelle and Stern go on to say:
> "Our results and criticsms, although casting considerable doubt on Brenner's results for Britain do not mean unemployment has no adverse health effects. Indeed it is as plausible that such effects do exist - but there is as yet no evidence which can be used to estimate their magnitude."

Indeed macro analysis cannot stand on its own because there are real problems of demonstrating causality and in fact the whole approach used may be questioned, but that is a separate issue (see Stern 1981 and Colledge 1982). As we said earlier Brenner's work can be more readily accepted if taken in the context of total communities rather than just unemployed individuals. Another approach is to take Brenner's analysis and that of others conducted in a similar vein as part of the evidence that unemployment damages health against the background of micro analysis which explores how the individual and their family are directly effected.

Micro analysis: social and psychological reactions

In micro analysis a number of themes emerge, which seem to interlock. First stress coupled with loss of self-esteem and purpose, this coinciding with the material deprivation and downward social mobility that often follows in the wake of unemployment, suggests a result in changing patterns of health of individuals, their families and the community. The results of stress are often reported in terms of mental disorder. Evidence of the stressful impact of unemployment goes back to the Great Depression. Komora and Clark examined the impact of economic decline on psychological wellbeing during the period 1929-1932 by measuring increases and decreases in psychiatric hospital admissions. Other studies have looked at the relationship between social classes and mental illness, and the issue of support during periods of economic downturn. Leim and Leim consider that social class should be seen as central in psychological dysfunction, suggesting that lower socio-economic groups are the most vulnerable. Numerous other studies have looked at stress, deterioration of interpersonal relations against a background of insecurity and unemployment (Myers et al., Catalona and Dooley, Coates et al.).

Studies of this kind have tried to bridge the gap between the macro analysis and life events at a family and individual level.

From a psychological perspective which examines directly the impact of unemployment on the individual and their families, three studies emerge that give an insight into the stages the unemployed move through. Hill describes three stages in the career of the unemployed. First the individual feels disbelief, but maintains a degree of optimism, regarding the fact of job loss as temporary: however the optimism soon runs out and the next stage is one of pessimism, finances are short, they are caught in the web of market forces which leads to an inability to act. This stage Hill calls the "unemployed identity". Moving to the third stage time loses its importance for the individual and the idea of being "unemployed" rather than "worker" is internalised.

A recent study by Nutman gives a similar picture and adds detail to the work of Hill by suggesting that at the beginning the individual finds difficulty in accepting redundancy however expected it has been. As one individual put it "It's like a kick in the stomach". Also for Nutman in the intermediate stage the individual although aware of the reality of unemployment does not want to accept or recognise their plight and distance themselves from the reality.

Fagin's study of twenty-two families in the United Kingdom and their experiences of unemployment emphasised an important point in that the stages the unemployed individual moves through and their experiences are mirrored in the rest of the family, having an effect on their general wellbeing and health. Spouses with previous histories of poor health suffered relapses and aggravation of their previous illness. Lack of work set into motion psychological changes leading to depression, sadness and self-blame. Also Fagin notes that health problems or an established illness relieves tension in unemployed male breadwinners and comments with the dictum "it is better to be sick and unemployed, than healthy and unemployed, seems to be true for the jobless man in our society".

Like macro studies, micro analysis also has difficulty in disentangling the effects of unemployment from other stresses occurring at the time or the effects of previous life histories, but rather suggests that unemployment is a paramount variable which effects the health of members of the community.

Conclusion

Given the difficulties outlined throughout this paper none of the studies overviewed stand on their own, but taken collectively present overwhelming evidence historically that the business cycle and economic uncertainty affect the health of given populations. For the working class who carry the main brunt of any depression through mass unemployment combined with previous social disadvantages (and the inevitable consequences that follow reduction in consumer durables, downward social mobility etc.). These material indignities combined with the assault on their selfesteem are surely the link between observable changes in mortality and morbidity following a recession.

TABLE 1

RATIOS OF UNEMPLOYED TO NOTIFIED VACANCIES
(EXCLUDING SCHOOL LEAVERS) AUGUST 1980

	SOUTH EAST REGION	NORTHERN REGION
Managerial & Professional	3.8	6.0
Clerical	3.8	14.2
Other Non-Manual	2.0	10.9
Craft Foremen	2.5	12.9
Semi-skilled	2.8	10.2
General Labourers	40.8	172.5
All	3.9	17.6

SOURCE — Pimlott B. The North East : Back to the 1930's Political Quarterly No. I 1981.

TABLE 2

STANDARDISED MORTALITY RATIOS OF MALES AGED 15-64 YEARS FOR SELECTED CAUSES OF DEATH ENGLAND AND WALES, 1961 (ALL CLASSES = 100)

CAUSE OF DEATH	SOCIAL CLASS				
	1 Professional	2 Intermediate	3 Skilled	4 Part Skilled	5 Unskilled
All Causes	76	81	100	103	143
Tuberculosis	40	54	96	108	185
Cancer, Stomach	49	63	101	114	163
Cancer, Lung	53	72	107	104	148
Coronary Disease	98	95	106	96	112
Bronchitis	28	50	97	116	194
Ulcer, Duodenum	48	75	96	107	173
Accidents (ex road)	43	56	87	128	193

SOURCE - Prevention and Health : Everybodys Business, HMSO 1976

TABLE 3

ESTIMATES OF THE TOTAL EFFECTS OF ONE PERCENT CHANGES IN UNEMPLOYMENT RATES SUSTAINED OVER A SIX YEAR PERIOD ON THE INCIDENCE OF SOCIAL TRAUMA*
(BASED ON UNITED STATES POPULATIONS OF 1965 AND 1970)

MEASURES OF SOCIAL TRAUMA (1)	INCIDENCE OF PATHOLOGY RELATED TO 1 PERCENT INCREASE IN UNEMPLOYMENT, BASED ON 1970 POPULATION (2)	INCIDENCE OF PATHOLOGY RELATED TO 1 PERCENT INCREASE IN UNEMPLOYMENT, BASED ON 1965 POPULATION (3)	TOTAL INCIDENCE OF PATHOLOGY, 1965 (4)
Total Mortality	36,890	35,040	1,828,000
Cardiovascular Mortality	20,240	19,228	1,000,787
Cirrhosis of Liver Mortality	495	470	24,715
Suicide	920	616	21,507
Homicide	648	874	10,712
State Mental Hospital 1st Admissions	4,227	4,045	117,483

SOURCE — Modified from Brenner H. (1977) International Journal of Health Services Vol. 7 No. 4

* Social trauma = bodily diseases brought about by social causes

TABLE 4

INDUSTRIAL STRUCTURE OF EMPLOYMENT IN THE NORTHERN REGION 1979 AND NORTH TYNESIDE 1976

	(a) NORTHERN	(b) NORTH TYNESIDE
Primary	4.9	2.16
Manufacturing	32.9	38.05
Construction	7.8	8.55
Public Utilities	1.7	3.67
Transport/Distribution	17.4	16.55
Professions & Service	35.3	31.02
	100.00	100.00

SOURCES - (a) Department of Employment Gazette
(b) North Tyneside Community Development Project

Modified from Jobless (1980) A Study of Unemployed Young People in North Tyneside by North Tyneside Into Work

TABLE 5

THE RELATIONSHIP OF LABOURERS TO TOTAL UNEMPLOYED IN NORTH TYNESIDE BY OFFICE AND LABOURING VACANCIES JANUARY 1981

EMPLOYMENT OFFICE	TOTAL ALL UNEMPLOYED	UNEMPLOYED		TOTAL	VACANCIES	
		Heavy Lab	Light Lab		Heavy Lab	Light Lab
North Shields	3481	565	283	848 (24%)	4	-
Wallsend	3313	613	355	968 (29%)	2	-
West Moor	2600	390	367	757 (29%)	-	-
Whitley Bay	2132	257	192	449 (21%)	-	-

SOURCE – Manpower Services Commission

TABLE 6

LENGTH OF UNEMPLOYMENT

TIME OUT OF WORK	UNEMPLOYED MEN	NORTHERN REGION	GREAT BRITAIN
3 months or less	18% (16)	34%	37%
Over 3-6 months	20% (18)	18%	19%
Over 6-12 months	24% (22)	19%	21%
Over 1-2 years	23% (21)	15%	14%
Over 2 years	15% (14)	14%	9%
	100% (91)	100%	100%

SOURCE – In and Out of Work, North Tyneside Community Development Project 1978

TABLE 7

NORTH TYNESIDE INFANT MORTALITY* AND PERINATAL MORTALITY COMPARED WITH ENGLAND & WALES

	INFANT MORTALITY RATE		PERINATAL MORTALITY RATE	
	England & Wales	North Tyneside	England & Wales	North Tyneside
1974	16	15	20	17
1975	16	12	19	15
1976	14.2	15.6	17.7	20.1
1977	13.8	17.4	17.0	20.9
1978	13.2	14.3	15.5	21.5
1979	12.8	13.0	14.7	20.9

SOURCE - OPCS   S.D. 52

TABLE 8

MORTALITY PROFILE NORTHERN REGION AND NORTH TYNESIDE AREA HEALTH AUTHORITY 1975 - 1979

(SMR* = 100)
(England and Wales)

		NORTHERN			NORTH TYNESIDE		
		Male	Female	Person	Male	Female	Person
	All Causes	112.24	109.08	110.69	114.53	112.20	113.37
1	Infectious & Parasitic Diseases	112.75	105.02	109.40	113.48	122.16	117.29
2	Neoplasms	111.52	102.25	107.23	122.56	113.45	118.26
3	Endocrine, Nutritional & Metabolic Diseases & Immunity Disorders	103.40	111.81	108.50	108.64	93.01	99.01
4	Diseases of Blood & Blood Forming Organs	122.55	108.28	113.47	126.80	108.10	114.68
5	Mental Disorders	130.58	141.33	137.51	133.48	90.29	105.07
6	Diseases of the Nervous System & Sense Organs	107.98	104.60	106.23	142.64	122.69	132.10
7	Diseases of the Circulatory System	112.80	113.31	113.05	110.96	115.33	113.18
8	Diseases of the Respiratory System	113.61	103.08	108.66	113.70	103.70	108.89
9	Diseases of the Digestive System	113.26	102.91	107.69	120.20	94.95	106.38
10	Diseases of the Genito-urinary System	104.33	107.51	105.87	113.64	106.27	109.96
11	Complications of Pregnancy, Childbirth and the Puerperium	0.00	143.50	143.50	0.00	72.46	72.46
12	Diseases of the Skin & Subcutaneous Tissue	54.00	102.58	87.98	45.24	55.68	52.65
13	Diseases of the Musculoskeletal System and Connective Tissue	90.51	79.23	82.13	35.27	53.74	49.14
14	Congenital Anomalies	95.68	98.01	96.79	69.19	108.72	88.21
15	Certain Conditions originating in the Perinatal Period	108.75	111.22	109.74	96.56	91.00	94.31
16	Signs, Symptoms & Ill-defined Conditions	114.26	103.81	107.82	111.13	82.90	93.33
17	Injury and Poisoning	112.81	123.66	117.43	119.34	141.26	128.94

SOURCE - Experimental Database Project

* SMR - Standardised Mortality Ratio

REFERENCES:

BRENNER, M.H.: Foetal, Infant and Maternity Mortality during periods of Economic Instability. International Journal of Health Services, Vol.3, No.2 (1973).

BRENNER, M.H.: Mental Illness and the Economy. Harvard University Press (1973).

BRENNER, M.H.: Health Costs and Benefits of Economic Policy. International Journal of Health Services, Vol.7, No.4 (1977).

BRENNER, M.H.: Mortality and the National Economy. A review, and the experiences of England and Wales, 1936-1976. The Lancet, September 15th (1979).

BRENNER, M.H.: Mortality and the National Economy II. Principal factors affecting post-war British mortality trends.(Mimeo) (1981).

BUNN, A.R.: Ischaemic Heart Disease Mortality and the Business Cycle in Australia. American Journal of Public Health, Vol.69, No.8 (1979).

CATALANO, R. and DOOLEY, D.C.: Economic Predictions of Depressed Mood and Stressful Life Events in a Metropolitan Community. Journal of Health and Social Behaviour, Vol.18 (1977).

COATES, D., MOYER, S. and WELLMAN, B.: Yorklea Study: Symptoms, Problems and Life Events. Canadian Journal of Public Health, Vol.60 (1969).

COLLEDGE, M.: Unemployment and Health.North Tyneside Community Health Council (1981).

COLLEDGE, M.: Economic Cycles and Health: towards a sociological understanding of the impact of the recession on health and illness. Social Science and Medicine,Vol.16 (forthcoming) (1982).

COOK, D.S., BARTLEY, M.J., CUMMINS, R.O. and SHAPER, A.S.: Health of Unemployed Middle-aged Men in Great Britain. The Lancet,June 5th (1982)

DRAPER,P., DENNIS, J., GRIFFITHS, J., PARTRIDGE, J. and POPAY, J.: Microprocession, Macro-economic Policy and Public Health. The Lancet (1979).

DURKHEIM, E.: Suicides: A Study in Sociology. Free Press 1952 (1897).

EMPLOYMENT GAZETTE April 1980, January 1981, February 1981.

EYER, J.: Does Unemployment Cause the Death Rate Peak in Each Business Cycle? International Journal of Health Services,Vol.7,No.4 (1977).

FAGIN, L.: Unemployment and Health in Families. DHSS (1981).

GARRATY, J.A.: Unemployment in History and Economic Thought and Public Policy. Harper Row, New York (1978)

GRAVELLE, H.S.E., HUTCHINSON, S. and STERN, J.: Mortality and Unemployment: A Critique of Brenner's Time Series Analysis. The Lancet (1981).

HILL, M.J., HARRISON, R.M., SARGEANT, A.V. and TALBOT, V.: Men out of Work. Cambridge University Press (1973).

HILL, J.M.M.: The Psychological Impact of Unemployment. New Society 19th January (1978).

HMSO: Everybody's Business. Prevention and Health (1976).

HMSO: Inequalities in Health (Black Report) (1980).

JAHODA, M., LAZARSFELD, P.F. and ZEISEL, H.: Marienthal, pub. 1977 Tavistock (1933).

KASL, S. et al: Changes in Serum Uric Acid and Cholesterol Levels in Men Undergoing Job Loss. Journal America Medical Association, 206:1500 (1968).

KASL, S. and COBB, S.: Blood Pressure Changes in Men Undergoing Job Loss: A Preliminary Report. Psychosomatic Medicine, Vol.32 (1970).

KOMORA, P. and CLARK, M.: Mental Disease in the Crisis. Mental Hygiene, Vol.19 (1935).

LEIM, R. and LEIM, J. Social Class and Mental Illness Reconsidered: The Role of Economic Stress and Social Support. Journal of Health and Social Behaviour, Vol. 19 (1978).

MORRIS, J.N. and TITMUS, R.M.: Health and Social Change: A Recent History of Rheumatic Heart Disease. Medical Officer (1944).

MYERS, J., LINDENTHAL, J. and PEPPER, M.: Social Class, Life Events, and Psychiatric Symptoms: A Longitudinal Study. In: Dohrenwend, B.S. and Dohrenwend, B.P. (eds): Stressful Life Events: Their Nature and Effects. Wiley, New York (1974).

NORTH TYNESIDE COMMUNITY DEVELOPMENT PROJECT: In and Out of Work (1978).

NORTH TYNESIDE COMMUNITY DEVELOPMENT PROJECT FINAL REPORT, Vol.1: North Shields: Working Class Politics and Housing 1900-1977. Vol.II: North Shields: Living with Industrial Change. Vol.III: North Shields: Organising for Change in a Working Class Area. Vol.IV: North Shields: Organising for Change in a Working Class Area. Vol. V: North Shields: Women's Work (1978).

NORTH TYNESIDE INTO WORK (eds): Jobless. A Study of Unemployment Young People in North Tyneside (1980).

NORTH TYNESIDE TRADES COUNCIL: Ship building - The Cost of Redundancy. Report (1979).

NUTMAN, P.: The Psychological and Social Aspects of Unemployment. Paper presented at the Unemployment and Health Workshop. The Nuffield Centre for Health Studies, (Mimeo), Leeds (1981).

PIMLOTT, B.: The North East: Back to the 1930s? Political Quarterly, No.1 (1981).

POPAY, J.: Unemployment a Threat to Public Health. In forthcoming C.P.A.G. Pamphlet (1981).

SINFIELD, A., SHOWLER, B. (eds): The Workless State. Martin Robertson (1981a).

SINFIELD, A.: What Unemployment Means. Martin Robertson (1981b).

STERN, J.: Unemployment and its Impact on Morbidity and Mortality. Centre for Labour Economics, L.S.E. Diss. Press 93 (1981).

TOWNSEND, P.: Poverty in the United Kingdom. Penguin, London (1979).

Part 2

RECENT EMPIRICAL RESEARCH:

INDIVIDUAL-LEVEL ANALYSIS

THE HEALTH EFFECTS OF ECONOMIC INSTABILITY: A TEST OF THE ECONOMIC STRESS HYPOTHESIS

Ralph Catalano, Ph.D.
David Dooley, Ph.D.

Public Policy Research Organization
Program in Social Ecology
University of California, Irvine
Irvine, California 92715

ABSTRACT

Longitudinal survey data describing 6,190 subjects are analyzed using log-linear methods to determine which, if any, of three hypothesized links between short-term community economic change and illness or injury is correct. The first possible link assumes that economic contraction increases the incidence of undesirable job and financial events that, in turn, increase the incidence of illness and injury. The second possible connection assumes that economic change per se increases the incidence of undesirable job and financial events and, therefore, the incidence of illness and injury. The third connection assumes that economic change per se increases the incidence of all job and financial events and therefore the incidence of illness and injury. The data support the first hypothesized connection, but the process is observed only in middle socio-economic status respondents. While undesirable job and financial experiences increase the likelihood of illness or injury for high and low SES groups, high SES respondents are less likely to experience such events during periods of contraction of the local economy than during expansion. The risk of low SES respondents having undesirable job and financial events did not vary longitudinally with the performance of the local economy.

THE HEALTH EFFECTS OF ECONOMIC INSTABILITY
A TEST OF THE ECONOMIC STRESS HYPOTHESIS

One of the reasons we seek economic security is to avoid illness. That fact, however, implies nothing for the question of whether the connection between the performance of the economy and the incidence of illness or injury is direct enough to yield a systematic relationship that can be modeled to advance either theory or practice. Attempts to answer that question have become more common in recent years but differences in approach have precluded convergence on a clear answer. The analyses described in this paper synthesize the approaches and suggest that the answer is yes.

Background

The literature most frequently cited as supporting the contention that changes in the economy affect the incidence of health problems can be separated into two groups defined by analytic approach. The first group uses economic characteristics of geographic areas (e.g., nations, states, metropolitan areas, catchment areas) to predict the incidence of health problems in the populations of those areas. These analyses, which are based on the correlation of aggregate time series, have yielded correlations between economic stability and rates of such diverse health indicators as age and sex-specific mortality and cardiovascular-renal disease mortality (Brenner, 1976); suicide (Mark, 1979; Marshall and Hodge, 1981; Pierce, 1967); infant mortality (Brenner, 1973); and ischaemic heart disease mortality (Brenner, 1971; Bunn, 1979). With few exceptions (e.g., Catalano, 1979; Dooley et al., 1981; Eyer, 1977), the typical finding of these studies is that intuitively undesirable economic phenomena (e.g., increases in unemployment, decreases in stock prices) are followed by increases in the rates of health problems.

These aggregate, time-series studies have been criticized on several conceptual and methodological grounds. The principal conceptual criticism has been that the literature lacks a clear theoretical base that specifies the mechanisms assumed to connect macro-economic events to disease processes in individuals (Kasl, 1979; Lew, 1979). The literature often refers to the possibility that bad economic times affect diet and life style and therefore influence risk factors (Brenner, 1976). The same studies also note that economic change creates "psychosocial stressors" that have been implicated in disease processes (Brenner, 1976, Bunn, 1979). The psychosocial stressor suggestion has led to empirical analyses that indicate that the aggregate incidence of stressful life events (Catalano and Dooley, 1977; Dooley and Catalano, 1979) and of psychosomatic disorder (Catalano, et al., 1981) vary with economic instability.

The methodological criticisms have ranged from statistical to design weaknesses but the most telling, which is related to the weak theory base, is the "ecologial fallacy" (Kasl, 1979; Dooley and Catalano, 1980). The fallacy, a threat to all aggregate studies, is the logical error of assuming that an association between two characteristics of a population aggregate (e.g., unemployment and mean hypertension) will generalize to those characteristics when measured across individuals.

A second group of studies often cited as evidence that health is affected by economic fluctuations tests the hypothesis that individuals who experience work stressors (e.g., unemployment or retirement) are at higher risk of exhibiting health problems than those who do not (Kasl and Cobb, forthcoming). This relatively small literature reports an association between adaptations to job changes and such outcomes as suicide (Breed, 1963; Theorell and Floderus-Myrhed, 1977), corticoid production (Theorell, 1974), dyspepsia, joint swelling and the use of antihypertensive drugs (Kasl, et al., 1975). As in the case of the aggregate, time-series studies, these individual based analyses have their weaknesses. Many are cross-sectional or retrospective and therefore are subject to the "reverse causation" rival hypothesis that an unmeasured psychological or physiological problem causes both the unstable employment or financial history and the measured outcome. The prospective studies, on the other hand, have been based on small, homogeneous samples that raise the issue of how general the effect might be (e.g., Kasl, et al., 1975).

Beyond the above criticisms, the individual-based literature is not very helpful in answering the question posed at the outset. The reason is that the findings imply little about how the economy, as opposed to work or financial stressors, affects people. This may sound like "hair splitting" but it should be noted that people lose jobs or income in the most expansive economies and that sluggish economies do not necessarily deprive people of either. The assumption that work or financial stressors vary over time with changes in the economy has not been tested. The individual level analyses therefore, have not addressed the question of interest, which is, do the measurable characteristics of the economy (i.e., the system of production and distribution of goods and services) have a systematic, modelable effect on health?

Hypotheses

Three conceptually different explanations of how the performance of an economy can affect the incidence of psychosocial stressors are implied by the literature alluded to above. The first assumes that the ability of an economy to provide secure employment is the crucial dimension of economic performance because the undesirable job and financial experiences associated with contracting economies (e.g., anticipated or real job loss, income reduction, difficulty in paying bills) are thought to be risk factors in illness and injury (e.g., Pearlin, et al., 1981).

The second explanation assumes that economic instability per se, whether intuitively good, bad, or indifferent, is more important than simple contraction or expansion of employment opportunities. This assumption is made because intuitively desirable economic processes (e.g., expansion of the labor force) can lead to undesirable job and financial experiences such as incurring imprudent new debts, assuming stressful job responsibilities, or the disruption of established social networks.

A third explanation also posits that economic instability per se is more important than contraction of employment opportunities but asserts this position because desirable or indifferent economic processes can increase the incidence of desirable or indifferent job and financial stressors (e.g., promotion at work) that may be risk factors in illness and injury (e.g., Eyer, 1977). While the literature concerned with psychological outcomes suggests that undesirable events are more predictive of pathology than are other events (Tausig, 1982), the research concerned with somatic illness or injury does not converge on the issue of desirability.

The relative accuracy of these three explanations can be estimated by accepting or rejecting each of the following hypotheses.

1. Undesirable job and financial life events will be positively related to illness and injury when the effect of all other stressful life events is controlled.

2. Desirable and indifferent job and financial life events will be positively related to illness and injury when the effect of all other stressful life events is controlled.

3. The odds of experiencing undesirable job and finanacial events will be positively related to periods of economic contraction.
4. The odds of experiencing undesirable job and financial events will be positively related to periods of economic change _per se_.
5. The odds of experiencing positive and indifferent job and financial events will be related positively to periods of economic change _per se_.

Each of the three competing explanations implies that a unique set of the above hypotheses will be accepted or rejected. The first explanation, that contracting economies increase the incidence of undesirable job and financial events that, in turn, increase the risk of illness and injury, implies that Hypotheses 1 and 3 will be accepted and that 2 and 4 will be rejected. Explanation 2, that economic change _per se_ increases the incidence of undesirable job and financial events and therefore the risk of illness and injury, assumes that 1 and 4 will be accepted and 2 rejected. The third explanation, that economic change _per se_ increases the incidence of job and financial events that increase the risk of illness and injury, implies that Hypotheses 1, 2, 3 and 5 are true.

METHODS

Survey Data

The hypotheses were tested using data collected in the Los Angeles-Long Beach Standard Metropolitan Statistical Area (co-terminus with Los Angeles County). The data were gathered in twelve quarterly surveys of 500 households (new households drawn each survey wave) conducted from 1978 through 1980. Respondents were interviewed by telephone and asked items that measured psychological symptoms, health status, social support, employment experiences, and the incidence of economic and other stressful life events.

Telephone numbers were randomly generated and up to twelve attempts were made to complete an interview. Up to four of the possible twelve calls were made to make initial contact. If contact was made, a respondent was chosen randomly using the Trodahl-Carter Method (1964). Up to four additional calls were made to reach a chosen respondent not available at the time of the original contact. An additional four calls would be attempted to complete the interview with the respondent. A refusal to cooperate or a termination was not considered final until a second attempt, by a different interviewer, was made to gain cooperation. Calls for each survey were spread over three weeks and divided into day and evening as well as weekend periods. Interviews were conducted in both English and Spanish. Completion rates (i.e., completions/completions + refusal + terminations) averaged about 68 percent for the 12 surveys analyzed below.

Variables derived from the survey items included frequency of recent (last three months) episodes of illness or injury, job and financial life events, other life events not involving health, job, or finances; sex, socioeconomic status, and age. The life event items were adapted for telephone use from existing scales designed for paper and pencil or face-to-face administration. While the results of the telephone interviews may differ from face-to-face interviews using the same items, recent research suggests that the results would be similar (Klecka and Tuchfarber, 1978; Rogers, 1976). No differences, for example, were found between scores on a psychological symptom scale, similar to that used in another component of this study, when administered by telephone and in person (Aneshensel, et al., 1982). Even if telephone interviewing yields more optimistic or socially desirable answers on sensitive questions, this bias should not affect the analysis of interwave variability (Jordan, et al., 1980; Groves and Kahn, 1979).

The job and financial event inventory included 36 items, listed in Table 1, drawn from the PERI Life Event Scale (Dohrenwend, et al., 1978), the Holmes and Rahe scale (Holmes and Rahe, 1967), and the Theorell "workload" scale (Theorell and Floderus-Myrhed, 1977) as well as original items devised for this study. The dichotomy between undesirable and desirable or indifferent events was based on empirical analyses (Dohrenwend et al., 1978) for the PERI items and on the author's judgment for the Theorell and original items. An "other" life event inventory was constructed from 25 items (a combination of desirable, undesirable and indifferent events) that do not involve health, job or finances. These items, also shown in Table 1, were drawn from the PERI and the Homes and Rahe inventories. This event inventory was used to control for "background" stressors that may covary with financial and work stressors and to reduce the threat, discussed below, of a response bias leading to a spurious association between work and financial events and illness or injury.

The count of life events was used in this analysis rather than the sum of adaptation weights because recent research has suggested that weights and counts yield essentially identical results (Ross and Mirowsky, 1979). An event recall period of three months (rather than 12 months, 24 months, or longer) was used following findings that more recent events are more impactful (Brown and Harris, 1978; Horowitz, et al., 1977; Rahe, 1974) and are more accurately recalled (Uhlenhuth, et al., 1977).

TABLE 1. LIFE EVENTS INCLUDED IN THE SURVEY INVENTORY

Job or Financial		"Other"
Undesirable	Desirable or Indifferent	Desirable, Undesirable or Indifferent
1. Mortgage Foreclosed	1. Move to better residence	1. Lost house through disaster
2. Car, Furniture or other item repossessed	2. Move to equivalent residence	2. Pregnancy in family
3. Decrease in wages	3. Remodel home	3. Robbed
4. Financial loss	4. Take out mortgage	4. Involved in law suit
5. Move to worse residence	5. Buy car, furniture or other item on installment plan	5. Arrested
6. Go on welfare	6. Increase wages	6. Released from jail
7. Difficulty paying bills	7. Financial gain	7. Went to jail
8. Change to worse job	8. Go off welfare	8. Acquitted of crime
9. Demoted at work	9. Start work for first time	9. Convicted of crime
10. Fired from job	10. Return to work after not working for a long time	10. Engaged to be married
11. Laid off from work	11. New job better than old	11. Marriage engagement broken
12. Unemployed more that 30 days	12. New job about the same as old	12. Married
13. Trouble with boss	13. Promoted at work	13. Separated
14. Trouble with fellow workers	14. Work conditions improved	14. Divorced
15. Business loss or failure	15. Workload increased	15. Relations with spouse worsened
	16. Workload decreased	16. Relations with spouse improved
	17. End an extra job	17. Trouble with in-laws
	18. retire	18. First child born
	19. Start a new business or profession	19. Later child born
	20. Begin school or training program	20. Person move in or out of household
	21. Graduate from school or training program	21. Child adopted
		22. Spouse died
		23. Child died
		24. Other family member died
		25. Close friend died

Frequency distributions of the life event variables were very skewed. While 19% of the total sample reported at least one undesirable job and financial event, only 5.3% reported more than one. The distribution for "other" events was similar in that 40% reported at least one but only 12.5% reported more than one. Desirable and indifferent job and financial events were more common than the other two categories. Seventy-three percent of the sample reported at least two such events but only 17% reported more than two. Given these distributions and the fact that previous research does not suggest a strong linear effect of life events on illness, each life event variable was scored dichotomously. Undesirable job and financial as well as other events were scored as none and one or more. Desirable and indifferent events were scored as less than two and two or more.

Socio-economic Status (SES) was calculated from education and occupation following Hollingshead and Redlich (1958). Because of incomplete responses or refusals to answer the occupation item, SES could not be calculated for 19 percent of the respondents. SES was estimated separately for respondents with complete data using regression formulae incorporating education and several other variables. The formulae then were used to estimate SES for respondents with missing data. The sample was divided into three SES categories: low, medium, and high.

Respondents also were categorized by age and sex. The age categories 18-28, 29-39, 40-55, and 56+ were used because they divided the sample into nearly equivalent groups.

The dependent variable was constructed from items that asked respondents if they had been physically ill or injured in the last three months. It should be noted that these self-reported illnesses and injuries may include relatively minor as well as serious problems. The illness and injury variable was scored dichtomously (was, or was not ill or injured).

An assumption of the analyses described below is that the adult population of Los Angeles county is represented in each of 12 different periods (conceptualized as 12 different economic environments). It therefore was necessary to determine whether the 12 samples were sufficiently similar demographically to allow any interwave differences to be attributed to environmental influences rather than to sampling error. No significant differences among the survey samples were found for sex or age. Variation in completion rates from wave to wave was found to be insignificant. Differences in the SES composition of the samples were small but statistically significant. These differences should not affect results because, as described below, SES had no main effects on the likelihood of experiencing an undesirable job or financial event or on the likelihood of being ill or injured.

Economic data

Four economic variables were chosen to measure the constructs of employment opportunity and economic stability assumed by the three models described above. The unemployment rate was included in the analyses as a measure of employment opportunity to ensure comparability with earlier research. The unemployment rate, however, does not necessarily measure the number of persons who have lost or gained jobs. The rate is the proportion, determined by survey, of the population that wants but does not have a job. The number of jobs available therefore can increase in the same month that the unemployment rate increases or the latter can decrease when the number of available jobs also decreases. To ensure that the actual employment performance of the Los Angeles-Long Beach metropolitan area was included as a second variable. This variable is called "employment change." The unemployment variable should be thought of as a measure of the economy's ability to satisfy the employment needs of the population whereas the employment change variable tends to measure job loss or gain in the population.

The second dimension of economic performance, change _per se_ rather than expansion or contraction, was measured by an additional two variables. The first of these, absolute change in the size and structure of the metropolitan workforce, sums the absolute monthly differences in the number of persons employed in each sector of an 89-sector classification of the metropolitan area's workforce. This absolute change variable has been reported to be predictive of the mean number of stressful life events experienced by population samples (Catalano and Dooley, 1977).

A fourth economic variable, structural change, was included in the analyses because it is likely to accelerate and become widespread as new technologies become increasingly common. Structural change refers to shifts in the relative size (in terms of number of employees) of the industries and services that make up a region's economy (Catalano and Dooley, 1977). Manufacturing, for example, has become a relatively smaller employment sector as services have expanded. Structural change was measured by summing the monthly absolute differences in the _proportion_ of the labor force employed in each sector of the 89-sector classification used to compute the absolute change measure.

Structural change varies conceptually from absolute change in that the latter axiomatically differs from zero when any sector of the economy increases or decreases in total employees. Structural change, however, assumes that such changes are important only when they represent a shifting of the relative sizes of employment sectors. This shifting is potentially "stressful" from an economic perspective because it means change in the work skills expected of the population as well as in the social and physical environments experienced by the community. Such changes could include the presence of new labor unions, a change in the mix of air, water, or noise pollutants, or new scheduling of leisure periods.

The mean of each of these variables was computed for 12 three-month periods corresponding to the 12 survey waves. The three-month periods included the month of the survey and the two preceding months. Each of the resulting series of 12 values was then divided into a categorical measure with low, medium and high levels.

The conceptual differences among the four variables are reinforced by the empirical distribution of the 12 survey quarters across the catagories of each. These distributions are shown in Table 2.

Analyses

The hypotheses to be tested imply a multivariate analysis. While the life-event measures were devised to yield continuous scores, their frequency distributions were, in fact, highly skewed. Given the nominal or ordinal nature of the other variables, the interpretive appropriateness of dichotomizing the criterion variables (e.g., were or were not ill or injured), and the large sample size, logit analysis, a method for analyzing multivariate categorical data, was chosen (Fienberg, 1978). The use of logit analysis for short time series is not unprecedented (Clogg, 1979).

Logit analysis models the natural logarithm of the odds of falling into one rather than another category of the criterion variable as a function of

TABLE 2. The Continuous (3 month average) and Categorical Scores for Each Economic Variable for the twelve survey quarters.

QUARTER	1	2	3	4	5	6	7	8	9	10	11	12
Unemployment Rate												
Score	7.7	7.4	6.4	5.7	5.8	5.2	5.9	4.8	5.7	6.4	7.1	7.1
Category	H	H	M	M	M	L	M	L	M	M	H	H
Change in Total Employment												
Score (in thousands)	22.9	7.77	24.63	9.93	10.33	8.43	16.17	-6.47	9.0	-14.4	11.33	6.46
Category	H	M	H	M	M	M	H	L	M	L	M	M
Absolute Change												
Score	433.7	503.7	657	521.3	456	380.3	599.7	520.7	400.3	348.7	593.3	466
Category	M	M	H	M	M	L	H	M	M	L	H	M
Structural Change												
Score	1.08	1.237	1.947	1.263	1.073	.993	1.703	1.247	.963	1.037	1.617	1.08
Category	L	M	H	M	L	L	H	M	L	L	H	L

the categories of the predictor variables. In this analysis logit coefficients are derived from log-linear analysis (BMDP3F, see Dixon & Brown, 1977). These coefficients are expressed in their multiplicative, effect-on-odds form following Swafford (1980). The resulting coefficients are interpretively similar to their regression and ANOVA counterparts (i.e., expressions for the magnitude and statistical significance of main and interaction effects and for the overall "fit" produced by the best parameters).

RESULTS

Hypothesis 1

The hypothesis that the probability of illness or injury is related to undesirable job and financial events was supported by the data. Table 3 shows the models fit to the contingency table formed by the variables ill or injured (H), age (A), sex (X), socio-economic status (S), "other" events (N), desirable and indifferent job and financial events (O), and undesirable job or financial events (L). Models 1 through 6 in Table 3 suggest that among the control variables only age and "other" life events are related significantly to the odds of being ill or injured. As demonstrated by the difference between models 5 and 8 (1DF, $X^2 = 71.49$, $\underline{p} < .05$), the undesirable job and financial events variable significantly improves the fit of the "controls only" model. As shown in Table 4, the model coefficients indicate that age is related inversely to illness and injury while the life event variables are related positively to illness and injury.

TABLE 3. Models for the Odds of Being Ill or Injured (H) as a Function of Age (A), Sex (X), Socio-Economic Status (S), "Other" Events (N), Positive or Indifferent Job or Financial Events (O), and Undesirable Job or Financial Events (L).

Model*		DF	LR $\underline{X}^2$	P
1	H	191	288.65	.00
2	HA	188	268.05	.00
3	HA, HX	187	267.92	.00
4	HA, HS	186	265.85	.00
5	HA, HN	187	251.19	.00
6	HA, HN, HO	186	248.54	.00
7	HA, HN, HO, HL	185	179.36	.60
8	HA, HN, HL**	186	179.70	.62

*LONASX implicit in each model
**Coefficients for this model shown in Table 4

TABLE 4. Coefficients for Model of Illness and Injury as a Function of Age, "Other" Events, and Undesirable Job or Financial Events

Term	Log-Linear Coefficients	Multiplicative Dummy-Logit Coefficient
Age Group		
18-28	.04	1.00
29-39	.05	1.03
40-55	-.04	.86
56+	-.05	.83
"Other" Events		
None	-.05	1.00
1 or more	.05	1.24
Undesirable Job or Financial Events		
None	-.17	1.00
1 or more	.17	1.95
Constant	-.71	.17

The effect of experiencing one or more undesirable job or financial events on the odds of being ill or injured can be inferred from the coefficients in Table 4. As described by Swafford (1980), log-linear coefficients can be converted to multiplicative, dummy-logit forms that allow expressing strength of effect as increase in the odds of experiencing the dependent phenomenon. The odds for each combination of levels of the control variables and independent variable are the product of the constant and appropriate coefficients in column 4. For example, the odds of being ill or injured for an 18 to 28 year old who had experienced neither an "other" event nor an undesirable job or financial event are the product of the constant (.17), the age-group coefficient (1.00), and the two no-event coefficients (1.00 and 1.00) or .17. Experiencing an undesirable job or financial event would nearly double the odds of illness or injury for the same group (.17 x 1 x 1 x 1.95 = .33). The doubling effect of experiencing an undesirable job or financial event is indicated by the 1.95 multiplicative, dumm-logit coefficient for experiencing one or more as opposed to no such events.

Hypothesis 2

The proposition that the odds of being ill or injured is related to desirable or indifferent job and financial events was not supported. Table 3 shows that this life event variable (O) did not significantly add to the fit model (8) that included age (A), "other" events (N) and undesirable job and financial events (L). No significant interactions of the desirable or indifferent job or financial events variable with any of the control variables was detected.

Hypothesis 3

The hypothesis that economic contraction has a <u>main</u>, positive effect on the likelihood of experiencing an undesirable job or financial event was not supported. Unhypothesized effects of the interactions of sex and socio-economic status and of the unemployment rate and socio-economic status on the odds of experiencing undesirable job or financial events were, however, discovered.

Table 5 shows the modeling of the contingency table formed by undesirable job and financial events (L), age (A), sex (X), socio-economic status (S), and unemployment (U). Models 1 through 6 indicate that only age has a <u>main</u> effect on the odds of experiencing and undesirable job or financial event. The interaction of sex and socio-economic status, however, is related significantly to such events as indicated by the difference between models 5 and 8 (DF = 2, x^2 = 15.32, <u>p</u> < .05). The coefficients shown in Table 6, suggest that for males the likelihood of having an undesirable job or financial event varies over SES in an inverted "J" pattern with high-status males least likely and middle-status males most likely to experience such events. The pattern reverses for females to form an upright "J."

The interaction of SES and the unemployment rate is shown by the differences between models 9 and 10 (4 DF, x^2 = 12.07, <u>p</u> < .05). The coefficients indicate that the middle-status respondents were more likely to report such events as the unemployment rate increased. High-status respondents were less likely to report such events as the unemployment rate increased. The odds of low status persons reporting such events was unrelated to the unemployment rate.

TABLE 5. Models for the Odds of Experiencing One or More Undesirable Job or Financial Event (L) as a Function of Age (A), Sex (X), Socio-Economic Status (S), and Unemployment (U)

Model*		DF	LR χ^2	P
1	L	71	308.77	.00
2	LA	68	83.96	.09
3	LA, LS	66	82.22	.08
4	LA, LX	67	83.83	.08
5	LA, LX, LS	65	82.14	.07
6	LA, LX, LU	65	82.85	.06
7	LA, LXU	63	79.16	.08
8	LA, LXS	63	66.82	.35
9	LA, LXS, LU	61	65.67	.32
10	LA, LXS, LUS**	57	53.60	.60

*UAXS implicit in each model
**Coefficients for this model used in Table 6

TABLE 6. Coefficients for Model of the Odds of Experiencing one or more Undesirable Job or Financial Events as a Function of Age, and of the interactions of SES with Sex and Unemployment

Term		Log-Linear Coefficients			Multiplicative, Dummy-Logit Coefficients		
Age							
	18-25	.25			1.00		
	26-39	.21			.92		
	40-55	-.05			.55		
	56+	-.41			.27		
Interactions		SES			SES		
		Low	Middle	High	Low	Middle	High
Sex							
	Male	.03	.06	-.09	1.00	1.00	1.00
	Female	-.03	-.06	.09	.89	.79	1.43
Unemployment Rate:							
	Low	.01	-.09	.02	1.00	1.00	1.00
	Middle	-.02	-.05	.05	.95	1.08	1.07
	High	.01	.13	-.06	.99	1.54	.86
Constant		-.73	-.72	-.79	.42	.37	.29

TABLE 7. Models for the Odds of Experiencing One or More Positive or Indifferent Job or Financial Event (O) as a Function of Age (A), Sex (X), Socio-Economic Status (S), and Structural Change (C)

Model*		DF	LR χ^2	P
1	O	71	806.49	.00
2	OA	68	126.06	.00
3	OA, OX	67	112.30	.00
4	OA, OX, OS	65	86.51	.04
5	OA, OX, OS, OC	63	68.10	.31

*CAXS implicit in each model

The interaction of the unemployment rate and socio-economic status was not replicated when change in employment was used to measure contraction of the economy. A three-way interaction of sex, socio-economic status and empolyment change was found to add significantly to models that included only main effects and two-way interactions. None of these models, however, fit the contingency table for which they were derived. The log-linear coefficients, moreover, did not form an interpretable pattern.[1]

Hypothesis 4

The hypothesis that the odds of experiencing an undesirable job or financial event would be related to economic change per se was not supported. There were no main or interaction effects of either absolute or structural change on the dependent variable.

Hypothesis 5

The hypothesis that the risk of experiencing a desirable or indifferent job or financial event is related to economic change per se was supported. Table 7 shows the results of fitting models to the contingency tables formed by structural change (C) and age (A), sex (X), socio-economic status (S) and the experience of one or more desirable or indifferent job or financial events (O). The table shows that age, sex and status all are related to the dependent variable and that structural change adds significantly to the fit of the model containing only the control variables. The difference between models 4 and 5 in Table 7 (2 DF, $X^2 = 18.41$, $p < .05$) shows that structural change add to the control variables to yield a fit model. The modeling for absolute change yielded essentially the same results as those shown in Table 7 for structural change.

The coefficients for the models using absolute and structural change were very similar. The coefficients suggest that age is related linearly and inversely to the odds of experiencing a positive or indifferent job or financial event. They also suggest that females are less likely than males to have such events, and that socio-economic status is related positively and linearly to such events. The effect of absolute change on indifferent or positive job or financial events appears to be "J" shaped with the medium level slightly less likely to yield such events than the low level. Periods of high absolute change increase the odds of one or more such events by 25% over the low and 30% over the medium periods. The effect of structural change appears to be linear and positive with high periods increasing the odds of experiencing such events by 15% over medium and 37% over low periods.

Summary of Results

Hypotheses 1 and 5 were supported fully while Hypotheses 4 and 2 were rejected. Hypothesis 3 was found to be true only for middle-SES respondents. The results, therefore, detract from two of the possible mechanisms assumed to connect macro-economic events to individual illness and injury. These are the claims that economic change per se can increase the risk of illness or injury by increasing the incidence of either undesirable or of all job and financial events. While change per se does appear to increase the risk of indifferent or positive events, these events are not related directly to illness or injury. While undesirable job and financial events are related to illness and injury, they are not more likely to occur during periods of high than during periods of medium or low change per se.

The mechanism that assumes that economic contraction affects the incidence of illness and injury by increasing the incidence of undesirable job and financial events was supported for middle-SES respondents. While having such events apparently increased all respondents' odds of being ill or injured, only the middle class had more such events during periods of high unemployment than during other periods.

DISCUSSION

Rival Explanations

The approach taken in this research avoids the ecological fallacy inherent in the aggregate research and makes the connection, lacking in the individual-based research, between individual experiences and the macro economy. Among the weaknesses of the approach, however, is that it does not <u>directly</u> control for any enduring, person-based characteristics (unrelated to age, sex or socio-economic status) that might cause respondents to experience undesirable job or financial events and to be ill or injured. This rival hypothesis is unlikely given that the 12 representative samples varied in both life events and in illness and injury. An enduring, person-based characteristic should not vary from one to another representative sample of the same population. One could argue that some transient, person-based characteristic caused respondents to have both life events and illness. This argument, however, requires an explanation of why, for middle- and high-SES respondents, this transient characteristic varied longitudinally with the unemployment rate.

Another type of person-based "third variable" that could cause a spurious association between undesirable job and financial events and illness or injury is a bias (unrelated to age, sex or socio-economic status) toward positive responses. This is not likely to be a serious problem in the analyses reported above for two reasons. The first is that response bias would not explain the finding that the odds of middle- and high-SES respondents reporting an undesirable job or financial event varies with the unemployment rate. The second is that the relationship of undesirable job and financial events to illness and injury was significant <u>controlling</u> for desired or indifferent job and financial events and for other events not involving health, job, or finances. Response bias, if present, should affect reporting of all three types of life events and its effect would therefore be removed through the use of any of the life event groups as a control variable.

A third rival explanation is the "reverse-causation" hypothesis that persons who are ill or injured are more likely to have undesirable job or financial events than are healthy people. This would be a more serious problem if a connection had not been found for middle- and high-SES repondents between the macro-economy and undesirable job and financial events. The parsimony of the reverse causation explanation is weakened by its logical extension to the position that the unemployment rate of the Los Angeles-Long Beach SMSA is affected by the number of persons 18 years of age or older who are ill or injured whether or not they are in the labor force. This improbable situation does not, however, weaken the reverse-causation hypothesis for low-SES respondents.

Individual Level Findings

The results of modeling the probabilities of being ill or injured yielded several counter-intuitive as well as expected results. The young, for example, were more likely to be ill or injured than the elderly. Sex or socioeconomic status, however, were not related to illness or injury. Having one or more events not involving health, job or finances increased the odds of being ill or injured by 24% whereas experiencing an undesirable job or financial event nearly doubled the odds of illness or injury. While the effect of undesirable life experiences on various psychological and health outcomes has often been described as weak (Rabkin and Struening, 1976), the doubling effect reported above impresses the authors as worth considering in attempts to understand the etiology of illness or injury.

The finding that positive and indifferent job and financial events were not related to illness or injury is consistent with the literature reporting that undesirable events are associated more strongly with symptoms of psychological disorder than are other events. These findings tend to weaken the argument that aggregate, time-series associations between economic expansion and several health indicators are due to the experience of positive and indifferent job or financial events (e.g., Eyer, 1977; Catalano, 1979).

As might be intuited, the odds of experiencing a desirable or indifferent job or financial event were related linearly and inversely to age and linearly and positively related to socio-economic status. The patterns shift for experiencing one or more undesirable job or financial event with socio-economic status taking on added importance. The young remain more likely to fall in the high category but the odds are highest for the low-status and decrease for the middle- and high-status young. While the probabilities decrease with age for all SES groups, the pattern across SES remains the same. Males are more likely than females to have such events for low- and middle-SES women but high-SES women are inexplicably likely to have more than males of the same class.

Findings Involving the Economic Environment

Testing for relationships between the economic environment and the likelihood of experiencing job or financial events produced both intuitive and counter-intuitive results. As hypothesized, the odds of experiencing desirable or indifferent job and financial events was highest during periods of high change *per* *se*. In contrast, however, the hypothesized and intuitive main effect of economic contraction on the odds of experiencing undesirable job and financial events was not found. What was found was that the effect of economic contraction, when measured by the unemployment rate, varied significantly across SES groups. The former interaction of SES and unemployment indicated that low-SES respondents were no more likely to experience these events in contracting than in expanding economies. This suggests two general categories of explanation that differ in the assumed direction of causation between illness and life experiences. The first would assume that the chronically ill are likely to have undesirable job experiences regardless of the economy. They therefore will have undesirable financial experiences and, in turn, be likely to have low income. The second would assume that low-income persons are either discriminated against, unskilled, or both and therefore at risk for undesirable job and financial events regardless of the performance of the economy. These events, in turn, are assumed to increase the probability of illness and injury. The data analyzed for this paper cannot discriminate between these two categories of explanations.

The economic well-being of middle-class respondents is probably tied directly to their access to employment since they are not as likely as the wealthy to have investment income. The likelihood of the middle-SES group experiencing undesirable events should be, and was, related to the unemployment rate.

The pattern for high-SES respondents, which indicates that they are less likely to have undesirable job and financial events as unemployment increases, can be explained if one assumes that the group is less likely to take employment and investment risks during sluggish than during improving economies. Because a proportion of high-risk ventures fail, failures should decrease in number as the number of ventures decrease. If risk-taking behavior is related positively to the status of the economy, high-SES respondents should experience fewer adverse job and financial experiences in sluggish economies.

Comparison with the Aggregate Findings

The fact that a main effect of economic contraction on undesirable job and financial events was not found is inconsistent with the most frequently cited aggregate literature that reports strong, pervasive effects of economic contraction (e.g., Brenner, 1976). While this lack of convergence may be due to methodological artifacts (e. g., Borgatta & Jackson, 1980; Firebaugh, 1978) it may also be that the aggregate, time-series methods capture effects not implied by the three explanations tested in this paper. At least three possible additional mechanisms could be at work. The first of these is that the economy may have a direct effect on illness and injury in addition to its effect _via_ undesirable job or financial events. This direct effect could take at least two forms. The first is a cognitive mechanism in which the anticipation of undesirable events may elicit stress reactions or increase the risk of injury by accident. The second is a contagion effect in that individuals who are ill with infectious syndromes or who are distracted in part because they experienced undesirable job or financial events may infect or become safety hazards for others who have not experienced or anticipated such events.

The direct-effect hypothesis was tested by modeling four contingency tables, each of which included one of the economic variables and sex, age, socio-economic status, total job or financial events, illness and injury, and other events not involving health, job, and finances. No effect of any economic variable was found, controlling for the demographic and life event variables, on the odds of being ill or injured.

A second reason why the results reported in this paper differ from those in the aggregate research may be that experiencing an undesirable job and financial event increases the odds of experiencing subsequent events not involving health, job or finances. These events, which were conceptualized as control variables in the above analyses, were found to be related to illness or injury. This explanation of the difference between the findings reported above and aggregate analyses is supported by the results of modeling a contingency table formed by the demographic and life-event variables. The odds of experiencing an event not involving health, job or finances are related significantly to the experience of an undesirable job or financial event when the effect of positive and indifferent job and financial events is controlled. The coefficients for this model indicate that the three life event variables are positively related. This association does not imply that undesirable job and financial events "cause" an increased risk of events not involving health, job or finances. The association however, is consistent with the argument that the discrepancy between the results described above and the aggregate research is due to such a causal relationship.

A third explanation for the apparent divergence of the findings reported in this paper and the aggregate-time series research is that the economy was too benign during the observed period to detect the intuitive effect of contraction on other than the middle-SES respondents. This is a plausible argument given that the economy of the Los Angeles-Long Beach SMSA did not exhibit any dramatic downturns during the three test years 1978 through 1980. It is possible that this analysis measures the effect of normal oscillations in economic activity rather than of societally significant economic dislocations such as the recession of 1981/82. This proposition cannot be tested with the current survey data set but, as noted below, data should soon be available to make such a test possible.

Implications

The findings reported above have implications for both theory and practice. The principal theoretical contribution of these analyses has been to test rigorously the proposition that economic phenomena affect health through psycho-social stressors. Of equal theoretical importance is that the analyses were designed to reinforce or discredit competing descriptions of the nature of the processes assumed to connect the economy to health. The proposition has passed the test. The nature of the connecting mechanism appears, at least for middle-SES respondents, to be that economic contraction affects the incidence of undesirable job and financial events that, in turn, increase the risk of illness and injury. The findings at the individual level converge with the existing theoretical and empirical literature dealing with stressful life events in general and with job and financial events in particular (Warr, 1982). They also extend that research by demonstrating that the incidence of life events may not be stochastic but may be related to community processes of long-standing interest to sociologists (e.g., Durkheim, 1897; McKenzie, 1926).

The findings involving the economic climate do not converge with the aggregate time-series research in the field in that economic contraction appears to affect the middle- and upper-SES groups in diametrically opposed directions while not affecting the low-SES respondents at all. This finding, while not hypothesized, is explicable and demonstrates that the most intuitively solid link in the assumed chain, that people have more undesirable job and financial events when the economy contracts, is not simple and requires as much analytic attention as the connection of life events to illness.

Literature has appeared describing the possible contributions of research such as this to primary prevention and the formation of public policy (e.g., Catalano and Dooley, 1981; Sclar, 1981). This literature argues, in essence, that policy decisions are based on explicit or implicit cost/benefit analyses and that the costs of policy alternatives may have been underestimated through an ignorance of the effects discovered in research such as this. It is argued that if the costs were better understood, more humane policies would be adopted thereby making the regulatory system a means of primary prevention.

It has also been noted that the implications of the findings for the provision of health services are potentially great (Catalano and Dooley, 1981; Liem, 1981). Should the research progress to the point that the effect of economic climate on health can be modeled, the health services community would be in an advantageous position to render preventive services as well as to plan the deployment of remedial services. Further research could identify those groups or geographic areas likely to be most affected by expected changes in public and private investment policies. Primary prevention programs could be targeted to those groups through labor unions or through geographically defined organizations (e.g., churchs). Even if preventive services were not fiscally possible or were ineffective, the ability to model the effect of economic change on health could allow institutions to increase the deployment of remedial services when needed and to decrease them when less likely to be used.

Future research should test the proposition that more extreme economic conditions than those observed during this study would yield more intuitive findings regarding the probability of experiencing undesirable job and financial events. The authors will soon have collected four additional survey waves of data. Three of these surveys were conducted in the first three quarters of 1981. The fourth wave will be conducted in the summer of 1982. The economic conditions during these surveys will be much more severe than during the three years sampled by the twelve surveys used in the analyses in this paper. These added data should allow a test of the severity hypothesis.

Future research needs to be more specific regarding health outcomes than are the analyses reported above. Among dependent variables of interest are days lost from work or reduced social activity due to health problems, as well as incidence of specific stress-related syndromes (e.g., gastrointestinal disorder). Additional research also needs to disaggregate the sample by ethnic group and by participation in the labor force. The effect of economic change on workers, for example, may be significantly greater than on a representative sample such as that used in this study. Worker samples also could be disaggregated by industrial sector to improve the ability to simulate the effects of industry-specific economic fluctuations.

FOOTNOTE

1. The log-linear coefficients suggested that low-SES respondents, regardless of sex, were unaffected by employment change. The likelihood of middle-SES males experiencing an undesirable job or financial event was not affected by a reduction in total employment, decreased with employment stability, and increased with employment growth. Middle-SES females were similarly unaffected by employment contraction but reaction to stability and growth was opposite that for males. The likelihood of middle-SES females experiencing an undesirable job or financial event increased with stability and decreased with growth. Neither sex of high-SES was affected by employment contraction. High-SES males reacted to stability and contraction identically to middle-SES females whereas high-SES females reacted identically to middle-SES males.

REFERENCES

Aneshensel, C. S., R. R. Frerichs, V. A. Clark, and P. A. Yokopenic
    1982   "Measuring depression in the community: A comparison of telephone and personal interviews." Public Opinion Quarterly 46:110-21.

Borgatta, Edgar, and David Jackson
    1980   Aggregate Data Analysis and Interpretation. Beverly Hills: Sage.

Breed, W.
    1963   "Occupational mobility and suicide among white males." American Sociological Review 28:179-88.

Brenner, M. Harvey
    1971   "Economic changes and heart disease mortality." American Journal of Public Health 59:1154-68.
    1973   Mental Illness and the Economy. Cambridge: Harvard University Press.
    1976   "Estimating the social costs of national economic policy: Implications for mental and physical health and criminal aggression." Paper No. 5., Report to the Congressional Research Service of the Library of Congress and Joint Committee of Congress. Washington, DC: U.S. Government Printing Office.

Brown, George W., and Tirrel Harris
    1978   Social Origins of Depression: A Study of Psychiatric Disorder in Women. New York: Free Press.

Bunn, A. R.
    1979   "Ischaemic heart disease mortality and the business cycle in Australia." American Journal of Public Health 69:772-81.

Catalano, R. A.

    1979   "Health costs of economic expansion: The case of manufacturing accident injuries." American Journal of Public Health 69:789-94.

Catalano, R. A., and C. D. Dooley

    1977   "Economic predictors of depressed mood and stressful life events." Journal of Health and Social Behavior 18:292-307.

    1981   "The behavioral costs of economic instability." Policy Studies Journal 10:338-49.

Catalano, R. A., C. D. Dooley, and R. L. Jackson

    1981   "Economic predictors of admissions to mental health facilities in a nonmetropolitan community." Journal of Health and Social Behavior 22:284-97.

Clogg, Clifford C.

    1979   Measuring Underemployment: Demographic Indicators for the United States. New York: Academic Press.

Dixon, W. J., and Morton B. Brown (eds.)

    1977   BMDP-77 Biomedical Computer Programs: P-Series. Berkeley: University of California Press.

Dohrenwend, B. S., L. Krasnoff, A. R. Askensy, and B. P. Dohrenwend

    1978   "Exemplification of a method for scaling life events: The PERI life events scale." Journal of Health and Social Behavior 19: 205-29.

Dooley, C. D., and R. A. Catalano

    1979   "Economic, life, and disorder changes: Time-series analysis." American Journal of Community Psychology 7:381-96.

    1980   "Economic change as a cause of behavioral disorder." Psychological Bulletin 87:450-68.

Dooley, C. D., R. A. Catalano, R. L. Jackson, and A. Brownell
  1981   "Economic, life, and symptom changes in a nonmetropolitan community." Journal of Health and Social Behavior 22:144-54.

Durkheim, Emille
  1897   Suicide: A Study in Sociology. Paris: Alcan.

Eyer, J.
  1977   "Prosperity as a cause of death." International Journal of Health Services 7:125-50.

Fienberg, Stephen E.
  1978   The Analysis of Cross-Classified Categorical Data. Massachusetts: MIT Press.

Firebaugh, G.
  1978   "A rule for inferring individual-level relationships from aggregate data." American Sociological Review 43:557-72.

Groves, Robert M., and Robert L. Kahn
  1979   Surveys by Telephone: A National Comparison with Personal Interviews. New York: Academic Press.

Hollingshead, August B., and Frederick L. Redlich
  1958   Social Class and Mental Illness. New York: Wiley.

Holmes, T. H., and R. E. Rahe
  1967   "The social readjustment rating scale." Journal of Psychosomatic Research 11:213-18.

Horowitz, M., C. Schaefer, D. Hiroto, N. Wilner, and B. Levin
  1977   "Life event questionnaire for measuring presumptive stress." Psychosomatic Medicine 39:413-31.

Jordan, L. A., A. C. Marcus, and L. G. Reeder
  1980   "Response styles in telephone and household interviewing: A field experiment." Public Opinion Quarterly 44:210-22.

Kasl, S. V.
  1979   "Mortality and the business cycle: Some questions about research strategies when utilizing macro-social and ecological data." American Journal of Public Health 64:784-88.

Kasl, S. V., and S. Cobb
  forth- "Variability of stress effects among men experiencing job loss."
  coming In L. Goldberger and S. Breznitz (eds.), Handbook of Stress. New York: The Free Press.

Kasl, S. V., S. Gore, and S. Cobb
  1975   "The experience of losing a job: Repeated changes in health, symptoms, and illness behavior." Psychosomatic Medicine 37:106-22.

Klecka W. R., and A. J. Tuchfarber
  1978   "Random digit dialing: A comparison to personal surveys." Public Opinion Quarterly 42:105-14.

Lew, E. A.
  1979   "Mortality and the business cycle: How far can we push an association?" American Journal of Public Health 69:782-83.

Liem, R.
  1981   "Unemployment and mental health: Implication for human service policy." Policy Studies Journal 10:350-64.

McKenzie, R.
  1926   "The ecological approach to the study of the human community." Pp. 63-80 in Robert Park and Ernest Burgess (eds.), The City. Chicago: University of Chicago Press.

Mark, M. M.

    1979   "The causal analysis of concomitancies in time series." Pp. 321-39 in Thomas D. Cook and Donald T. Campbell (eds.), Quasi-Experimentation: Design and Analysis Issues for Field Settings. Chicago: Rand McNally.

Marshall, J. R., and R. W. Hodge

    1981   "Durkheim and Pierce on suicide and economic change." Social Science Research 10:101-114.

Pearlin, L. I., M. A. Lieberman, E. G. Menaghan, and J. T. Mullan

    1981   "The stress process." Journal of Health and Social Behavior 22:337-56.

Pierce, A.

    1967   "The economic cycle and social suicide rate." American Sociological Review 32:457-62.

Rabkin, J. G., and E. L. Struening

    1976   "Life events, stress, and illness." Science 194:1013-20.

Rahe, R. H.

    1974   "The pathway between subjects' recent life changes and their near-future illness reports: Representative results and methodological issues." Pp. 73-86 in Barbara S. Dohrenwend and Bruce P. Dohrenwend (eds.), Stressful Life Events: Their Nature and Effects. New York: Wiley.

Rogers, T. F.

    1976   "Interview by telephone and in person: Quality of responses and field performance." Public Opinion Quarterly 40:51-65.

Ross C. E., and J. Mirowsky

    1979   "A comparison of life event-weighting-schemes: Changes, undesirability, and effect-proportional indices." Journal of Health and Social Behavior 20:166-77.

Sclar, E.

    1981   "Social costs minimization: A national policy approach to the problems of distressed economic regions." Policy Studies Journal 10:235-47.

Swafford, M.

    1980   "Three parametric techniques for contingency table analysis: A nontechnical commentary." American Sociology Review 45:664-90.

Tausig, M.

    1982   "Measuring life events." Journal of Health and Social Behavior 23:52-64.

Theorell, T.

    1974   "Life events before and after the onset of premature myocardial infarction." Pp. 101-17 in Barbara S. Dohrenwend and Bruce P. Dohrenwend (eds.), Stressful Life Events: Their Nature and Effect. New York: Wiley.

Theorell, T., and B. Floderus-Myrhed

    1977   "'Workload' and risk of myocardial infarction: A prospective psychological analysis." International Journal of Epidemiology 6: 17-21.

Troldahl, V. C., and R. E. Carter

    1964   "Random selection of respondents within households in phone surveys." Journal of Marketing Research 1:71-76.

Uhlenhuth E. H., S. J. Haberman, M. B. Balter, and R. S. Lipman
    1977   "Remembering life events." Pp. 117-34 in John S. Straus, Haroutun M. Babigian and A. M. Roff, (eds.), The Origins and Course of Psychopathology. New York: Plenum Press.

Warr, P., and G. Parry
    1982   "Paid employment and women's psychological well-being." Psychological Bulletin 19:498-516.

This research was supported by a grant from the Center for the Study of Work and Mental Health of NIMH (MH# 28934-10A1). The authors acknowledge the contributions of Arlene Brownell, Robert Jackson, Norman Jacobson, James Wichelman, James Hayes, and Mary Komarnicki. Reprints available from first author.

HEALTH PROBLEMS AND PSYCHO-SOCIAL STRAINS OF UNEMPLOYED
A Summary of Recent Empirical Research in the
Federal Republic of Germany

Christian Brinkmann

Institute of Employment Research of the Federal Employment Institute
Nuremberg, Federal Republic of Germany

1. Preface

Since the end of the 50's unemployment was not a serious problem in the Federal Republic of Germany. Until the early 1970's - due to high rates of economic growth and a declining potential labor force - a growing shortage of domestic labor led to a rising number of foreign workers. The economic recession of 1966/67 was short and relatively mild. The average number of unemployed reached its lowest points in 1965 and 1970 (about 150 000 unemployed, less than 1% of the employed).

In terms of international comparison, this labor market situation was quite atypical. It has changed, however, much to the worse since the "First oil crisis" and the recession of 1974/75. In the long term perspective the economic growth rate declined and the demographic situation reversed; until about 1990 about 1 million additional persons will enter the potential domestic labor force, also the second and third generation of foreign workers in Germany will lead to a higher supply of labor. According to long-term projections only in the 1990's may there be a reversal in the overall labor market situation. Until then - without appropriate economic and labor market policy efforts, especially including measures reducing working time - the rise in the number of unemployed will almost be certain. The present recession level: about 1 1/4 million are registered as unemployed and an estimated additional 800 000 so-called "Silent reserve" (discouraged workers not officially registered as unemployed). All the figures in this paper refer to registered unemployed only; it should be kept in mind, however, that the second group may be subject to health problems, too.

As a regular source of information about the structure of registered unemployment, the Federal Employment Institute, starting in 1973, provides at least once a year detailed statistics, also on "health problems relevant to re-employment efforts". If there is an officially certified reduction in working capability ("Minderung der Erwerbsfähigkeit", relevant to insurance benefits), this fact is also noted in addition. In most other cases, information about these health problems comes from the unemployed himself.

In addition to these regular unemployment statistics - supplemented recently by inflow and outflow statistics - a few respresentative unemployment surveys were undertaken, especially a follow-up study in 1975 by our institute (short: IAB-study) and a follow-up study in 1978 by Infratest institute (short: infratest study), the latter requested by the Federal Ministry of Labour. Most research results cited in this paper were gained from these two studies.

2. Unemployed reporting health problems relevant to re-employment efforts: amount and development

Between 1975 (bottom of the recession) and 1979 the proportion of unemployed with health problems rose continously from 20% to 34% (figure 1). Selection processes resulted in a rising number of unemployed with health problems (by some 50.000 to about 250.000 persons) while overall unemployment figures were reduced somewhat.

Prior to the current labour market crisis, however, on a much lower level of unemployment, the proportion of unemployed with health problems was already quite high [32% in September 1973 (70.000 persons)]. The labour market slack in its first recession phase (1974) reduced this proportion considerably, even though absolute numbers of those unemployed climbed up, too. Selection processes unfavorable to this group of unemployed mainly take place later on during the up-swing phases and in long periods of labour market slack.

Accordingly, at the present recession time in Germany the relative situation of unemployed with health problems seems to ease somewhat, signalling no general change, however, it just means a below average risk of losing jobs, mainly due to a job protection law for seriously disabled (Schwerbehinderte) and to a wide spread protection against dismissal for older workers being part of many labour agreements. Upon becoming unemployed, chances for re-entry into the employment system are much below average. It is the latter fact which proves to be the main problem for persons with health problems.

The development of unemployment was more unfavorable for those with severely reduced working capability than for other unemployed with health problems (figure 1). It has to be recognized, however, that at least part of this results from a change in legal definition: In 1974 legislation led to a still rising number of persons with officially certified reduction in working capability.

3. Consequences of health problems to unemployment patterns

I mentioned already unfavorable selection processes for persons with health problems; empirical evidence on this will be cited in this section. The next section will deal with the question how far unemployment additionally leads to strains of health.

In 1975 IAB-study showed that one year after drawing the sample only 22% of registered unemployed with health problems relevant to re-employment efforts were back in work, as compared 43% of those without. Even considering the different age structures of both groups - elderly unemployed generally having heavily reduced reintegration chances - the marked differences in re-employment ratios between both groups remained at the same level (figure 2).

Other studies showed similar results, especially the infratest-study of 1978 which also yielded supplementary information by questionning personnel of local employment bureaus and employers: 1*)

- According to a representative sample of placement, personnel health problems (besides lack of qualification or job experience) play a leading role in respect to occupational reintegration problems of long-term unemployed - a greater role than older age and a much greater role than other factors (family situation, occupational attachment, motivation to work, etc.)
- Unemployed themselves have a similar view; they think that personal difficulties in finding a new job are mainly connected with their special occupation, their age, their special need or wish of getting a part-time job, health problems and lack of qualification.
- Employers, however, see things differently; according to them health problems and age just play a minor role (places 14 and 15 out of 18 possible reasons). Reintegration problems would mainly be due to

---

1 *) Infratest, 1978, pp. 89

"lack of qualification", "not reliable", "fluctuation too high", "didn't want to work", "lack of experience".

Considering re-employment ratios as well as the dominant and quasi neutral view in employment bureaus, this just means that factual discrimination of unemployed with health problems in the hiring process is one thing, giving reasons obviously another.

At the same time, there is a strong connection between health problems and the duration of unemployment spells, as figure 3 shows (tree analysis with dichotomous splits on the basis of maximal reduction of between-group variance). In this analysis, the main causal direction cannot be seen immediately. A supplementary tree analysis (health problems relevant to re-employment efforts being the dependent variable) indicates however, that dominant influences on the occurrence of such health problems happen prior to the incidence of unemployment: According to the IAB data in very many cases health problems were of importance already at the time unemployed lost or quitted their last job (reduction of variance 14%, much more than by any other single factor). Age and occupational status prior to unemployment also played a role (reduction of variance 6% rsp. 4%). In addition, the duration of unemployment exerts some but no very strong influence (reduction of variance in the first stage of analysis 4%); this influence is - as far as could be seen from the material - partially independent form other factors. In connection with these results it has to be kept in mind that basis of the analysis were self-reported health problems relevant to re-employment efforts, not however, the whole scale of possible physical or psychical strains or sickness.

4. Consequences of unemployment to health problems

The infratest unemployment panel study went much more into details of health problems, double-questionning the unemployed using the same items (figures 4 and 5; drawing the sample in the fall of 1977, first interviews early 1978, second interviews in the fall of 1978). First of all, factors characterizing working place and occupational history prior to unemployment were found in this study to have a significant influence on the occurrence of diverse aspects of bad health. Unemployed with health problems had "above average bad conditions in their last working place such as unsuitable, cramped position, monotonous, uninteresting work, unfavorable weather conditions, increased danger of accidents, noise, bad air, heavy physical work, shift work, piece work." 1*)

Among unemployed who at the second time of interviewing still or again were registered as unemployed there was - as expected - a higher proportion of those with reduced working capability, diverse health problems and also (on a subjective basis) a feeling of bad health. The research team found it "plausible to assume that negative consequences of the occupational history prior to unemployment and the direct influence of unemployment would cumulate to a higher risk on health." 2*)

Surprisingly, no signigicant differences on health problems showed up for those (long-term) unemployed who where registered as such at both times of interviewing (figures 4 and 5). As interviews took place for the first time at least several months after unemployment started, this result may not be over interpreted, however, changes possibly happening just in the first months of unemployment could not be measured because of the chosen research design.

Changes from in-between employment (T1) to renewed unemployment (T2) were found to worsen health problems, on the other hand movements from unemployment out of the labour force or going out of the labour force as in the case of housewives were found to ease health problems. The main conclusion of the authors:

"The strongest visible influence on the (subjective) state of health is not exerted - as often is assumed on the basis of cross-sectional comparisons - by the relative duration of unemployment, but by the <u>employment status</u> itself and its <u>change</u> in time. This will be seen especially in psycho-somatic dimensions: unemployed still or again in this status at the end of the follow-up period show at the end more sleeping disturbances and stomach pains; re-employed people, however, indicate less nervous restlessness, yet at the same time <u>more</u> stomach pains, states of exhaustion and of being tired and of being worn out as compared to early 1978. This illustrates the bias of argumentations now and again being heard of, which emphasize the dangers to health connected with unemployment and which neglect the proven health hazards connected with

---
1*) Büchtemann, Rosenbladt, 1981, p. 31
2*) P. 32

the working process, especially in the initial phase at a new working place." 1*)

5. Psycho-social consequences of unemployment

Unemployment, especially long-term unemployment, not only means financial restraints, but also may lead to severe psycho-social problems. These problems may be different for different groups of unemployed and they need to be viewed in a dynamic manner, since failure in attempts to find a new job may change motivation to work and attitudes toward unemployment and employment.

At present, a single and operationalized way to measure psycho-social strains of unemployed does not exist. The IAB-study used the concept of <u>social roles</u> to structure the problem area:

In the first place unemployment means a disturbance of the work role and - complementary - the "leisure role", with changing time perspectives and losing control over fields of action. Additionally, social ties (to colleagues, neighbours, friends) may be disrupted. Changing interaction patterns (especially within the family) may conflict with role expectations, disrupted work contacts may result in isolation, societal attitudes toward unemployment may lead to a lower self-esteem of the unemployed and even stigmatize them. In the last consequence, due to strains on all social ties, serious crises of personal identity may be the result of unemployment.

As a matter of fact, the study showed that - in general, young unemployed were an exception, for instance - psycho-social strains were felt to be a greater burden by the unemployed than financial strains. Increase in leisure time as a result of unemployment proved to be a major problem. Half of the unemployed felt that "staying at home got on their nerves", the same proportion felt "absolutely useless sometimes" (figure 6).

Unemployment, indeed, also means a great strain on social relations: For half of the unemployed "it was not easy" to tell friends and acquaintances that they were out of work. This clearly indicates (the fear of) negative reactions of the environment. The fact that one third of the unemployed did not visit their friends and acquaintances as frequently as they used to before they were out of work indicates problems

---

1*) Büchtemann, Rosenbladt, 1981, p.34

of isolation. One third of the unemployed reported more aggravation in the family than usual. Only a comparatively small part of the unemployed (17%) blamed themselves for being out of work (indicator for problems involving crisis of identity).

As the supplementary table (7a) shows, the statements may be - by factor analysis - reduced to three dimensions:
Factor 1: strains on social relations (social well-being dimension of health according to WHO definition).
Factor 2: positive aspects dominating over strains
Factor 3: strains on personal identity (mental well-being dimension of health according to WHO definition).

At a first glance no continuous relationship can be seen between <u>duration of unemployment</u> and psycho-social strains. This has to be viewed partially as a methodological problem, since in this case only cross-sectional comparisons are possible (between groups of short-term and long-term unemployed having quite a different structure according to age, sex, qualification, etc.)

Generally and especially in this connection one important finding was that unemployed having <u>socially and financially acceptable alternative roles to employment</u> (older unemployed qualifying for early pension schemes after one year of unemployment; married women taking over the role of a full-time housewife more or less voluntarily; youngsters having the chance of re-entering in the educational system, etc.) showed up with considerably fewer strains than unemployed without such aternatives (figures 6 and 7). If we restrict the analysis to the latter group (male unemployed who after one year were either back in work or still/ again unemployed), a certain, though not very strong influence also of the duration of unemployment on persons with fewer problems especially in the group unemployed for 3 months or less, will be seen.

A supplementary tree analysis not yet published comes to a similar result (figure 8). <u>Dominant</u> influences in psycho-social strains in general (apart from special dimensions, using an index on the basis of the <u>numbers</u> of problems indicated on the questionnaire) are financial strains, alternative roles, sex and marital status, <u>not</u> however duration of unemployment.

Figure 6 also contains some new findings for unemployed with health problems: For them psycho-social strains - as well as financial strains - are somewhat higher than for other unemployed. It has to be noted however that differences are not as marked as should have been assumed on the basis of their reduced re-employment chances. This obviously is connected with the fact that an above average proportion of these unemployed leave the labour market (figure 2); in case of such alternatives there should be relatively fewer strains, in contrast to the unemployed with health problems but without alternatives who will be in a much more difficult situation.

6. <u>Depression, "anxiety in social situations", "expectation of failure", fatalism, resignation, status uncertainty, change in consumption of cigarettes, alcohol and drugs</u>.

In some other recent studies <u>validated scales</u> were used to measure special aspects of psychical burdens of unemployed:

<u>Mohr</u> and <u>Frese</u> investigated a smaller group of unemployed male blue collar workers above the age of 45 in respect to depression (prospective panel with double interviewing using the same scale).
They found out that "unemployment causes depressive signs. It could be seen that variables like <u>control</u>, <u>activity</u> and <u>financial strains</u> are important moderating variables". 1*) To what extent did the length of unemployment exert a direct influence was not reported, probably because of the relatively small empirical basis (147 persons in the sample). It also remains a question of how far does this result also hold for other groups of unemployed (figure 9).

The <u>infratest-study</u> used scales on "anxiety in social situations" and "expectation of failure", analysing results from both interviews at the beginning and the end of the reference period, like <u>Mohr</u> and <u>Frese</u> mainly using changes in employment status as basis for their interpretation (figure 10). Results are quite differentiated: Changes from unemployment to employment or to full-time house work have relieving effects, equally the staying of formerly unemployed persons in work.

Remaining unemployed (or being unemployed again) leads to <u>higher</u> "expectation of failure", but at the same time also to <u>less</u> "anxiety in social situations", the latter meaning adaption and getting used to the unemployment situation. In different strain dimensions unemployment obvious-

---

1*) Mohr, Frese, 1978, p. 192

ly may have different or even reverse consequences. In addition the authors state explicitly that in no way may a "natural law-linear" influence of unemployment on the psycho-social constitution be assumed: the reported changes are net changes of group averages; behind them partially reverse changes may be found for single persons or subgroups of unemployment, as may be seen from figure 11.

In this connection it should further be mentioned that a further unemployment study of the ISO-institute - Mr. Fröhlich reports from this study on this symposium - concentrated, among other research areas, on the connection between unemployment and fatalism. According to their findings male and female long-term unemployed (12 months or longer) score significantly higher on a fatalism scale than short-term unemployed and employees in work; because of the cross-sectional research design, the existing cross-tabulations leave the question of causal direction somewhat open, however. 1*)

Heinemann, Röhrig and Stadié studied women unemployed and not unemployed, double-questionning them after half a year. Among other physical problems and psycho-somatic strains resignation was shown to be a result of unemployment (figure 12): There is a considerable reduction of it after re-employment, and a certain increase for long-term unemployed. Somewhat different from results of Fröhlich (for unemployed men), at least for women, "connection to work" and "work orientation" do not seem to play a central role in this connection; they also seem to be somewhat influenced by unemployment themselves, but problems of operationalization may play a role in this respect.

On the basis of group dynamic theory and stigmatization concepts Reinke-Dieker developed and tested (on a very small sample of about 100 unemployed) the hypothesis that unemployment mainly leads to status uncertainty . This seems to be quite plausible, more so than the general thesis of status reduction or downgrading: according to empirical studies in Germany unemployment may result in upward mobility as well as in downgrading.

A representative cross-sectional study of 1800 unemployed in special urban areas undertaken by a research team in Göttingen (Sozialwissen-

---

1*) Hentschel, Möller, Pintar, 1977, pp. 210
   Fröhlich 1979, pp. 98

schaftliche Arbeitsgruppe WAL) developed a typology of psychical dispositions of unemployed using statements about suffering because of unemployment, depression and signs of worthlessness. These dispositions partly depend on financial strains, and they are very strongly related to self-reported physical sickness during unemployment, change in consumption of cigarettes, alcohol and drugs (figure 13). These interdependencies should be considered in regression analyses.

7. Concluding remarks

Recent empirical research on the consequences of unemployment lead to the general conclusion that one picture of the unemployed with his problems and his ways of dealing subjectively with his situation cannot be drawn. Instead, physical and psycho-social consequences of unemployment - as well as financial strains - may be very different for certain groups of unemployed.

Even though there is a lot of information available on such strains, detailed analyses of the psycho-dynamic processes connected with unemployment still remains to be undertaken. Also many questions remain open in relation to the very high proportion of people with physical health problems among the unemployed.

All studies reported here were restricted to a reference period of one to two years; long-term consequences of unemployment therefore remained out of the scope of these pieces of research. Probably even more important, high unemployment also may have severe negative consequences on physical health as well as on psycho-social well-being of those not actually unemployed but working permanently or for a long time under the more or less concrete threat of possible future unemployment: If, for instance, the proportion of such employees in companies is lower in times of a recession, this may imply additional health hazards in the long run perspective. Present studies allow no conclusions in this respect.

Figure 1: Registered unemployed 1973-1980 with health problems relevant to re-employment efforts and officially recognized reduction in working capability, in %

Unemployed	1973	1974	September 1975	1976	1977	1978	1979	1980
(1) with health problems, together	31,9	23,5	20,2	24,7	26,8	29,4	33,9	32,2
among them: (2) without official recognition of reduction in working capability	24,4	19,0	16,7	19,8	21,0	22,2	24,3	22,7
among them: (3) with official recogn. of reduction in working cap ability	7,4	4,5	3,5	5,0	5,8	7,2	9,7	9,5
(4) - reduction 80% and more	.	.	0,4	0,6	0,7	1,0	1,4	1,5
(5) - reduction 50% to under 80%	.	.	2,2	3,4	3,9	4,9	6,5	6,3
(6) - red. 30% to u. 50%, considered as "seriously disabled" (Schwerbehind.)	.	.	0,8	0,3	0,4	0,4	0,5	0,4
(7) - red. 30% to under 50%, else (without Gleichstellung)	.	.		0,7	0,8	0,9	1,3	1,3
(8) sum "seriously disabled" (Schwerbehinderte) (4) - (6)	.	.	2,8*	4,4	5,0	6,3	8,3	8,2
(9) without such health problems	68,1	76,5	79,8	75,1	73,2	70,6	66,1	67,8
Sum	100	100	100	100	100	100	100	100
Overall number of unemployed	219 105	556 876	1 006 554	898 314	911 257	864 243	736 690	822 701
among them: number of unemployed with health probl. (corresponds to row 1)	69 856	130 898	202 861	223 368	244 048	254 115	249 808	265 310

Source: Brinkmann, 1981, on the base of official unemployment statistics

Figure 2: German unemployed of September 1974, according to age, health problems relevant to re-employment efforts and employment status in September 1975, in %

Employment status in Sept.75	All			Under 35 years			35-55 years			55 years or older		
	health problems			health problems			health problems			health problems		
	no	yes	sum	no	yes	sum	no	yes	sum	no	yes	sum
Registered unemployed	29,6	44,6	33,5	25,5	41,2	27,6	38,4	52,4	43,4	27,4	33,1	30,0
Employed	43,3	21,9	37,7	48,3	30,4	45,9	43,9	24,7	37,0	13,5	7,9	11,0
Education or further education	5,1	5,1	5,1	7,7	12,8	8,4	1,8	3,6	2,4	-	-	-
Else	22,0	28,4	23,7	18,5	15,6	18,1	16,0	19,3	17,2	59,1	59,0	59,1
Among them: housewife (fulltime)	11,9	7,9	10,8	13,7	9,5	13,1	11,2	9,8	10,7	4,3	2,7	3,6
Among them: pensioner	5,7	15,6	8,4	0,1	1,1	0,2	0,8	4,8	2,2	51,2	51,4	51,3
Sum	100	100	100	100	100	100	100	100	100	100	100	100
Number of cases	5064	1757	7024	3009	454	3495	1522	859	2381	533	444	980

Source: Brinkmann, Schober-Gottwald, 1976, p.100

Figure 3: Duration of spell of unemployment (at the end of registration, in months) as dependend variable
GERMAN UNEMPLOYED 20 YEARS OR OLDER, of September 1974
Tree analysis, R= reduction of variance in % of total variance
x= average duration of unemployment in months
n= number of cases

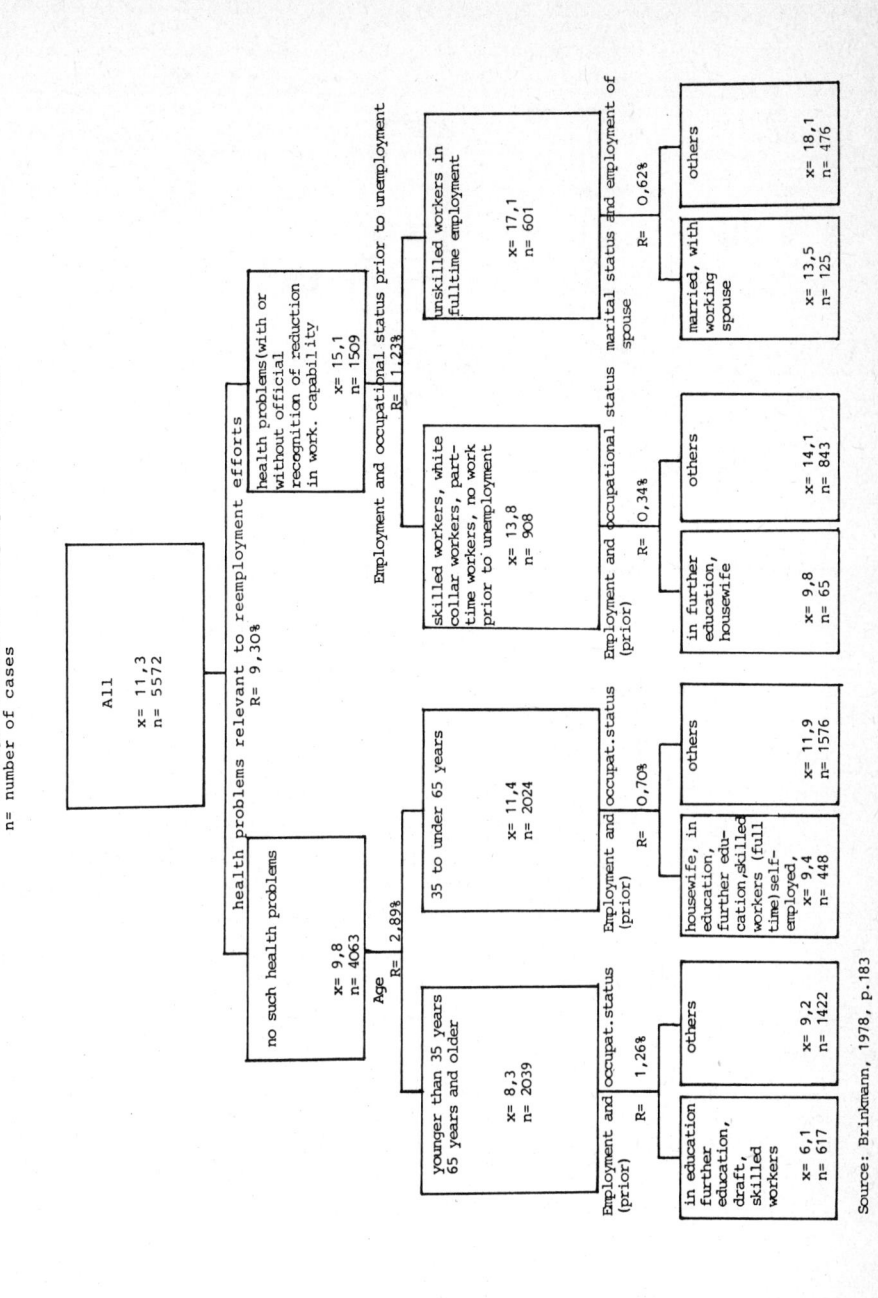

All
x= 11,3
n= 5572

health problems relevant to reemployment efforts
R= 9,30%

- no such health problems
  x= 9,8
  n= 4063

  Age
  R= 2,89%

  - younger than 35 years 65 years and older
    x= 8,3
    n= 2039

    Employment and occupat.status (prior)
    R= 1,26%

    - in education, further education, draft, skilled workers
      x= 6,1
      n= 617
    - others
      x= 9,2
      n= 1422

  - 35 to under 65 years
    x= 11,4
    n= 2024

    Employment and occupat.status (prior)
    R= 0,70%

    - housewife, in education, further education, skilled workers (full time), self-employed,
      x= 9,4
      n= 448
    - others
      x= 11,9
      n= 1576

- health problems (with or without official recognition of reduction in work. capability
  x= 15,1
  n= 1509

  Employment and occupational status prior to unemployment
  R= 1,23%

  - skilled workers, white collar workers, part-time workers, no work prior to unemployment
    x= 13,8
    n= 908

    Employment and occupational status (prior)
    R= 0,34%

    - in further education, housewife
      x= 9,8
      n= 65
    - others
      x= 14,1
      n= 843

  - unskilled workers in fulltime employment
    x= 17,1
    n= 601

    marital status and employment of spouse
    R= 0,62%

    - married, with working spouse
      x= 13,5
      n= 125
    - others
      x= 18,1
      n= 476

Source: Brinkmann, 1978, p.183

Figure 4: Proportion of unemployed and formerly unemployed (fall of 1977) with subjective feeling of bad health at the beginning and the end of the reference period, according to employment status at both times

Employment status		Proportion (%)
February 1978	November 1978	
employed	unemployed	13 / 19
employed	employed	9 / 8
unemployed	employed	16 / 16
unemployed	unemployed	32 / 32
unemployed	housewife	16 / 12
housewife	housewife	9 / 5

▓▓▓ proportion with subjective feeling of bad health in February 1978

☐ proportion with subjective feeling of bad health in November 1978

Source: Büchtemann, Rosenbladt, 1981, p.33

Figure 5: Proportion of unemployed and formerly unemployed (fall of 1977) with pains and signs of sickness within the last three months at T1 (beginning of reference period) and T2 (end of it), in %

T1 February 1978
T2 November 1978

pains and signs of sickness within the last three months	All unemployed at the time		T1 unemployed T2 unemployed at the time		T1 employed T2 unemployed at the time		T1 unemployed T2 employed at the time		T1 unemployed T2 housewife at the time		T1 employed T2 employed at the time	
	T1	T2	T1	T2	T1	T2	T1	T2	T1	T2	T1	T2
Basis of proportion (=100%)	1966	1966	404	404	50	50	366	366	151	151	531	531
Head ache	26	26	27	28	20	21	24	28	29	29	28	26
Rheumatism	7	8	12	11	4	3	7	8	6	9	4	6
spinal affection	13	15	20	20	10	13	12	14	13	16	9	11
Sleeping disturbances	13	13	20	20	8	15	13	12	20	11	7	8
nervous restlessness	15	16	22	24	21	16	18	14	15	16	11	13
Bronchitis	7	6	10	9	9	4	7	6	4	5	4	4
stomach pains	11	12	16	17	6	13	10	14	7	7	11	10
Abdominal pains	5	5	8	5	6	6	6	5	4	6	3	3
Heart aches	8	8	13	12	5	4	6	6	11	7	3	5
Blood circulation problems	21	21	28	26	14	24	22	22	27	23	12	15
High blood pressure	6	7	9	9	5	4	6	6	5	4	4	4
Diabetes	2	2	2	3	–	3	2	3	4	1	1	1
state of exhaustion and of being tired	9	11	13	14	5	5	6	11	10	11	7	8
Being worn out	8	10	10	10	15	9	7	13	7	8	7	11
Liver-/gall-bladder pains	5	5	9	9	4	2	5	4	3	4	3	3
feeling like feeding fishes	3	3	5	5	4	1	2	4	4	3	2	2
pains connected with the kidneys	5	4	6	6	3	4	6	3	4	4	3	3
pains connected with the uterus	5	4	6	5	4	2	5	3	6	6	2	3
skin diseases	3	3	2	3	4	7	3	2	3	5	3	3
phlebitis	4	4	6	6	–	4	2	3	7	6	2	2
pains connected with accidents	4	7	5	8	4	6	5	9	3	3	3	5
No such pains/diseases	22	26	21	18	24	19	24	27	17	22	25	32

Source: Büchtemann, Rosenbladt, 1981, p.33

Figure 6: German unemployed (20 years or older) of September 1974 according to psycho-social strains during unemployment, in %, base of the row proportions at the end of the row (=100%)

	very anxious getting a new job	felt absolutely useless sometimes	staying at home got on my nerves	missing contacts with colleagues	it was not easy to tell friends and acqu. about it	more aggravation in the family than usual	did not visit friends and acquaintances as often	often blamed myself for being out of work	unemployment seemed to me not as bad as I thought before	I used the time doing things I like	It was not bad to have more time for the family	number of cases (basis for proportions)
	1	2	3	4	5	6	7	8	9	10	11	12
All unemployed	71,3	55,3	55,0	52,6	44,9	31,8	31,5	17,4	29,7	45,7	47,0	4965
Males	75,2	62,4	65,0	46,0	54,5	42,6	38,9	23,9	23,4	39,6	35,3	2451
Females	67,2	47,4	43,9	59,4	34,7	20,5	23,5	10,6	36,1	52,3	58,9	2389
Without health problems relevant to re-employment	69,9	52,9	52,9	53,5	42,5	31,1	29,5	18,2	29,9	47,8	48,7	3549
With health problems, no off. recogn. of reduct. capability	75,5	61,6	60,8	49,7	51,8	33,6	37,3	16,1	28,6	39,2	42,7	1017
With health problems, with off. reduct. of work capability	72,9	58,5	56,1	52,5	49,6	33,6	32,9	12,2	30,4	44,0	41,9	273
With health problems (sum)	75,0	60,6	59,8	50,3	51,3	33,6	36,3	15,3	29,0	40,2	42,5	1290
Age 20 -under 25 years	66,5	31,3	54,0	53,5	35,4	35,7	25,3	20,3	30,2	51,2	46,5	911
25 -under 35 "	72,3	53,6	53,1	55,4	41,2	34,0	29,4	22,5	30,3	47,9	47,8	1356
35 -under 45 "	76,8	55,9	58,0	52,4	50,5	34,0	34,3	15,8	26,1	41,2	49,8	1010
45 -under 55 "	77,8	62,3	61,1	51,8	53,8	29,0	37,0	13,2	27,9	39,7	43,9	907
55 years or older	57,7	52,2	45,5	47,0	44,9	20,8	31,6	10,5	35,3	49,2	47,0	655
Employment status Sept. 75												
Employed	75,1	55,4	58,6	53,1	44,3	33,7	29,4	18,7	24,2	46,7	44,3	1866
Unemployed	80,9	65,0	64,0	51,9	53,8	37,6	39,1	19,9	26,3	38,8	40,4	1757
thereof: renewed spell	83,5	66,6	68,7	50,5	60,0	44,9	39,2	25,1	23,9	40,7	40,9	375
without interruption	80,2	64,4	62,8	52,3	52,3	35,6	39,0	18,7	27,0	38,4	40,2	1396
education,further education	65,1	54,9	53,7	47,4	36,3	35,0	25,6	21,0	30,9	51,0	39,6	215
Housewife	49,6	32,6	28,6	62,0	24,2	15,1	18,1	8,2	49,6	55,7	73,9	595
thereof:												
-"discouraged worker"	64,1	40,1	40,2	72,1	32,4	18,6	19,6	12,9	39,3	49,8	67,0	219
- no longer interested in work	23,9	15,7	10,0	41,2	11,1	8,2	9,3	4,5	63,3	66,7	82,9	114
- pensioner	43,0	42,9	34,5	45,6	39,8	17,7	29,3	7,7	41,3	55,7	54,5	330
Duration of unemployment:												
less than 1 month	58,4	39,4	45,5	41,4	38,8	20,9	20,6	20,6	21,1	41,2	39,7	137
1- less than 3 months	64,4	47,0	54,0	48,2	40,2	28,0	27,4	20,0	24,3	48,6	40,2	483
3- less than 6 "	73,0	54,5	58,9	51,0	41,6	33,2	28,2	16,5	26,7	50,3	47,7	581
6- less than 9 "	72,9	55,5	53,9	52,9	42,8	35,4	29,0	16,3	29,5	47,1	48,7	591
9- less than 12 "	67,6	53,0	49,5	56,1	39,6	27,8	29,3	15,8	35,3	52,9	53,5	678
12- less than 15 "	69,8	56,0	52,7	56,5	46,5	27,9	31,2	16,4	32,2	44,3	51,0	1087
15- less than 18 "	77,8	56,6	57,3	57,0	51,4	35,8	35,9	19,3	30,6	42,3	43,8	446
18- less than 24 "	78,7	62,8	61,2	47,9	50,2	39,7	39,8	18,9	29,1	41,8	41,8	493
24 months or more	75,5	66,0	64,1	49,0	56,4	38,1	41,5	17,6	26,3	32,9	37,4	269
Duration of unemployment for males "without status alternatives" (being in work or unemployed in September 75)												
less than 3 months	70,2	52,0	59,1	44,8	48,2	33,0	30,9	25,3	22,5	41,7	36,6	315
3 -under 9 months	83,8	61,1	67,8	45,3	54,0	47,7	36,1	23,5	20,2	41,1	36,9	469
9 -under 12 "	80,9	69,7	72,0	47,1	57,4	51,5	38,8	25,3	23,8	38,7	31,0	178
12 -under 18 "	83,7	71,5	74,1	52,1	63,6	47,0	46,2	29,2	17,9	30,6	30,4	314
18 months or more	80,9	72,7	73,8	43,4	59,3	47,8	48,2	22,3	21,9	32,5	29,4	404
Occupational status prior to unempl.												
unskilled blue collar worker	73,9	56,4	56,8	47,9	48,0	34,1	32,9	16,7	32,8	45,2	50,9	1539
skilled blue collar worker	72,1	60,3	63,2	48,9	50,1	39,5	33,7	18,3	26,6	43,4	42,1	720
white-collar worker in low or middle position	69,8	52,3	48,3	62,2	39,9	24,9	28,5	16,1	32,7	48,7	50,0	1260
white-collar worker in higher or leading pos.	72,9	57,1	60,0	59,8	53,2	31,9	37,6	20,4	22,8	41,4	38,7	516
During unemployment no great financial problems	44,6	36,4	35,9	46,8	29,0	14,3	19,6	12,0	46,0	59,4	59,8	854
During unemployment greater financial problems	83,8	67,5	69,1	53,0	55,9	49,4	45,8	25,5	20,2	38,9	39,3	1491

Source: Brinkmann, 1976, p.408

Figure 7: German unemployed (20 years or older) of September 1974, according to psycho-social strains during unemployment, duration of unemployment (at the end of registration, selected groups) and employment status in September 1975 (selected groups)

1. very anxious getting a new job
2. felt absolutely useless sometimes
3. staying at home got on my nerves
4. missing contacts with colleages
5. it was not easy to tell friends and acquaintances about unemployment
6. more aggravation in the family than usual
7. did not visit friends and acquaintances as often as before
8. often blamed myself for being out of work
9. unemployment seemed to me not as bad as I thought before
10. I used the time of unemployment doing things I like
11. It was not bad to have more time for the family

Duration of unemployment:
All ———
less than 1 month ― ― ―
2 years or longer ·······

Employment status September 1975:
employed
renewed spell of unemployment
still unemployed
housewife, no longer interested in work
pensioner

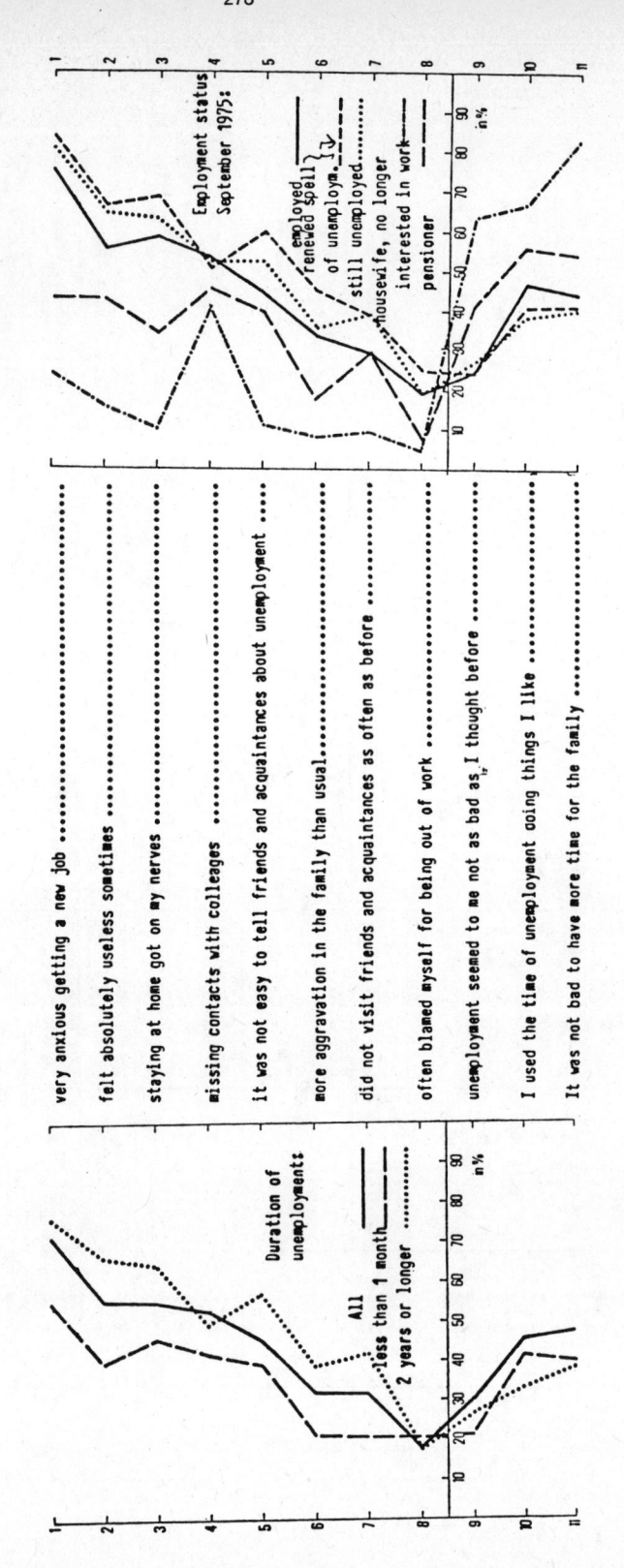

Source: Brinkmann, 1976, p. 410

Figure 7a: Factor analysis of <u>psycho-social strains</u> during unemployment
- German unemployed of Sept. 1974 (20 years or older) -

Total correlation matrix (description of dimensions see below)

TOW/COL=	1	2	3	4	5	6	7	8	9	10
1	1.00000									
2	-0.04216	1.00000								
3	0.08554	-0.18004	1.00000							
4	0.07651	-0.10507	0.25481	1.00000						
5	0.13879	-0.19482	0.22994	0.17264	1.00000					
6	0.16770	-0.22373	0.28960	0.24497	0.42803	1.00000				
7	-0.04833	0.25625	-0.15468	-0.10706	-0.26681	-0.25659	1.00000			
8	0.07974	-0.15911	0.23164	0.27124	0.30281	0.33179	0.17455	1.00000		
9	0.02215	0.37554	-0.15725	-0.08211	-0.18042	-0.22572	0.27494	-0.17177	1.00000	
10	0.16094	-0.29620	0.31566	0.21434	0.35898	0.49705	-0.26229	0.30291	-0.33131	1.00000
11	0.04400	-0.04102	0.18184	0.13981	0.14192	0.17624	-0.06018	0.17961	-0.08860	0.15536

Factor analysis:
Varimax rotated factor matrix
(normalized solution)

	ROW/COLUMN	1	2	3
missing contacts with colleages	1	0.07902	0.01810	0.26635
I used the time of unemployment doing things I like	2	-0.10866	<u>0.55768</u>	-0.07575
more aggravation in the family than usual	3	<u>0.43750</u>	-0.18624	0.17781
did not visit friends and acquaintances as often as before	4	<u>0.48893</u>	-0.05811	0.11360
very anxious getting a new job	5	0.23942	-0.24215	<u>0.48560</u>
felt absolutely useless sometimes	6	0.32464	-0.27323	<u>0.58845</u>
unemployment seemed to me not as bad as I thought before..	7	-0.10240	<u>0.39916</u>	-0.21332
it was not easy to tell friends and acquaintances about <u>un</u> employment	8	<u>0.43111</u>	-0.17557	0.25416
it was not bad to have more time for the family	9	-0.11014	<u>0.65167</u>	-0.01366
staying at home got on my nerves	10	0.30759	-0.41659	<u>0.44067</u>
often blamed myself for being out of work	11	0.30946	-0.04652	0.10309

	Factor Contributions
Factor 1 : strains on social relations	1.01007
Factor 2 : positive aspects dominating over strains	1.27323
Factor 3 : strains on personal identity	1.01838
<u>Sum</u>	3.30168

Figure 8: Amount of psycho-social strain during unemployment (index 0-8 according to number of dimensions indicated) as dependend variable; GERMAN UNEMPLOYED (20 years or older) of September 1974
Tree analysis, R= reduction of variance in % of total variance
x= group average (index)
n= number of cases

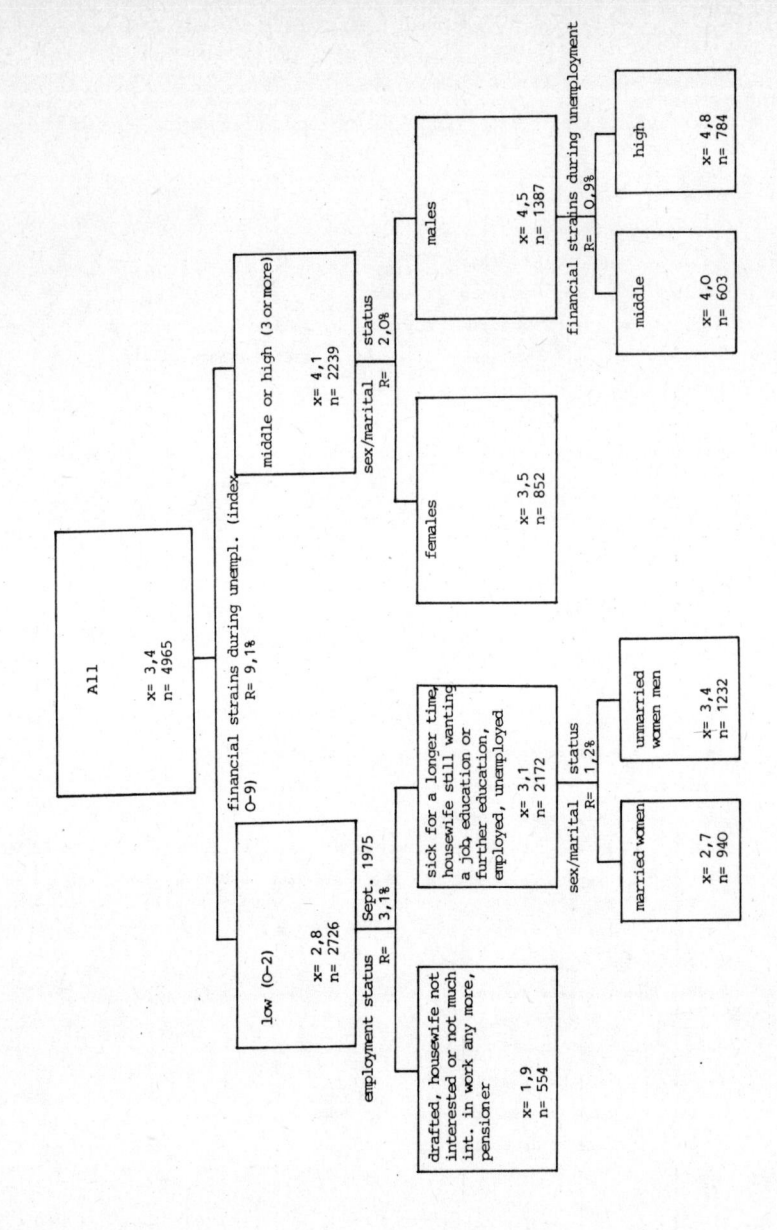

```
                              ┌─────────────┐
                              │    All      │
                              │   x= 3,4    │
                              │   n= 4965   │
                              └──────┬──────┘
                    financial strains during unempl. (index 0-9)
                                R= 9,1%
              ┌──────────────────────┴──────────────────────┐
        ┌─────────────┐                              ┌─────────────┐
        │  low (0-2)  │                              │ middle or high (3 or more) │
        │   x= 2,8    │                              │   x= 4,1    │
        │   n= 2726   │                              │   n= 2239   │
        └──────┬──────┘                              └──────┬──────┘
    employment status Sept. 1975                    sex/marital status
             R= 3,1%                                      R= 2,0%
    ┌────────┴────────┐                          ┌────────┴────────┐
┌─────────────┐ ┌─────────────┐            ┌─────────────┐ ┌─────────────┐
│ drafted,    │ │ sick for a  │            │  females    │ │   males     │
│ housewife   │ │ longer time,│            │   x= 3,5    │ │   x= 4,5    │
│ not         │ │ housewife   │            │   n= 852    │ │   n= 1387   │
│ interested  │ │ still want- │            └─────────────┘ └──────┬──────┘
│ or not much │ │ ing a job,  │                          financial strains during unemployment
│ int. in work│ │ education or│                                R= 0,9%
│ any more,   │ │ further edu-│                          ┌────────┴────────┐
│ pensioner   │ │ cation,     │                     ┌─────────────┐ ┌─────────────┐
│   x= 1,9    │ │ employed,   │                     │   middle    │ │    high     │
│   n= 554    │ │ unemployed  │                     │   x= 4,0    │ │   x= 4,8    │
└─────────────┘ │   x= 3,1    │                     │   n= 603    │ │   n= 784    │
                │   n= 2172   │                     └─────────────┘ └─────────────┘
                └──────┬──────┘
            sex/marital status
                  R= 1,2%
         ┌────────┴────────┐
    ┌─────────────┐ ┌─────────────┐
    │  married    │ │ unmarried   │
    │  women      │ │ women men   │
    │   x= 2,7    │ │   x= 3,4    │
    │   n= 940    │ │   n= 1232   │
    └─────────────┘ └─────────────┘
```

Source: IAB-study 1974/75

Figure 9: Change in _depressivity_ according to change in employment status
Male blue collar workers above the age of 45, all of them being unemployed at first time of interviewing (1975)

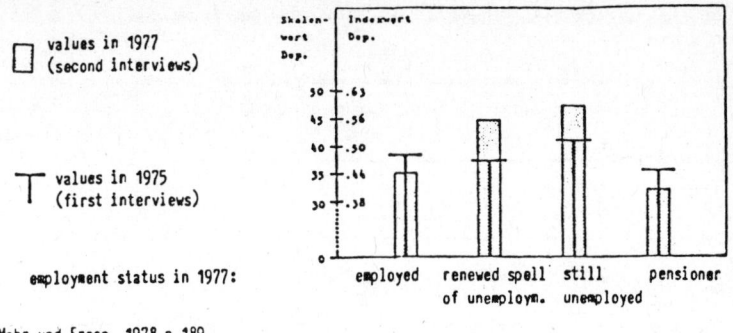

☐ values in 1977 (second interviews)

⊤ values in 1975 (first interviews)

employment status in 1977:   employed   renewed spell   still   pensioner
                                         of unemploym. unemployed

Source: Mohr und Frese, 1978, p.189

Figure 10: "Expectation of failure" and "anxiety in social situations" of unemployed and formerly unemployed (fall of 1977 at the beginning and at the end of the reference period, according to employment status at both times

Employment status		Expectation of failure (index 0-6)	Anxiety in social situations (index 0-9)
February 1978	November 1978		
employed	unemployed	1,6 / 2,2	3,0 / 3,0
employed	employed	1,4 / 1,3	2,6 / 2,5
unemployed	employed	2,0 / 1,6	3,0 / 2,6
unemployed	unemployed	2,1 / 2,3	3,1 / 2,9
unemployed	housewife	1,1 / 1,0	2,8 / 2,6
housewife	housewife	1,1 / 1,0	3,0 / 2,7

6-4: very high   9-6: very high
3-2: high   5-3: high
0-1: low   0-2: low

values in February 1978   values in November 1978

Source: Büchtemann, Rosenbladt, 1981, p.29

Figure 11: Gross changes in "expectation of failure" between both times of interviewing (T1,T2) according to selected groups of employment status at T1 and T2, in % (unemployed and formerly unemployed of fall of 1977)

Expectation of failure at:	T1 and T2 unemployed expectation of failure at:			T1 unemployed, T2 employed expectation of failure at:			T1 and T2 employed expectation of failure at:		
T2	T1 very high	T1 high	T1 low	T1 very high	T1 high	T1 low	T1 very high	T1 high	T1 low
very high	61	24	11	33	17	5	28	9	5
high	21	45	26	35	31	22	38	39	19
low	18	32	63	32	52	73	34	52	77
sum	100	101	100	100	100	100	100	100	101

Source: Büchtemann, Rosenbladt, 1981, p.30

Figure 12: Resignation of women in employment, unemployment, and household (full time) at T1 (summer of 1978) and T2 (after half a year), in %

Source: Klaus Heinemann, Peter Röhrig, Rolf Stadié, table 46

RESIGNATION		Employed/Employed (N=323) %				Unempl./Employed (N=227) %				Unempl./Unempl. (N=528) %				Unempl./Household (N=155) %				Househ./Househ. (N=330) %			
		T1	T2	S	S	T1	T2	S	S	T1	T2	S	S	T1	T2	S	S	T1	T2	S	S
TOTAL (N)		20	15	39	91	46	25	42	91	49	52	72	67	45	28	52	91	26	24	42	82
DURATION OF UNEMPLOY-MENT	less than 1 month					42	22	38	89	49	50	68	67	75	15	-	85				
	1-2 months					48	20	35	94	47	45	63	72	65	48	54	63				
	3-5 months					48	27	55	100	52	53	69	65	37	18	49	100				
	6-11 months					52	25	35	86	41	46	70	70	45	32	59	90				
	12-23 months					39	36	56	76	56	66	82	54	54	33	52	91				
	24 months and more					16	17	0	80	57	65	89	67	47	23	42	93				
AGE	20-29 years	15	7	21	95	42	21	38	91	41	41	59	72	37	19	40	94	23	23	53	86
	30-44 years	18	17	43	89	46	25	47	94	48	54	68	59	48	36	57	82	31	21	39	88
	45-60 years	29	26	52	86	54	31	42	82	64	70	89	64	53	34	58	94	24	30	34	72
QUALI-FICATION	low	35	25	47	88	52	35	49	81	62	63	86	60	53	44	67	81	47	36	39	66
	middle	18	15	30	88	53	25	37	89	52	53	69	65	44	24	48	96	22	33	78	79
	high	12	11	34	93	24	9	31	97	32	35	54	74	36	18	34	91	17	13	27	90
FAMILY ORGANI-SATION	youngest child under 3 years	19	9	0	89	30	-	-	100	35	38	70	78	34	18	34	91	16	21	58	86
	youngest child 3-5 years	31	10	23	96	42	22	27	82	45	54	62	53	50	19	23	85	28	27	42	79
	youngest child 6-15 years	13	13	40	91	51	33	57	92	57	60	77	63	51	37	64	91	27	21	36	85
	youngest child over 16 years	19	30	83	82	34	32	70	87	51	57	81	67	28	20	46	90	25	30	22	68
	with spouse	19	9	28	96	39	15	29	94	50	49	60	62	33	25	57	91	37	21	41	92
	with others	18	17	64	93	63	32	40	82	71	78	76	16	50	50	100	100	-	-	-	100
	alone	22	19	30	84	57	22	29	89	49	52	75	71	91	60	66	100	50	50	71	72
CONNEC-TION TO WORK	household	18	21	50	86	53	24	34	87	48	54	75	66	37	23	54	96	27	29	42	76
	equivocal	18	14	29	89	38	31	58	86	48	55	72	62	43	35	51	78	11	19	40	84
	work	20	12	39	95	47	21	39	95	50	49	70	71	59	30	48	95	32	31	61	84
WORK ORIEN-TATION	extrinsic	27	21	51	90	54	35	47	78	57	65	79	53	59	49	65	74	37	26	28	75
	equivocal	22	17	35	88	56	29	45	92	50	56	69	56	36	22	52	94	28	28	75	90
	intrinsic	11	9	37	94	20	10	26	97	40	35	61	83	40	16	32	94	25	20	33	85

S: Proportion not changing score on "resignation" (stable group)

Figure 13 Psychical Dispostion and self-reported sickness, change in consumption of cigarettes, of alcohol and drugs, in %

		total	Psychical disposition: type					
			I	II	III	IV	V	VI
sickness during unemployment	NO	76.1	97.0	94.4	80.8	60.8	61.3	43.2
	YES	23.3	3.0	4.7	18.8	39.2	38.1	56.4
change in cigarette consumption	NO	71.7	85.6	79.4	73.5	66.9	60.2	56.2
	YES	27.8	14.4	19.9	26.5	33.1	38.7	43.8
change in alcohol consumption	NO	88.6	91.7	96.0	88.9	88.6	80.7	81.9
	YES	11.0	8.0	4.0	10.9	11.4	18.2	18.1
change in drug consumption	NO	91.5	98.9	99.1	95.5	89.2	84.0	76.9
	YES	8.5	0.8	0.9	7.3	10.8	14.9	22.7
Total	base number	1755	264	322	547	166	181	260
	%	(100.0)	(100.0)	(100.0)	(100.0)	(100.0)	(100.0)	(100.0)

Source: Sozialwissenschaftliche Arbeitsgruppe (WAL) p.207

MAIN LITERATURE:

(1) BRINKMANN, C.: Finanzielle und psycho-soziale Belastungen während der Arbeitslosigkeit. In: Mitteilungen aus der Arbeitsmarkt- und Berufsforschung MittAB 4 (1976)

(2) BRINKMANN, C.: Strukturen und Determinanten der beruflichen Wiedereingliederung von Langfristarbeitslosen. In: MittAB 2 (1978)

(3) BRINKMANN, C.: Zur Arbeitsmarktsituation von Behinderten und Leistungsgeminderten: Arbeitslosigkeit, berufliche Rehabilitation, arbeitsmarktpolitische Perspektiven. In: MittAB 3 (1981)

(4) BRINKMANN, C.; SCHOBER-GOTTWALD, K.: Zur beruflichen Wiedereingliederung von Arbeitslosen während der Rezession 1974/75. In: MittAB 2 (1976)

(5) BÜCHTEMANN, C.F., ROSENBLADT von, B.: Arbeitslose 1978: Die Situation in der Arbeitslosigkeit. In: MittAB 1 (1981)

(6) FRÖHLICH, D.: Psycho-soziale Folgen der Arbeitslosigkeit. Eine empirische Untersuchung in Nordrhein-Westfalen. Cologne: Institut zur Erforschung sozialer Chancen 23 (1979)

(7) HEINEMANN, K.; RÖHRIG, P.; STADIE, R.: Arbeitslose Frauen im Spannungsfeld von Erwerbstätigkeit und Hausfrauenrolle. Melle/St.: Augustin (1980)

(8) HENTSCHEL, U.; MÖLLER, C.; PINTAR, R.: Zur Lage der Arbeitslosen in Nordrhein-Westfalen - Eine erste Darstellung und Interpretation von Befragungsergebnissen. Cologne: Institut zur Erforschung sozialer Chancen 11 (1977)

(9) INFRATEST SOZIALFORSCHUNG/WIRTSCHAFTSFORSCHUNG, SÖRGEL, W.: Arbeitssuche, berufliche Mobilität, Arbeitsvermittlung und Beratung. Forschungsbericht im Auftrag des Bundesministers für Arbeit und Sozialordnung Bonn. Social research publication series of the Labor Ministry No.5 (1978)

(10) KUTSCH, T.; WISWEDE, G.; (Eds.): Arbeitslosigkeit II: Psychosoziale Belastungen. Soziale Probleme der Gegenwart Bd.2. Königstein/Ts. (1978)

(11) MOHR, G.; FRESE, M.: Arbeitslosigkeit und Depression. Zur Langzeitarbeitslosigkeit älterer Arbeiter. In: Vom Schock zum Fatalismus. Soziale und psychische Auswirkungen der Arbeitslosigkeit (Ed.: A. Wacker). Frankfurt/Main (1978)

(12) REINKE-DIEKER: Ins Abseits. Eine gruppendynamische Bestimmung sozialer Ausgrenzung von Arbeitslosen. Cologne (1980)

(13) ROSENBLADT von, B.; BÜCHTEMANN, C.F.: Arbeitslosigkeit und berufliche Wiedereingliederung. Erster Teilbericht über Ergebnisse einer repräsentativen Längsschnittuntersuchung bei Arbeitslosen und Abgängern aus Arbeitslosigkeit in der Bundesrepublik Deutschland 1977/78. In: MittAB 4 (1980)

(14) SATERDAG, H.: Situationsmerkmale von Arbeitslosen 1975 und Voraussetzungen für die Aufnahme einer neuen Beschäftigung. In: MittAB 2 (1975)

(15) SCHOBER, K.: Arbeitslose Jugendliche: Belastungen und Reaktionen der Betroffenen. In: MittAB 2 (1978)

(16) SOZIALWISSENSCHAFTLICHE ARBEITSGRUPPE (WAL) UNIVERSITÄT GÖTTINGEN (BRÖDEL, R.): Die soziale und psychische Lage der Arbeitslosen. Ansatzpunkte für Weiterbildung. Göttingen (1978)

(17) WACKER, A.: Arbeitslosigkeit - soziale und psychische Voraussetzungen. Frankfurt, Cologne (1976)

(18) WACKER, A.: Vom Schock zum Fatalismus? Soziale und psychische Auswirkungen der Arbeitslosigkeit. Frankfurt/Main (1978)

UNEMPLOYMENT: A PSYCHIATRIC PROBLEM AS WELL?

Leonard Fagin

Claybury Hospital, Woodford Bridge, Woodford Green
Essex, Great Britain

The spate of suicides and riots in unemployment-stricken towns has recently brought to the public attention a feature of joblessness which had not figured in the minds of those that thought it would only have financial and probably minor social consequences. Since then, a flurry of interest has been spurred by the media who regularly report on studies that show some association between unemployment and ill health, quite often, and not surprisingly, to make party political meal of a long-term problem that is bound to have implications for health provision in this country, at least over the next two decades. As psychiatrists we all know the central role played by regular, satisfying employment in the mental health of our patients, and I am sure many of us are affected by our total inability to secure adequate rehabilitation alternatives on which we are sure our patients' future, and that of their families, depend to a great extent. Some of us may also have been aware of the increased demand on mental health resources over the past few years and of the worrying tendency for admissions into psychiatric hospitals to be prolonged as a result of the time it takes for an ex-psychiatric patient to re-enter the labour force.

Despite this, and until recently, unemployment has been virtually ignored by the British health care profession as a possible pathogenic force. This is surprising when one considers that other major life changes, mostly involving loss, appear to be associated with alterations in psychological and physical well-being. Studies have shown how, for example, bereavement, immigration and loss of limbs, are followed by psychological phases of adjustment and sometimes long lasting emotional and physical problems. Other writers have found that, when these loss experiences are unresolved, they may be at the core of many psychosomatic disorders, such as asthma, ulcerative colitis and psoriasis. This neglect is all the more surprising when one finds that evidence has slowly been accumulating since the 1930's associating unemployment and increased morbidity. Marie Jahoda (1) and Eisenberg and Lazarsfeld (2) described the three psychological phases following unemployment which have been corroborated by later researchers and which follow a similar pattern to other experiences of loss. Briefly, the first phase amounts to a denial of the situation, a feeling of relief and sense of holiday, with an increase in the activities which had to be postponed because of the work routine, such as house repairs and decoration, car maintenance etc. The second phase is experienced with increasing distress as the ex-worker is confronted by the seriousness of his situation when he sucessively fails to regain employment and with the prospects of poverty and inability to provide for his family. Job seeking during this time is done in earnest. In the third phase the ex-worker is broken and resigned, adjusting to an unemployed style of life, dropping his efforts in job seeking and courtailing his social interests, spending most of his time at home, in front of the T.V. set and even isolated from his family circle.

These phases are obviously an abstraction and there are many exceptions to the rule. One or two of them may be entirely missed or they will vary in length and degree according to, among others, the worker's past job record, previous experiences in unemployment, his attachment to his job and status, the way in which he lost his job (i.e. whether it was voluntary or forced, massive or individual), age and marital status how chances of re-employment are personally assessed and the level of unemployment in his area. It is perhaps relevant here to mention that these phases apply to men rather than to women in our society. No studies have looked at the plight of the unemployed woman, although one suspects that the adaptability of the woman's role may render her more capable of sustaining the pressure to regain employment.

Kasl and Cobb (3) found increases in physiological measures, such as blood pressure, cholestrol and uric acid levels, in workers undergoing job loss in factories in Detroit, all these measures indicating how the body might be responding to the stress associated with redundancy. Professor Brenner's (4) studies, correlating over long periods of time a group of economic indices (such as growth rates, employment rates, decline in per capita real income and rate of inflation) and health indices (such as suicide and homicide rates, admissions to psychiatric hospitals, mortality rate, cardiovascular disease mortality rate, cirrhosis rate), have shown that there is an association in timing between these factors, often with lags of one to three years. Although Brenner's findings have recently been the subject of some controversy, they are impressive and need to be corroborated. A United Kingdom study, done at Queen Mary's College, will be out shortly and, hopefully, answer some of the criticism to Brenner's work, mostly centered on the way he has interpreted the different lag periods when he correlated various indices. One thing that Brenner does not answer in these macrostatistical studies is whether it is the unemployed who are experiencing the brunt of the variation of health problems during business cycles, and leaves us with the suspicion that those at work may equally suffer from economic instability and the threat of redundancy during hard times. Especially worrying is Brenner's assertion that societies which experience increases of unemployment of one million over five years, are likely to have 50.000 more deaths by general illnesses, 167.000 more deaths by heart diseases and 63.900 more admissions into psychiatric hospitals. In the U.K. unemployment has risen by over a million in one year and, since 1972, the rate of increase has been far higher than any other industrialised country. At the moment of writing 11.4% of the workforce are jobless, with those out of work for over 6 months accelerating in proportion. (Unemployment Unit Bulletin 5)

In 1978, when the rate of unemployment took a massive upward swing, there were very few researchers looking at the psychological response to joblessness, and none at all focusing on the family as the unit of observation. With this in mind, we approached the DHSS in the hope of getting a sample of 22 unemployed male workers from a national unemployment survey they were undertaking (3000 respondents) so that we could interview them and their families while undergoing the experience of unemployment. We selected married breadwinners who registered as unemployed in October 1978, who had dependents and had not been out of work in the year prior to registration. We interviewed groups of families in South Wales, Midlands, Tyneside, and the North East and in the Greater London area. Each family was interviewed twice, 6 months and one year after the male breadwinner registered as unemployed. The interviews consisted of a structured questionnaire, going into detail into family life, past history, life events, job and medical records and dependency on health and social services; a time-schelude questionnaire, in which we explored how use of time had been affected prior and after unemployment; a Malaise Inventory, a modification of the Cornell Medical Index Health Questionnaire; and an unstructured taped interview in which we explored changes following unemployment. Although we did not set out to write on health and unemployment in families, health matters seemed to be so important during our interviews that we decided to focus on these.

The main findings from this pilot study (6) was that health in the families deteriorated following the event of unemployment and that these subjective changes in health were not restricted to the breadwinner but were also experienced by the wives and children. Some husbands and wives showed clinical features of moderate to severe depression, taking anti-depressants, tranquillisers or sleeping pills supplied by their doctors. Quite often their General Practitioners were unaware of the main breadwinners unemployment. People who had experienced previous psychosomatic disorders, such as asthma, psoriasis, gastro-intestinal complaints, insomnia and headaches, and had not been bothered by them for some time, had recurrences of these illnesses. Disabled people who had managed to keep their disabilities at bay throughout their working lives, suffered serious and rapid decline in their physical handicaps.

The "ill role" appeared to be something many of the male breadwinners turned to, as an unconscious way of justifying their joblessness when they felt under family and societal pressure to regain employment, more so in those people who irrationally blamed themselves for being out of work. The children of the families also experienced a variety of disorders, many of them stemming from feeling neglected by their parents, who were totally taken over by the experience of being out of work and worrying about how they would provide. A number of children from our sample deteriorated in their performance at school, experienced more incidents of truancy and wandering, and sometimes showed uncharacteristic behaviour such as stealing from their mother's handbag or becoming more infantile and demanding. Some children were taken to their doctor because of refusal to eat, tummy upsets, earaches, or general unmangeability. In the marital relationships there was also evidence of sexual difficulties, violence and a number of families separated permanently following the onset of unemployment.

In a small but interesting number of cases, subjective and objective experiences of health improved. This was the case for a man who was chronically disgruntled with his job, and for wives who assumed a central wage-earning role to supplant that lost by her husband. Those families where no health problems were reported were more likely to be mutually supportive where the husband retained some authority despite his joblessness, where the wife was already at work prior to husband's registration or where the husband had other interests to turn to whilst he was on the dole. Social class did not appear to be a crucial factor, as far as one can tell from the size of the sample, and if anything, those in higher status jobs appeared to suffer more dramatically in the months immediate to their unemployment. If unemployment is a cause of illness, how is it mediated? In the thirties, the prevailing thoughts were that the misery caused by unemployment, such as nutrition, poverty and inactivity, would all contribute to ill health. Although one can by no means dismiss these factors, there was no doubt that the families we interviewed experienced severe distress, that this had a lot to do with present social attitudes towards the unemployed, and that factors such as loss of identity, loss of family role, loss of wage earning capacity, reduction in socialisation, inability to control one's affairs, loss of skill, inability to fill one's time, all contributed to these feelings of distress.

Since this pilot study was finished, other researchers have found associations between unemployment and minor psychiatric morbidity, in adults as well as in school-leavers, and most agree that the area is a complex one to study but that unemployment and employment seem to be major contributory factors in determining well being. Although more research is warranted, there is a great deal of concern for those masses of unemployed workers currently experiencing distress and especially those at risk of developing health problems. These appear to be the jobless in their fifties, the disabled, those with previous records of physical or mental ill-health, the non-achieving school leavers and those in ethnic minorities. Those in the health care professions must be alerted to the fact that unemployment can manifest itself in terms of ill health, and be aware of their educative and counselling role. Many of the unemployed are oblivious to the possible effects the experience of unemployment has in store for them and their families and preparing them for it may have preventative results. This is particularly important in view of the finding that "unemployment leaves scars which remain even after re-employment" in terms of irreparable damage to self confidence and self-esteem. (Daniel 7)

Lastly, we must not be expected to be able to patch up ills that are generated by decisions made by social planners, economists and government, who often lose sight of the human response to their actions. Although this moves medical practitioners into the political field, my opinion is that it is part of our practice and responsibility to make representation to those in power and create a lobby of resistance for the sake of our present and future patients.

REFERENCES:

(1) JAHODA, M., LAZARSFELD, P., ZEISEL, H.: Marienthal: The sociography of an unemployed community. (1933) London: Tavistock (Re-published 1972)

(2) EISENBERG, P., LAZARSFELD, P.: The psychological effects of unemployment. Psychological Bulletin 35, 358-390 (1938)

(3) KASL, S., GORE, S., COBB, S.: The experience of losing a job. Reported changes in health, symptoms an illness behaviour. Psychosomatic Medicine 37, 2, 106-122 (1975)

(4) BRENNER; M.H.: Mental illness and the economy. Cambridge: Harvard University Press (1973)

(5) UNEMPLOYMENT UNIT BULLETIN No.1, 1981. London: Tress House (1981)

(6) FAGIN, L.: Unemployment and health in families. London: Dept. of Health and Social Security (1981)

(7) DANIEL, W.W.: Strategies for displaced workers. PEP Broadsheet 38, 517 (1970)

ECONOMIC DEPRIVATION, WORK ORIENTATION AND HEALTH
CONCEPTUAL IDEAS AND SOME EMPIRICAL FINDINGS

Dieter Fröhlich

Institut zur Erforschung sozialer Chancen
Cologne, Federal Republic of Germany

This article deals with two problems. First, I want to develop and elaborate an analytic frame of reference to help us answer the following basic questions: Why does unemployment affect the unemployed negatively, in particular their health status? Which aspects of the loss of work cause negative effects of unemployment and under what circumstances are these consequences reinforced or reduced? More technically speaking, the question of independent and intervening variables will be raised. The question itself is not new at all. But in my opinion it did not get enough attention by theorists and researchers in the discipline of sociology who deal with the problem of unemployment on a micro-level.

Second, these conceptual considerations will lead to some hypotheses which I will test with my own empirical data (roughly 950 interviews with unemployed males in 1976). In accordance with the general theme of this conference I have chosen three effects of unemployment, three dependent variables, that can - with some good-will - be considered as aspects of the three dimensions of health in the broad definition of the WHO: physical, mental and social well-being. The empirical test will lead us to a reformulation of some theoretical assumptions. I want to point out that the empirical findings - although they might prove to be interesting in themselves - are in the context of this paper secondary to the theoretical reasoning. The theoretical considerations will hopefully lead us to somewhat refined concepts in unemployment research and to a better understanding of the unemployed and their problems.

Theory I

Unlike Brenner (1973), sociologists interested in problems of unemployment and doing research on the micro level spent surprisingly little thought about the problem of cause and effect when dealing with the problems of the unemployed. Thus, social research has come up with many results about the consequences of unemployment which are certainly interesting, but which too often remain on a descriptive level of analysis and reasoning. An enumeration of negative effects might describe the situation of the unemployed and their living conditions in vivid terms. But it does not tell us why these negative effects have come into being apart from the fact that all these people have lost their jobs. When researchers have purposely constructed a hypothetical causal order, especially economic deprivation has been put forward as the main independent variable to affect the unemployed mentally and socially. The authors of the famous Marienthal-study (Jahoda, Lazarsfeld and Zeisel 1933) hint at this causal chain when they state a clear relationship between the weekly available financial resources and mental health: The "unbroken" have the highest financial resources while the "apathetic" dispose of the least financial means. Similarly, Aiken, Ferman and Sheppard (1968) found a definite relationship between economic deprivation, anomia and political extremism. In newer German research Frese and Mohr (1977) state a close connection between lack of money and depressiveness. Similar results are to be found with Saterdag (1975) and Brinkmann (1978).

One can say that the economic, material functions of work have been properly identified as one factor to cause negative effects for the unemployed in various dimensions of attitudes, health and behaviour. But work has never been defined in financial and economic terms only, and all theorists and researchers agree that there is more to work than just the "bread-winning" aspect. Work has a number of non-material functions, and their loss through unemployment will lead to mental, social and physical deprivations that might even be more devastating than the effects caused by the material problem in unemployment.

Some of these non-material functions of work in industrial societies are:

- the potential to structure time: daily, weekly, yearly time, and - through the social definition of age - even life-time.

- This biographical aspect points to the integrating function of work: young people get socialized into society, grown-ups are socialized and integrated in society, and old age is often defined as a process of gradual desocialization of a person, beginning at retirement.

- Work is connected with different occupations, and they give social status and prestige and locate persons and their families in different social strata with the equivalent material and non-material benefits and life chances.

- In industrial societies, occupations and the equivalent social status can - in principle - be achieved through own efforts, and this achievement principle can act as a powerful means for personal identity.

- Achievement in work can make for feelings of mastery over circumstances, over material and social surroundings and can lead to feelings of competence.

Apart from the fact that such non-material functions of work imply a heavy male bias that restricts the usefulness of this approach mainly to the problems of men, it is fairly easy to hypothesize the loss of these non-material functions through unemployment to have grave consequences for the unemployed. This kind of reasoning is certainly useful and appropriate. But the problems lie in the conceptual and the measurement level: The non-material functions of work have rarely been consciously operationalized and measured as independent variables. Their existence and their influence have only indirectly been "proven" by certain measured effects on attitude, behavior and health of unemployed people. The logic of this "proof" might be described as follows: Take the (negative) effects of unemployment and deduct that part of the variance explained by the loss of the material functions of work (economic deprivation) and some demographic data. The unexplained variance must then be caused by the loss of the non-material functions of work. Thus, the non-material functions have been taken into account only indirectly; they have never been consciously measured and operationalized as independent variables.

The reasons for these shortcomings might be the lack of a theory of work which would permit us to break up the broad category "non-material functions of work" into different analytic dimensions, to operationalize them and to deduce hypotheses as to their effects on people in the event of unemployment. Such a theory is not at hand, and I cannot offer one either. But bits and pieces of such a theory do exist and have always been used in theory and research on unemployment without being fully aware of this fact: Some of the so-called demographic data have the quality of operationalized non-material functions of work.

Take age, for instance: Age in industrial society is mainly defined through involvement in the working process. A young person is someone who is still in the training process for taking an active role in the working world. Youth ends by entering the working sphere with the supplementary conditions that a person can fully support himself and possibly others (his or her family) through his work.[1] Old age means that a person is no more active in work either by force of circumstances like failing health or by legal definition. This sociological definition is intimately connected with the idea of societal integration: A young person in this sense is not yet fully integrated into society; an old person tends to pull himself out of society or gets pushed out (the desocializing effect of retirement). - Another aspect of age that is tied up with the concept of work is the problem of personal identity: A young person is still a learner; a grown-up has the (self-) image of being active, applying what he has learned. An old person is harvesting the fruits of his activities and rests upon the material and non-material laurels of his activity phase - or is just considered "ready for the scrap heap".

The combination of age with marital status brings out the aspect of social integration even more clearly: To be young and unmarried normally does not mean a very intensive degree of integration. In contrast, the status of being married and having children normally entails the highest degree of integration into society. The sociology of the family tells us that parents with children at home have intensive neighborhood contacts, are interested in the school system, later in the system of professional training and in the future of different jobs and professions, and they follow "big politics" more intensely than anyone else.

Sex is another variable directly related to the world of work via the role concept. Especially when dealing with problems of unemployment one automatically differentiates between men and women and expects women to suffer less from the loss of work than men do. For explanations one points out the centrality of the work role in the lives of men, while women dispose of socially accepted alternative roles as housewife and mother.

Finally, occupation is that demographic variable most directly related to the working sphere. As the best single indicator for social status it links the working world to very important structures of society, like social class and social stratum and to material and non-material life styles.

All this is, of course, not new. But what might be new is the view of certain demographic data as operationalized, non-material functions of work. I do not want to dwell on this topic any further, and I abstain from trying to develop the "theory" behind the demographic data. Nevertheless, it was necessary to point out their quality as operationalized, non-material functions of work as their worth and their importance have been demonstrated by Brenner. In his analyses he finds a definite relationship between economic instability (measured by rates of employment) and hospitalization, but at the same time he states that economic instability alone is of relative little influence on hospitalization. Only when "important side effects" or "secondary effects" are taken into account, strong relationships between economic instability and hospitalization show up (Brenner 1979, p. 117; quoted from the German translation). According to Brenner, these secondary effects are age, marital status, ethnic background, economic status and education, thus mainly demographic data which he interprets in the theoretical context of role theory, status, prestige and social mobility. Within his net of causal reasoning he treats them as intervening variables and - as said before - attaches more explanatory potential to them than to economic instability itself.

Taking Brenner literally, one might as well change the causal ordering of the variables: The non-material functions of work - no matter how they are defined and operationalized at the moment - might become the true independent variables while economic instability or economic deprivation get the status of an intervening variable that mediate the effects on attitude, behavior and health of unemployment.

Theory II

My plea to see certain demographic data in a new light and to regard them as elements of a hidden theory about the non-material functions of work should not be misunderstood as a call to use these demographic data as the most important or the only independent variable. For such an approach, their theoretical potential is not sufficiently developed. So far the demographic data can only be used as additional independent variables, additional to other approaches of which I want to introduce one now.

The non-material functions of work could be introduced and measured as the subjective evaluation of the working sphere, especially as an evaluation of the centrality of work for one's own life, by the employed and unemployed themselves. The reasoning behind this approach is the idea that one can expect a person to react differently to the working sphere and to loss of work according to the value which he attaches to work and occupation in his life. If work is central to a person's life, work and occupation will be valued for themselves, as an end, not just as a means to other ends that are located outside the working world. Other people might evaluate work exactly in the latter sense, as a means for bread-winning and for material security which form the base to persue other aims.

Both attitudes are know as expressive and as instrumental work orientation. They stand for two sets of motivation which (hypothetically) lead to different reactions in the event of unemployment: One can expect a person with an expressive work orientation to suffer comparatively much as this person loses a goal, an end in itself. On top of the already high level of frustration a high degree of economic deprivation may aggravate the person's situation further. But the additional influence of the economic situation will be comparatively slight because it concerns only a secondary aspect of work. The situation of a person with an instrumental work orientation will be different: As work is regarded mainly as a means to other ends, unemployment will have less negative effects on this person to begin with (because only a means is threatened, not a goal). In addition, this person's reaction to unemployment will be modified by the degree to which the means is treatened: The higher the degree of economic deprivation the more negative the evaluation of the situation (and reverse). But on the whole, one can expect the more instrumentally oriented unemployed to be less negatively affected than males with an expressive work orientation.

Before these hypotheses are confronted with empirical data I want to briefly discuss a possible objection to my concept of non-material functions of work. It could be argued that the definition and measurement of these functions on a subjective level is not appropriate, that one should define further dimensions of the concept and should try to find more "objective" indicators for them. I would agree that a further differentiation of the concept "non-material functions of work" will be necessary. And there is certainly some truth when objecting against the subjective approach to measure work orientation. But I consider this approach a progress compared to the hitherto used way to leave the non-material functions of work undefined and unmeasured.

Or to give the answer a more positive twist: The subjective evaluation of the situation very likely will have consequences for attitudes and behavior according to the Thomas-Theorem: When people define a situation as real, it is real in its consequences. Finally I think that the worth of this approach cannot only be discussed and proven theoretically; its worth has to come out in empirical research.

Data and Methods

The data consist of questionnaire interviews with 1.300 unemployed and an equal number of employed persons as control group (the latter group will not be taken into account in this paper). The interviews were carried out in mid-1976 in three pre-selected regions of Northrhine-Westphalia, representing the main economic structures of that state. Within these regions a random selection was planned but could not be carried out. The selection was restricted to persons of German nationality above the age of 18. This limitation was achieved during interviewing. Not achieved was a 50 : 50 distribution of sex. In the end, there were approximately 70 % males and 30 % females interviewed in both groups. In comparison to the unemployment statistics of the three regions, unqualified workers are underrepresented in our sample. In addition, we have all reasons to believe that by the method of interviewee selection the problem cases of unemployment are somewhat underrepresented. These limitations make descriptive generalizations impossible. But the data permit non-descriptive, explanatory conclusions, i. e. the testing of hypotheses. - The following data analysis will be confined to unemployed men only, the reason being the male bias of theories about the non-material functions of work which in many ways do not fit the situation of women.[2]

When putting forward hypotheses about the influence of work orientation I used the word "suffer" to denominate negative effects of unemployment. The deterioration of health is one aspect of "suffering". The WHO discriminates three dimensions of health: physical, mental and social well-being. On the basis of this definition my data permit to operationalize these three dimensions, although my measures cannot be regarded as "hard" indicators:

<u>Physical health</u> was measured as self-reported change of health to the better or to the worse (or "no change") during unemployment (for similar measurement see Freese 1978, p. 19).

<u>Mental health</u> was measured by five statements that formed one factor in factor analyses. These statements are about the feeling not to be useful anymore, to be redundant to society, to be a charity seeker; that the hours of a day slip by, that the day drags along. These five statements were turned into an index.

<u>Social well-being</u> has been measured by two questions about social activities with friends and acquaintances during unemployment. Turned into an index it shows social activities as intensified, same or reduced.

These three indicators are certainly "soft" measurements of the three dimensions of health, and they are open to debate. To my opinion, the mental health index taps the personal dimension of worthlessness and depression too little and stresses too much the societal aspect, i. e. the emotional relationship between the person and society. Anomia might be a more appropriate label for that index. Likewise, social well-being might be too narrowly measured, and I suggest to name that index social contacts to reduce its broad meaning. Only physical health is properly and narrowly defined, but here the question is whether this subjective self-reported health status can serve as a reliable indicator.

With these limitations in mind we come to percentage distributions of health effects in unemployment (see tabel 1). They cannot be taken as descriptions about health effects in our three regions: We have all reasons to believe that by the specific way of finding the interviewees the deprived unemployed are underrepresented and that the percentages of men with worsened physical health, with high anomia and reduced social contacts are higher than our data show. The value of our data is only obtained

Table 1: Percent-distribution of the dependent variables

physical health	%	anomia	%	social contacts	%
improved	21.4	low	37.9	intensified	40.6
same	54.3	medium	34.6	same	42.8
worsened	24.3	high	27.5	reduced	16.6
% =	100.0		100.0		100.0
N =	891		879		858
no answer	75		87		108

by confronting them with our independent variables, when asking causal questions.

Economic deprivation, the loss of the material functions of work, has been identified as the most widely used independent variable. As is the case with the dependent variables, one gets into measurement problems here, too. How does one define and measure economic deprivation? Two different approaches are feasible: to define the economic situation from the income or from the consumption side.

A definition of economic deprivation from the income side would entail:
- the loss of income of the interviewee through unemployment, i. e. the difference between the last salary and unemployment compensation. But this in itself does not mean very much:
- Important is the percentage of loss. Again, this percentage alone is not very informative: it can be a great loss for a person having had an income near existence level; it may mean a comparatively slight loss for a person with a previously high income.
- In addition, several demographic characteristics have to be taken into account to render such figures meaningful: stage in family life cycle, number of persons in the household that have to be supported and that contribute to the income of the household.[3]

Further, we know that questions regarding income generally belong to the "touchy" questions and possibly even more so during unemployment: In the interview situation of 1976 there were quite a few chances for moonshining in the three regions, and as extra earnings are not permitted when receiving unemployment compensation, an unknown proportion of the interviewees might have had good reasons to hesitate in giving true information as to their real income during unemployment. There are still additional problems to measure income during unemployment properly[4], and all of them make it advisable not to base economic deprivation on the income side of the material situation.

Much less problematic is measurement mainly on the consumption side. If one develops a measure that takes into account the change of expenditure and consumption patterns of a household during unemployment, one circumvenes the problem of demographic characteristics like marital status, size and composition of household, stage in the family life cycle. At the same time questions about the restructuring of consumption patterns, of indebting oneself or using up savings are far less problematic for the interviewees to answer than questions regarding income.[5]

In view of our data I have developed an index of economic deprivation that takes into account the following items: indebtedness; renunciation of holiday trips and of purchase of durable goods; savings in the purchase of food, clothes and weekend expenditures; selling of car, spending of savings. The items were weighed[6] and summed up to an index ranging from 0 to 21 with the latter figure standing for highest economic deprivation. Reduced to three values we get the following percentage distribution of economic deprivation:

Table 2: Percent distribution of economic deprivation

low econ. deprivation	36.7 %
medium econ. deprivation	46.7 %
high econ. deprivation	16.6 %
% =	100.0
N =	891
no answer	75

It should be remembered again that these figures are not apt to describe the economic situation of the unemployed in our three regions in general. Very probably families with high economic deprivation are underrepresented in our sample.

Work orientation is our second independent variable. Our questionnaire holds six statements, three of them stressing the importance of work for one's own life, the other three stressing the importance of family life and spare time. The interviewees were asked to bring these statements into an order according to their personal preferences. The index "work orientation" is constructed in a way that someone who did not put any of the work centered items on one of the first three ranks is regarded as "not work oriented". With one of the work centered items on the first three ranks he is regarded as "low on work orientation", with two items "medium", and with all three items he is "highly work oriented". The distribution of work orientation is as follows:

Table 3: Percent distribution of work orientation, unemployed men

not work oriented	12.5 %
low on work orientation	30.1 %
medium on work orientation	36.0 %
highly work oriented	21.4 %
% =	100.0
N =	880
no answer	86

We are now in the position to examine our hypotheses concerning the relative impact of work orientation and economic deprivation on health during unemployment.

Results

Earlier I had advanced the hypothesis that males with an expressive work orientation are more negatively affected by unemployment than instrumentally oriented males, the reason being that the former lose a goal, an end in itself while instrumentally oriented males only lose a means to an end. In other words, when regarded separately, work orientation will have a stronger effect on males than economic deprivation. Or, in still a different formulation: The kind of work orientation explains the health effects of unemployment better than economic deprivation. The figures pertaining to these statements are in table 4.

The influence of both independent variables can best be shown in the case of anomia (table 4 b). The degree of anomia is particularly low with males who are not work oriented at all (the true instrumentally oriented), and this percentage increases when one gets to the medium and high work orientation groups (the difference being 37 %). Although not as strong, the opposite pattern shows up in case of high anomia: Only 12.9 % of the instrumentally oriented men are highly anomic, but 36.9 % of the interviewees with a definite expressive work orientation. In contrast, the relationship between economic deprivation and anomia is by far not as close and not even linear for the highly anomic group: The largest difference is 10 % between low and medium economic depriva-

Table 4: The separate influence of work orientation and economic deprivation on the three dimensions of health; unemployed men

a) physical health	work orientation				economic deprivation		
	not work oriented	low	medium	high	low	medium	high
better	19.6	26.6	22.5	16.8	23.8	16.2	23.7
same	65.7	54.9	50.3	50.2	57.1	56.8	46.0
worse	14.7	18.5	27.2	33.0	19.1	27.0	30.3
% =	100.0	100.0	100.0	100.0	100.0	100.0	100.0
N =	102	244	298	185	303	389	139
	$p < .001$; CC = .16; gamma = .17				$p < .01$; gamma = .13; CC = .13		

b) anomia	work orientation				economic deprivation		
	not work oriented	low	medium	high	low	medium	high
low	66.3	39.8	29.1	29.6	44.6	35.7	32.1
medium	20.8	38.6	37.6	33.5	32.7	31.7	37.3
high	12.9	21.6	33.3	36.9	22.7	32.6	30.6
% =	100.0	100.0	100.0	100.0	100.0	100.0	100.0
N =	101	251	306	179	294	398	134
	$p < .001$; gamma = .28				$p < .05$; gamma = .15		

c) social contacts	work orientation				economic deprivation		
	not work oriented	low	medium	high	low	medium	high
intensified	48.5	43.3	40.6	37.3	47.5	33.9	37.6
same	43.7	40.0	41.6	40.8	43.7	47.0	31.2
reduced	7.8	16.7	17.8	21.9	8.8	19.1	31.2
% =	100.0	100.0	100.0	100.0	100.0	100.0	100.0
N =	103	240	286	169	284	381	138
	$p < .13$				$p < .001$; gamma = .24; CC = .22		

tion. In case of low anomia the percentages decrease from 44.6 % in the low economic deprivation group to 32.1 % in case of high economic deprivation (12 % difference). The weaker influence of economic deprivation in comparison to work orientation is exemplified by a lower level of significance and a lower gamma, too.

Basically the same pattern appears when looking at physical health: Among the highly instrumentally work oriented only 14.7 % report the worsening of their health, but in the (high) expressive orientation group exactly one third feels worse in terms of physical well-being. As a trend, economic deprivation has a similar effect. But while here the maximum difference is 11 %, it is 28 % between the two extreme groups of work orientation.

As to the status of the variable "physical health" a note on method is in order. It seems that self-reported health measures only on the negative pole. Self-reported improvement of health does not follow any recognizable pattern, and one could imagine that health improvements during unemployment and an unchanged health status somehow belong together. Differences between both aspects might result from very idiosyncratic personal characteristics. As a consequence, we probably do not have a true ordinal variable, and altogether one gets the impression that this way of measuring physical health is not too convincing.

Similar methodical reserves might be appropriate in case of "social contacts" where intensification during unemployment might lie on the same level as "no change in social contacts". One structural aspect stands out though: Intensification of social activities during unemployment is in our data fairly typical for young and unmarried men - somewhat a commonsense result. From a theoretical point of view social retreat is the real interesting sub-dimension in the variable as there is no normal, commonsense reason why people should reduce their social activities unless they are compelled to do so by some reasons specific to the situation of unemployment.

Compared to physical health and anomia we find a very different pattern when looking at the development of social contacts. Here there is just a slight (statistically not significant) trend in the relationship between work orientation and social retreatism, with the highly work oriented males showing the highest percentage of social withdrawal. But - unlike the other two health dimensions economic deprivation plays a definite role in whether a person reduces his activities with friends and acquaintainces: Social retreatism is low in case of low economic deprivation (8.8 %) and high (31.2 %) in case of high economic deprivation. This result, the dominant influence of the material situation, does not conform to our observations so far, and it will be shown later that this is not just coincidence or due to poor measurement.

So far we have looked at the influence of work orientation and economic deprivation on the three dimensions of health separately. The next step will be to look for the influence of one independent variable under control of the other. Tables 5-7 show the relationship of work orientation and the health dimensions controlling for economic deprivation.

Table 5: The relationship between work orientation and physical health, controlling for economic deprivation; unemployed men.

	low economic deprivation				medium/high economic deprivation			
	work orientation				work orientation			
physical health	none	low	medium	high	none	low	medium	high
better	28.6	23.8	27.8	18.0	9.8	24.8	16.9	16.2
same	64.3	60.0	51.5	54.1	68.6	55.0	49.7	49.6
worse	7.1	16.2	20.7	29.9	21.6	20.2	33.4	34.2
% =	100.0	100.0	100.0	100.0	100.0	100.0	100.0	100.0
N =	42	80	97	61	51	149	177	117
	p<.20				p<.05; gamma = .14; CC = .18			

It turns out that under conditions of low economic deprivation the deterioration of physical health is fairly dependent on the work orientation: The more the work orientation tends to the expressive type the

larger the percentage of unemployed males who report a worsening of
their physical health. Basically the same holds true under conditions
of medium and high economic deprivation: The level of health deterioration is higher to begin with. But in addition, the percentages of
men with health problems are markedly higher in the two work oriented
groups than in the two groups with low work orientation.

Table 6: The relationship between work orientation and anomia,
controlling for economic deprivation; unemployed men

anomia	low economic deprivation				medium/high economic deprivation			
	work orientation				work orientation			
	none	low	medium	high	none	low	medium	high
low	70.5	42.9	39.2	32.1	63.5	39.9	24.9	27.6
medium	22.7	40.5	36.1	25.0	19.2	34.6	34.6	36.2
high	6.8	16.7	24.7	42.9	17.3	25.5	40.5	36.2
% =	100.0	100.0	100.0	100.0	100.0	100.0	100.0	100.0
N =	44	84	97	56	52	153	185	116
	$p < .001$; gamma = .34				$p < .001$; gamma = .25			

The same pattern is particularly prominent in regard to anomia. Under
conditions of low economic deprivation there is a very strong rise in
anomia dependent on work orientation, and an equally strong decrease in
percentages of low anomia. Again, the level of anomia is generally
higher in case of a poor material situation during unemployment, and it
rises further in the groups with stronger work identification (with a
corresponding decrease of percentages of low anomia). Yet, deteriorated
health and strong anomia is almost equally high in the expressive work
orientation groups under all conditions of economic deprivation, rendering the material situation as rather obsolete for the explanation of
negative health effects. Work orientation seems to explain the way men
are affected by unemployment much better than economic deprivation.

Table 7: The relationship between work orientation and social contacts, controlling for economic deprivation; unemployed men

social contacts	low economic deprivation				medium/high economic deprivation			
	work orientation				work orientation			
	none	low	medium	high	none	low	medium	high
intensified	67.4	45.0	47.1	41.1	30.2	39.3	34.8	34.9
same	27.9	43.8	44.8	46.4	60.4	39.3	40.4	36.8
reduced	4.7	11.2	8.1	12.5	9.4	21.4	24.8	28.3
% =	100.0	100.0	100.0	100.0	100.0	100.0	100.0	100.0
N =	43	80	87	56	53	145	178	106
	$p < .20$				$p < .05$; gamma = .08 CC = .16			

This latter interpretation is only valid for the dimensions of physical health and anomia. It does not apply to social activities and social withdrawal: There is virtually no effect of work orientation on social retreat in case of low economic deprivation; the percentage of social withdrawal remains equally low in all work-orientation-groups. In the medium/high economic deprivation category the shares of social withdrawal are markedly high beginning already in the group of men who are low on work orientation. This result stresses the idea that social retreat is basically not influenced by the kind of work orientation but by economic factors. Again, in its relationship to the independent variables this dimension of health is not compatible with the other two dimensions measured.

Before we make a final test as to the relative dominance of one of the two independent variables we have to remember the possible other influences in the realm of the non-material functions of work that have been traditionally controlled: the demographic data. In comparison to work orientation their influence is fairly weak. Physical health is somewhat related to marital status with married males showing a 10 % higher share of deteriorated health; to age: the middle-aged groups have somewhat more health problems; and to professional training and to occupational status: the better the training and the higher the occupation, the smaller the share of self-reported health deterioration. None of these relationships exceed the correlational strength of .11.

Anomia is basically related to age, again showing the middle-aged as being more anomic than the younger and the older unemployed. The number of persons in the household is of the same significance, and both demographic characteristics - age and size of household - seem to point into the direction of the life-cycle-concept according to which middle-aged men with family responsibilities are more severely hit by unemployment than younger ones (without families) or older ones where children possibly have left home already.

Quite in line with our previous results, social activities follow a very different pattern: They are fairly strongly dependent on age ($r = .21$) with the young unemployed showing a marked intensification of social activities while the older groups tend more towards social retreatism. Marital status, too, seems to be of some significance: Here it is not the married but the divorced, widowed and separated males that form the problematic group.

For physical health and social contacts the duration of unemployment seems to be of some significance: The longer the duration of unemployment the higher the shares of deteriorated physical health and social withdrawal (maximum $r = .18$). - To sum up: The classical "independent variables" representing the non-material functions of work are of comparably small significance in explaining the health effects of unemployment when compared to the kind of work orientation.

Slight as these influences may be, they still might somewhat affect the relationships between our three dimensions of health and work orientation and economic deprivation. In a final test I will take professional training, occupational status, size of household and duration of unemployment into account as intervening variables. As we use partial correlation for this test (see table A in the Appendix), marital status and age will not be controlled, the variable "marital status" being only of nominal quality, and age because of its curvi-linear relationship with the health dimensions.

There are two ways of partialling out the influence of one of our two main independent variables: One can keep work orientation (and other variables) constant or the influence of economic deprivation is partialled out. I have done both steps with the following results (table 8):

Table 8: Partial correlations of the main variables involved (for complete zero order correlations see table 4 A)

a) Relationship between work orientation and	zero order coefficients: direct relationships	partial correlation coefficients under separate control of:					under common control of b-f
		professional training	occupational status	size of household	duration of unemployment	economic deprivation	
	a	b	c	d	e	f	g
physical health	.12^{+++}	.14^{+++}	.13^{+++}	.12^{+++}	.11^{+++}	.12^{+++}	.12^{+++}
anomia	.23^{+++}	.24^{+++}	.24^{+++}	.22^{+++}	.22^{+++}	.22^{+++}	.23^{+++}
social contacts	.10^{++}	.12^{+++}	.11^{+++}	.09^{++}	.08^{+}	.09^{+}	.09^{+}

b) Relationship between economic deprivation and						work orientation	
	see above	see above	see above	see above	see above		see above
	a	b	c	d	e	f	g
physical health	.08^{+}	.08^{+}	.08^{+}	.08^{+}	.05	.07^{+}	.05
anomia	.10^{++}	.10^{++}	.10^{++}	.10^{++}	.10	.09^{++}	.09^{+}
social contacts	.17^{+++}	.17^{+++}	.17^{++}	.17^{++}	.14^{+++}	.17^{+++}	.13^{+++}

+ significant on 5%-level
++ significant on 1%-level
+++ significant on .1%-level

Table 8a, column a, shows quite a strong relationship between work orientation and anomia, a weaker relationship with physical health and an even weaker one with social contacts. The variables controlled (columns b - f) have practically no effect on the direct relationship, not even economic deprivation. In the end (column g) the correlational strengths remain basically the same, only social contacts are slightly affected, mainly by duration of unemployment.

The reverse test (table 8 b), partialling out the influence of work orientation is revealing: The direct relations between economic deprivation and physical health and anomia are much lower to begin with. When controlling for duration of unemployment and work orientation, the relationships become insignificant in case of physical health and are slightly reduced in case of anomia (through work orientation). Only social activities follow a different pattern again. Here the direct relationship to economic deprivation is comparatively strong (.17). By controlling duration of unemployment it gets weaker in the end (.13), but still stands out markedly among the three dimensions of health measured. A surprising result in both tables is the almost nonexistent effect of the three demographic variables (of which size of family was used as a substitute variable for marital status).

Discussion

On the whole, the empirical findings presented above are somewhat heterogenous. There is a relationship between physical health, economic deprivation and work orientation, but it is not very close. Social contacts, particualarly the aspect of social withdrawal, does not conform to the hypothetical expectations in that they are only connected to economic deprivation but not to work orientation. Only our construct of anomia is consistently and convincingly related to our two independent variables.

For this somewhat blurred picture two explanations are possible: Operationalization and measurement were poor or the theory behind the data might be faulty. Both possibilities need serious attention.

As I have stated above, of all three dimensions of health only the anomia-index measures on both ends, on the positive and on the negative side. Physical health and social contacts seem to measure only on the negative pole, that means only the worsening of physical health and social retreatism probably are useful indicators for (negative) effects of unemployment. An improvement in physical health and an intensification of social activities do not necessarily indicate positive effects of unemployment. Thus, future research should develop measures that are built on the extension and refinement of the negative end of these two variables.

Another question is whether physical health and social activities have been adequately operationalized and measured at all. As a contrast one should have a look at the anomia-index: Anomia has been measured very indirectly, and this might account for the discriminating power of the variable. Physical health, on the contrary, is measured only by one direct question about the subjective assessment of one's health during unemployment. Very likely this is too gross a measure, leaving too much room for every kind of rationalization. The best measurement would certainly consist in medical tests in the tradition of Kasl, Cobb and Brooks (1968), Kasl and Cobb (1970), Cobb (1974) and Kasl, Gore and Cobb (1975). But this approach is not feasible in survey research where the aim is to gather information from large numbers of unemployed that enable generalized results. The next best method would be to apply techniques used in psychology to find out psychosomatic symptoms like headaches, sleepnessness, unrest etc. The quality of such measurements would probably lie inbetween medical tests and our direct question, and such an indirect approach might have the discriminating power of our construct of anomia.

An indirect approach might also be feasible in case of social well-being, particularly in regard to social withdrawal and the reduction of social activities. But in this case we might not only be dealing with measurement problems but touch upon questions of theory and concepts. Poor as my operationalization might be, social withdrawal consistently falls out of the pattern observable with physical health and anomia: Here economic deprivation "explains" social retreat far better than the kind of work orientation. As to my knowledge, there is no other research to check this result because work orientation has not been used as an independent variable.[7]

This deviant finding might be explained and interpreted through the concept of reciprocity of social contacts: Seeing friends, acquaintances and relatives is connected with financial expenditure for the ones who are visited, and unwritten norms prescribe that one cannot see others repeatedly without inviting and entertaining them in return. When money gets scarce in unemployment one could stop seeing others just because one is no more able to uphold these norms of reciprocity (see Bakke 1940, p. 10; Bahnmüller 1978). Such an interpretation of social withdrawal would be of different quality compared to the usual interpretation of social retreat in terms of shame and depressiveness. Interpreted in my way, social retreat would mean a much less problematic effect of unemployment than explaining it in terms of a shaken personal identity.

This interpretation might also attach a question mark to the WHO definition of health. If social well-being as one dimension of health is mainly operationlized through the development of social activities and if such activities are reduced mainly because of financial reasons, while physical and mental health are mainly affected by the loss of the non-material functions of work, then it looks that the health definition does not only tap three different dimensions, but that these dimensions are not even on the same level of abstraction. If such be the case the health definition would need more additional theoretical attention and sophistication.

To take up another problem: In the research literature there are findings that go - at first sight - contrary to my results and interpretations. The Marienthal-study states a clear linear relationship between income and optimistic or pessimistic attitudes. Aiken, Ferman and Sheppard (1968, p. 67, 69) write: "Economic deprivation was the best predictor of anomia ... it was not the length of unemployment or unemployment experiences per se that produced feelings of anomia, but rather, the decline in the economic integrity of the worker and his family." Frese and Mohr (1977, p. 677, 679), in a longitudinal study with unemployed males in Germany, come to the conclusion that the outstanding finding was the very close relationship between lack of money and depressiveness (r = .46). These results are certainly not in accord with my interpretations about the paramount importance of the non-material functions of work as compared to the material side of the working sphere.

But even in full knowledge of these "contradictions" one can still keep to the interpretation I have offered, simply because of the fact that the (possibly) more important independent variable, work ethic or work orientation, has not been controlled in the studies cited above. In my data there are also clear relations between economic deprivation, physical health and anomia. But they are definitely weaker than the relationships with work orientation.

In principle, my data conform to the results of Brenner who states - with a different method though - an obvious relationship between economic instability and hospitalization. At the same time he points out that economic instability in itself is of comparably small importance. Only when taking additional variables into account this basic relationship really becomes prominent. These additional factors are some demographic variables which I have previously interpreted as latent operationalizations of non-material functions of work and occupation. Thus, there are parallels between Brenner's and my results insofar that both of us locate an influence of economic factors on health, but that the non-economic, the non-material factors play the more prominent role in explaining health effects of unemployment. As a conclusion in regard to theory I would therefore suggest to change priorities in the ordering of the variables, taking the non-material functions of work as the main independent variables and treating economic deprivation, the material aspect of work, more as an intervening variable.

In contrast to Brenner's results, the demographic characteristics are of comparatively slight importance in the data and findings presented here. This might partly be due to the fact that my construct "work orientation" is somewhat dependent on at least two demographic characteristics of the unemployed: on professional training (r = .24) and on occupational status (r = .22), thus being in itself in a way an indicator for these demographic characteristics. But these relationships are not strong enough to regard work orientation as a substitute variable for professional training and/or occupation.

This brings me to a final point concerning the future use of hitherto "important" demographic data. The question is how useful our old, traditional categories of explanation will be in coping with the problems of the unemployed in the future. To a certain extent unemployment today can hardly be compared with the situation several decades ago. Marie Jahoda, one of the authors of the Marienthal-study, has recently (1979) observed that due to largely improved social welfare systems the unemployed on the whole no longer suffer acute physical deprivation. According to Jahoda this fact might have boosted their general morale. She further notices a decline of the Protestant work ethic which should influence reactions to the loss of work, too. In more secular terms this problem of a changed work ethic, with work and occupation losing their towering moral grip on people, is discussed as value change (see Inglehart 1977). The general notion in this discussion is that of a hedonist trend in the highly industrialized societies where self-actualization is sought and found more and more outside the working world.

If these observations turn out to be correct we can expect less problematic consequences of unemployment in cases where an instrumental work orientation predominates and a sufficiently high standard of living is guaranteed one way or the other. As a decline of the traditional work ethic can be watched even in occupational groups who have traditionally been the bearers of this ethic, we might be forced to reorient ourselves as to "firm" knowledge about who is going to be hit hardest by unemployment. Already today Bakke's famous dictum "The higher they rise, the deeper they fall" does not seem to be in line with social reality anymore. In our data it is the members of the higher occupational groups who suffer least from unemployment. Jahoda (1979, p. 493) has stated the same trend.

If these observations have a solid base in reality one has to focus future attention more and more on the determinants of the work ethic when trying to evaluate the situation of the unemployed and to prognose effects of unemployment. In my opinion, the little information we have so far about the impact of the work ethic points to the importance and fruitfulness of this approach when dealing with the problems of the unemployed.

Notes

1. Accordingly, the sociological definition of youth cannot follow specific age cuts, and youth is mainly a function of the duration of the educational phase. Compare for instance the term of advantaged/disadvantaged adolescence.

2. In our days we see a change as to the importance of work for both men and women: The work role of men softens up while women get more involved in work. It would be beyond the scope of this article to investigate this aspect further.

3. Proper measuring must also consider weighing problems: The size of family and its composition must be taken into account as fixed costs decrease with the size of the family. For an early example of handling this weighing problem see Jahoda, Lazarsfeld and Zeisel 1975, p. 39 (first 1933).

4. Even subjectively precise information about income could objectively be incorrect. Exact calculations must include governmental transfer payments and tax refunds which probably will be overlooked by the interviewees. See BMAS 1978, p. 58.

5. Furthermore, it has been shown in recent German research that the "consumption approach" explained psycho-social problems of the unemployed far better than the "income approach". See Wal 1978, p. 151, 173 - 174.

6. It would exceed the scope of this paper to go into details as to the weighing procedure. For details see Fröhlich 1979, p. 180 - 191; for a similar but simpler approach see Aiken, Ferman and Sheppard 1968, p. 51 - 61.

7. Aiken, Ferman and Sheppard (1968, p. 77 - 78) state the same clear relationship between economic deprivation and social integration, using frequency of visiting relatives as an indicator. Unfortunately, work orientation was not used as a variable in that study, so its relative weight cannot be cross-checked.

APPENDIX

Table A: Zero order coefficients of main variables

	1	2	3	4	5	6	7	8	9
1 economic deprivation	—								
2 work orientation	.05	—							
3 physical health	.08$^+$	.12^{++}	—						
4 anomia	.10^{++}	.23^{+++}	.19^{+++}	—					
5 social contacts	.17^{+++}	.10^{++}	.14^{+++}	.17^{+++}	—				
6 professional training	-.04	.20^{+++}	-.07	-.05	-.08$^+$	—			
7 occupational status	-.01	.20^{+++}	-.05	-.03	-.07$^+$	.61^{+++}	—		
8 no. of persons in family	.04	.05	.07$^+$	-.09^{++}	.10^{++}	-.16^{+++}	-.15^{+++}	—	
9 duration of unemployment	.19^{+++}	.10^{++}	.13^{+++}	.02	.18^{+++}	-.05	-.07$^+$	.04	—

+ significant on 5%-level
++ significant on 1%-level
+++ significant on .1%-level

LITERATURE:

(1) AIKEN, M., FERMAN, L.A., SHEPPARD, H.L.: Economic failure, alienation and extremism. Ann Arbor, Mich., USA (1968)

(2) BAHNMÜLLER, R.: Arbeitslose als politisches Konfliktpotential? In: Vom Schock zum Fatalismus? Soziale und psychische Auswirkungen der Arbeitslosigkeit. (Ed.: A.Wacker). Frankfurt, New York (1978)

(3) BAKKE, E.W.: Citizens without work. 1940. New Haven, Conn., USA (reprinted 1968)

(4) BMAS BUNDESMINISTER FÜR ARBEIT UND SOZIALORDNUNG (Ed.): Motivation von Arbeitssuchenden, Hemmnisse für die Einstellung von Arbeitslosen, Effektivität von Vermittlung und Fortbildung und Mobilitätsbereitschaft von Beschäftigten. Bonn (1978)

(5) BRENNER, M.H.: 1973: Mental illness and the economy; in German: Wirtschaftskrisen, Arbeitslosigkeit und psychische Erkrankung, München, Wien, Baltimore (1979)

(6) BRINKMANN, Ch.: Belastungen durch Arbeitslosigkeit. Finanzielle und psycho-soziale Probleme der Arbeitslosigkeit. In: Arbeitslosigkeit II: Psycho-soziale Belastungen. (Eds.: Th. Kutsch, G. Wiswede) Königstein/Ts. (1978)

(7) COBB, S.: Physiologic changes in men whose jobs were abolished. Journal of Psychosomatic Research 18, 245-258 (1974)

(8) FRESE, M.: Arbeitslosigkeit, Depressivität und Kontrolle. Eine Studie mit Wiederholungsmessung. Bielefelder Arbeiten zur Sozialpsychologie Nr. 29 (1978)

(9) FRESE, M., MOHR, G.: Die psychischen Folgen der Arbeitslosigkeit: Depression bei älteren Arbeitslosen. In: WSI-Mitteilungen 11, 674-679 (1977)

(10) FRÖHLICH, D.: Psycho-soziale Folgen der Arbeitslosigkeit. Eine empirische Untersuchung in Nordrhein-Westfalen. Institut zur Erforschung sozialer Chancen, Köln Nr. 23 (1979)

(11) INGLEHART, R.: The silent revolution. Changing values and political styles among western publics. Princeton, N.J., USA (1977)

(12) JAHODA, M.: The psychological meanings of unemployment. New Society, 6. Sept. 1979, 492-495 (1979)

(13) JAHODA, M., LAZARSFELD, P.F., ZEISEL, H.: Die Arbeitslosen von Marienthal. Ein soziobiographischer Versuch über die Wirkungen langanhaltender Arbeitslosigkeit (1933) Frankfurt (new edition 1975)

(14) KASL, S.V., COBB, S., BROOKS, G.W.: Changes in serum urin acid and cholesterol levels in men undergoing job loss. Journal of the American Medical Association 206, 1500-1507 (1968)

(15) KASL, S.V., COBB, S.: Blood pressure changes in men undergoing job loss. A Preliminary Report. Psychosomatic Medicine 32, 19-38 (1970)

(16) KASL, S.V., GORE, S., COBB, S.: The experience of losing a job. Reported changes in health, symptoms and illness behavior. Psychosomatic Medicine 37, 106-122 (1975)

(17) SATERDAG, H.: Situationsmerkmale von Arbeitslosen Anfang 1975 und Voraussetzungen für die Aufnahme einer neuen Beschäftigung. In: Mitteilungen aus der Arbeitsmarkt- und Berufsforschung 2, 136-148 (1975)

(18) SOZIALWISSENSCHAFTLICHE ARBEITSGRUPPE (WAL) UNIVERSITÄT GÖTTINGEN: Die soziale und psychische Lage der Arbeitslosen. Ansatzpunkte für Weiterbildung. Göttingen (1978)

UNEMPLOYMENT AND LIFE-STYLE CHANGES

Niels Beckmann and Klaus-Dieter Hahn

Arbeitsgemeinschaft für Angewandte Psychologie
Hamburg

1. The life-style concept and its determinants

We are a group of psychologists who, for the purpose of our Ph.D. theses, have specialized on the topic of life styles. These theses were part of a project carried out at the Institute of Psychology at the University of Kiel under the direction of Dr. Berbalk. The project included the development of a dynamic life-style model which will be presented below.

For the last two years we have been mainly dealing with the problem of unemployment, in particular long-term unemployment.
We held several four-week-courses with different groups of unemployed persons in the north of Germany.
General aim of such courses according to German laws concerning the tasks of the Employment Institute (Arbeitsförderungsgesetz) is to improve personal situations of the participants in order to increase their chances of employment.
Our task is to focus on the individual situations and personal problems of the participants within the courses.
To understand the individual ways of living and coping with the fact of unemployment it is necessary to refer to a psychological concept that represents subjective and objective aspects of life as well as interrelations and dynamics of these aspects.
We regard our dynamic life-style model as a useful concept in the above mentioned way. This model and its deviations and similarities to other psychological and sociological life-style concepts has been published by Berbalk & Hahn in 1980. Explaining also the importance of this model for clinical intervention, we consider it helpful to give a brief outline of it.
Describing the dynamic of and all important influences on a life-style we suggest five main determinants. Each determinant represents a number of variables.

I. **The objective environment** consisting of
   - individual conditions as intellectual capacities or physical handicaps
   - environmental conditions as working conditions, housing, material aspects of standards of living
   - social-cultural and political conditions including laws, traditions, possibilities for social life and personal growth.

II. **The subjective view of oneself and the world**
   - personal life goals, self-images and self-esteems
   - perceived environmental chances for action and personal growth
   - values and attitudes towards life and how it should be organized.

III. **All the behaviour patterns and abilities** an individual has in order to cope with everyday life
   - i.e. cognitive abilities as life-planning, task recognition, problem-solving or applications of information
   - social abilities as solving conflicts, giving and receiving feed-backs and other skills of communication
   - emotional abilities as accepting and expressing emotions
   - and manual abilities necessary for different tasks or different jobs.

IV. **The various criteria of efficiency in life**
   - psychological criteria as being free of mental illness, having feelings of happiness, satisfaction and/or well-being. Furthermore indices of competence, personal growth and self-actualization.
   - social criteria as social integration, adaption or adjustment, role fulfillment
   - biological criteria, i.e. indices of physical health.

V. **The individual life-history and its dynamics**
   i.e. the historical dimension including the development of society wherein a certain life-style is growing as well as the individual family background and learning history leading to this very life-style.

2. The interviews and the procedure used

To use this concept within the courses we had to achieve an instrument which a) helps to assess and understand important aspects of personal life-styles and b) includes criteria according to those we can evaluate the results of these courses.
In addition to that some diagnostic instruments are helpful in developing an individually orientated plan for the intervention within the four weeks of the courses.
Besides, psychosocial criteria are necessary for the evaluation for the courses mentioned above. This basic criterion, if a person is employed, unemployed or in further education after having passed a course is not sufficient to measure individual success as intended by the law.
In cooperation with the Institute of Psychology at the University of Kiel, in particular with Professor Grau, we developed a semi-structured interview which gave us information on the aspects as follows:
- the extent of social integration in family, friendship and neighbourhood
- the educational background and work-experience
- the personal way of coping with problems of life
- the financial, social and emotional experiences after having lost the job
- the actions undertaken to get a job
- the personal explanation: why has oneself lost the job
- the support, the pressures and the perceived expectancies within social relations

Apart from our personal experiences the interviews described above are the first step to a life-style based systematic analysis of the psychosocial problems in the forefield and field of unemployment.
The interviews were made during the second part of the course by specially trained undergraduate students, who have participated throughout the course. The interviews were made in a private setting and took about one to one and a half hours. We choose the semi-structured form as a compromise between standardized questions about special subjects and the chance for an individually orientated talk in confidental atmosphere .
In accordance with the basic aspects of 'action research' we took into consideration the personal interests and questions of the participants. Thus we afterwards fed back some of the results and impress-

ions of the interviews during the practical part of the course, in group situations or in personal talks.
In this way the interviews helped us to plan individual interventions within a course.
At the moment we are analysing the interviews in order to develop a more specialized pattern of questions which can be divided into modules. These modules of questions will be used in different moments and stages during a course.

3. Results, discussions and application of the life-style concept

We would now like to present one way to analyze the individual information of the interview.
All interviews of a course were taken together, hierarchical orders of the participants concerning different variables were made by ratings and than scatter plots were drawn out of two variables each.
For example: the first scatter plot shows on the ordinate the extent of social integration in neighbourhood, friendship and family, on the other axis the extent of actions undertaken in order to find a job - we call it efforts.
Every spot on the chart represents the two ordinal positions of one person concerning the two variables. A clear interrelation cannot be recognized, that will be interpreted later on.
The second scatter plot shows on the ordinate the extent of perceived social pressures towards work and employment, on the horizontal axis again the efforts.
Again there is no evident relation between the social pressures and actual efforts.
Now - as can be seen on the third scatter plot - if one constructs a combined hierarchy of social integration and social pressure on one hand and efforts to get a job on the other a nearly clear relation is evident.
This ordinal correlation, though not yet statistically tested, helps to describe one problem in the field of unemployment. Beyond this description an explanation or understanding based on the life-style model and on motivational theory can be attempted:

- Concerning the first scatter plot, social integration in a peer-group or subgroup of unemployed persons (I)* will reinforce the pursuit of unemployment, a corresponding value system (II) and life-style instead of pushing toward working life.
- Concerning the second scatter plot social pressure without social integration is not linked with efforts if a person either has experienced internal attributed failures (IV) and/or is unable to plan concrete actions (III) out of uncertain job interests (II) and/or is missing abilities (III) to search and use labour market information.
- Social integration may support hope for success and reduce fear of failure, that is increasing motivation (Heckhausen, 1965). This can lead to personal efforts on the labour market if the social environment is also representing work values (I). This linkage between social pressure and social integration probably leads to the efforts as shown on the third scatter plot.

Another scatter plot (4) shows a relation between the concrete form of future orientation and actual efforts.

To understand this result different explanations can be made:
- According to the assumptions of Stone & Schlamp (1971) material insecurity as a result of unemployment reduces the possibilities of long-range life planning. In addition short-sighted living will reduce actual efforts.
- According to motivation theory, loss of future orientation is closely linked to loss of expectancies which is supposed to be a result of internal attribution of experienced failures.
- According to our life-style concept further questions arise before intervention may be planned:
  For example no efforts and no future planning concerning the labour market may be the consequence in a realistic view (II) of objective personal chances in a regional economically, socially and politically given situation (I).

---

* Figures I-IV refer to determinants I-IV of the life-style model described above.

Concrete life-planning is a congnitive ability to bridge the gap
between objective given environmental chances and subjective life
goals and interests. A lack of this ability reduces the probability
of successful acting, coping and finally leading to passivity.
A negative self-image as a result of cumulated negative experiences
may lead to a wrong estimation (II) of either real chances given (I)
or one's own abilities (III) or both.
Some persons live in a very dominating social environment including
family, friends and representatives of social institutions. Their
life-styles are characterized by other-directedness. For these
persons personal life-planning is not useful, personal actions or
efforts are unnecessary.

Thus the life-style concept is helpful to extend the view of different
psychological theories in order to consider all important influences
on the life of an unemployed person and to consider possible effects
of interventions.

Based on our life-style concept we regard the problem of unemployment
on one hand as a multicaused symptom of society, on the other hand as
only one step in a personal lifespan development.
Although every unemployed person has its own specific work history
and way of coping with the problem of unemployment, we came across
some typical problems.
These problems can be described as deficits on different levels in
order to plan individually orientated interventions, but of course the
system of life-style allows and demands intervention within the given
environment as well. We will now concentrate on individual levels of
deficits in order to describe interventions in the forefield of
clinical intervention.

(1) The level of cognitive abilities

Life planning is one of these. This includes being able to build up
a hierarchy of personal interests and to deduce realistic immediate
objectives out of personal life goals.

A lack of this ability may lead to unemployment. For example:
someone is unable to adapt to changing working conditions as it
often occurs in the white-collar-sector, or someone has to look

for a new job because of health reasons but is unable to change orientation.

Furthermore , many people in our courses had great difficulties in finding information, expecially concerning the labour market, in understanding the unemployment office's demands as well as their suggestions in making full use of it in order to plan life perspectives and immediate actions. Evidently unemployment demands more and other cognitive abilities than these people had to have during their working life as an unskilled or semi-skilled worker.

A persons's first experience at the unemployment office are very often characterized rather by administrative aspects instead of consulting and helping aspects. Expecially nowadays with the constant number of clerks in the unemployment office being confronted with a growing number of jobless people.

The fewer cognitive abilities people have the more they get the feeling of being powerless and having no influence on what happens to them within this big institution.

In return the unemployed person may lose hope and motivation to discuss personal interests, problems and handicaps with the clerk in the jobcentre. Thus the talks reduce completely to formal procedures, mistrust and fear. This it to be understood as a development or cycle depending at least on personal coping styles and abilities of both participants and of institutional problems.

These experiences become personally more important if someone, for many years, was used to gain all his self-esteem and self-worth out of his working-life. Most of the participants in our courses are adherent to the Protestant Ethic ideals and the social environment normally represents the same tradition. In reference to our lifestyle model the congruence of given ethical traditions (I) and personal value systems (II) leads especially for male persons to a loss of nearly all self-esteem sources at the beginning of unemployment.

This includes a loss of the traditional 'breadwinner-role' within the family as described by Stone & Schlamp (1971). They analyzed the interviews of roughly 300 families belonging to the lower social class.

In our courses especially many middle aged males reported feelings of erosion in their family role. In some cases sexual problems up to impotence occurred.

Furthermore these cultural traditions mentioned above lead to
a minor ego-involvement in other areas of life as for example
leisure-activities. For them success in such activities contributes little to perceived self-esteem.
The personal and social value system often leads to internal
and stable causal attributions of unemployment with the consequences of a growing negative self-image.

(2) The level of social abilities
Members of the lower social class as well as members of the
lower white-collar-sector very often have a few skills of communication. This may be one reason for a ritualized and formalized
communication style within social institutions. People out of job
have less chances to succeed within the social institutions and
to keep social relations with friends and neighbours when social
discrimination and blame starts.
As stated by Satir (1980), there seems ot be a close linkage
between self-image, self-esteem (II) and communication skills (III)
Thus a loss of sources for self-esteem may lead slowly into a
growing social isolation via an increasing negative self-image.
These assumptions are in accordance with Jones et al. (1981) -
they interviewed 465 persons. They described lonely and isolated
persons rating themselves more negatively and reporting deficits
in social skills and self-concepts.
Some of these lacks in social abilities are very closely linked
with cognitive capacities. Listening carefully to understand another
person depends on memory capacities as well as on the ability to
exchange points of view. Especially this basic empathy seems to be
very difficult for many un- or semi-skilled workers.
A lack of social abilities (III) and/or the estimation of these (II)
is very often one of the most important reasons for staying in the
town people ever lived in. Regional mobility especially for singles
seems to be extremely dependant on former experiences being made
in foreign social environments.

(3) The level of emotional abilities
This includes the abilities to accept one's own feelings of joy as
well as of anger or fear and to express these feelings adequately.
Very often fear and anger are transformed into aggression or
avoidance which is leading to failure.
This seems to be very important for the experience in social

institutions with difficult and hardly understandable structures. Furthermore the ability to stand personal feedback, achievement evaluation and interpersonal criticism in order to make full use of it belongs to this level.

(4) The level of motivation

Many newspapers and even many very important political persons recently have taken the view of several people out of work being unwilling to work and misusing social aids. In many cases we too hit this phenomenon of no motivation to work and sometimes alongside with responding cognitive concepts. In most of the cases this appearance is to be looked at as a changeable result of a long cycle of experiences, interpretations of experiences and reactions by social institutions. Up to now we have never experienced a person who changed his life-style to hedonism with all its consequences. Most of these so-called 'unwilling persons' just have given up the attempt to fulfill their social role as a worker. Their value system was mostly quite traditional and under the surface of an open hostility against society a negative self-concept and sometimes social isolation and suffering existed. Apart from reasons we mentioned explaining our first scatter plot some people just have lost any hope to get a job. But nobody will attempt anything without any hope to succeed.
Other persons were really afraid and doubted that they could succeed to become reintegrated into the labor force. For them unwillingness was an expression of avoidance.
We think, the unwillingness to work has to be regarded as a mainly motivational fact with complex reasons, and as a personal way of coping - whether adequate or not.

4. Intervention points

Finally we are going to give an outline of points where intervention within the courses starts and which we regard as preclinical interventions.
(The latter will be remarked by *)

deficits of ...	examples for interventions within the courses

1. <u>Cognitive level</u>:

- looking for information
- making use of information
  - <u>group-discussions</u>: how to get relevant information
  - <u>activities</u>:
    - reading of vacancies in newspapers, leaflets of the unemployment office
    - making interviews with companies
    - video-based interview training
    - training of decision-making skills and problem-solving

- concrete life-planning
  - <u>group-discussions</u>: life-perspective of every participant
  - <u>discussion and evaluation</u> of working-life-experiences

- adaption to changing working conditions
  - <u>visiting</u> different companies and factories
  - confrontation with <u>different tasks</u> during the practical parts

- expressing own interests
  - talks with members of social institutions and especially the job-centre
  - <u>decision-making</u> skills

- successful discussion
  - video-based <u>group-discussion</u>

* - internal and controllable attributions of success as sources of self-esteem and future expectancies
  - giving chances for <u>activities</u> especially during the practical part with <u>process-orientated</u> support and discussion of the following causal attributions
  - <u>feed-back</u> within the group

- consciousness of values
  - <u>revaluating</u> of activities outside working-life
  - search for new meaningful activities (Goodman, 1969)

deficits of ...	examples of interventions within the courses
* - consciousness of social role expectancies and the extent of internalization	- discussions and <u>client-centered</u> talks - interviews in the street
2. Social abilities:	
- skills of communication	- <u>conflict solution</u>, training of different <u>social skills</u> method: ·small-group-discussion ·controlled dialog ·role-play ·modelling see: linkage - self-esteem and communication
* - social relations	- four week <u>group-experience</u> and initiation of future self-organization
3. Emotional abilities:	
* - self-disclosure	- verbalization of emotions (modelling) - video-self-confrontation - feed-back - talks with members of social institutions
4. Motivational level:	
- instrinsic and extrinsic motivation	- questioning and doubting individual cognitive concepts - differentiation of extrinsic/instrinsic incentives, rewards and reasons to work - consideration of handicaps, fears and interests - estimation of personal abilities and chances - reevaluation of interview-experiences

deficits of ...	examples for interventions within the courses
* 5. <u>Innerdirectedness:</u>	- encouragement of personal statements - setting of personal standards for the activities during the practical part - discussion about dependancy on persons, institutions and drugs - help and preparation of self-leading-groups - facilitating the step into therapeutic institutions

Of course the interventions mentioned above within the courses differ from course to course and lead to different effects, varying from participant to participant.

Apart from skill training during the last courses we more and more concentrated on fighting social isolation and, according to recent psychological research, on personal evaluation and attribution of success and failure. This includes normally the understanding and questioning of very limited cognitive concepts of oneself and the world which we regard as one important factor on the road to depression, aggression, delinquency and/or dependancy.

Our intention today was to present a system-view of life-style and to explain how this concept may help to understand the problem of unemployment. Individually oriented interventions may be deduced but it will also be possible to suggest political and economic interventions and their expected influences on personal life-style changes.

5. <u>Outlook</u>

Finally we will give a brief outlook on problems and open questions for our future research:

- How can individual ways of coping better be assessed?
  (see: Prystav, 1981)
  perhaps by: - improvement of the interview and development of modules of questions
  - video-presented open-ending life-situations which have to be completed within role-plays

- How can be prevented that people feel powerless, helpless, afraid and/or angry in social institutions?
  perhaps by: - training of clerks of the unemployment office
  - changing structures of these institutions in order to make them understandable and in order to allow confidental talks as well as personal influence on what is going on
  - change consuming habits and attitudes toward the unemployment office into the willingness and capacity to help organize one's own things within and outside the institution.

- How can interventions lead to more stability of life-style changes beyond the end of the course?
  perhaps by: - longer courses
  - more stress on training of self-organization
  - concepts of family-centered interventions

- How can cooperation with therapeutic institutions be improved without causing further prejudices against unemployed persons?
  perhaps by: - integrated concepts of public care (including more street-work).

THE FIVE DETERMINANTS OF LIFE-STYLE:

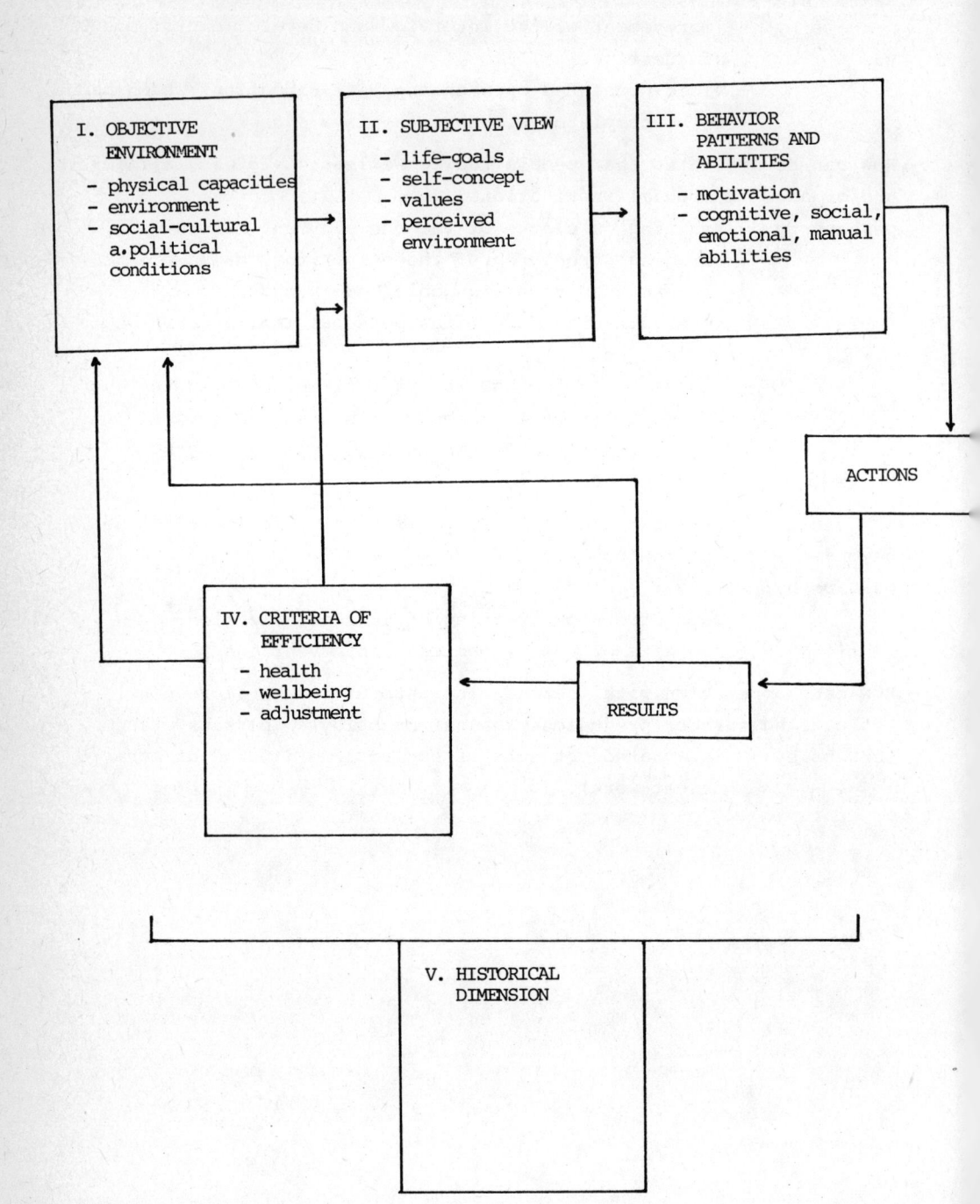

I. OBJECTIVE ENVIRONMENT
- physical capacities
- environment
- social-cultural a. political conditions

II. SUBJECTIVE VIEW
- life-goals
- self-concept
- values
- perceived environment

III. BEHAVIOR PATTERNS AND ABILITIES
- motivation
- cognitive, social, emotional, manual abilities

ACTIONS

IV. CRITERIA OF EFFICIENCY
- health
- wellbeing
- adjustment

RESULTS

V. HISTORICAL DIMENSION

SCATTER PLOT 1

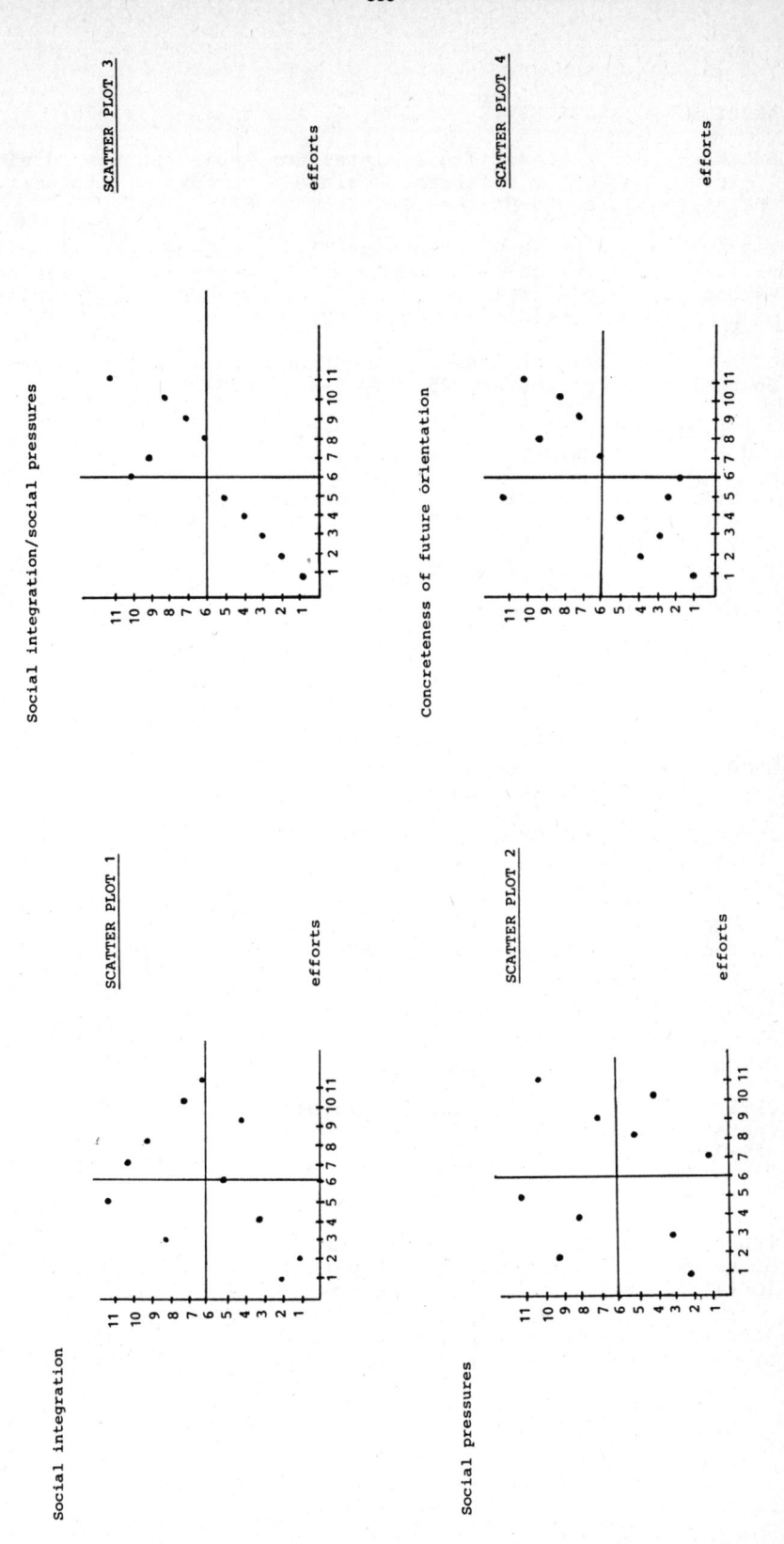

Social integration / efforts

SCATTER PLOT 2

Social pressures / efforts

SCATTER PLOT 3

Social integration/social pressures / efforts

SCATTER PLOT 4

Concreteness of future orientation / efforts

LITERATURE:

(1) ARBEITSFÖRDERUNGSGESETZ der BRD, 5. AFG-Änd.Ges. (1979)

(2) BECKMANN, N.: Lebensstil als Mittel der Anpassung an individuelle Ziele und subjektiv erfahrene soziale Erwartungen. Diplomarbeit, Christian-Albrechts-Universität Kiel (1980)

(3) BERBALK, H., HAHN, K.-D.: Lebensstil, psychisch-somatische Anpassung und klinisch-psychologische Intervention. In: Klinische Psychologie - Trends in Forschung u. Praxis Bd.3 (Eds.: U. Baumann et al.) Stuttgart: Huber (1980)

(4) CHRZANOWSKI, G.: The genesis and nature of self-esteem. American Journal of Psychotherapy 35, 1, 38-46 (1981)

(5) FIEDLER, P.A., HÖRMANN, G.: Aktionsforschung in Psychologie und Pädagogik. Darmstadt: Steinkopff (1978)

(6) FORSYTH, D.R., Mc. MILLAN, J.H.: Attributions, affect, and expectations. A test of Weiner's three-dimensional model. Journal of Educational Psychology 73, 3, 393-403 (1981)

(7) GOSWICK, R.A., JONES, W.H.: Loneliness, self-concept, and adjustment. Journal of Psychology 107, 237-240 (1981)

(8) HAAN, N.: Coping and defending. New York: Academic Press (1977)

(9) HAHN, K.-D.: Ziele in Arbeit und Freizeit als Aspekte des Lebensstiles. Diplomarbeit, Christian-Albrechts-Universität Kiel (1980)

(10) HECKHAUSEN, H.: Leistungsmotivation. In: Handbuch der Psychologie Bd.2 (Ed.: H. Thomae) Göttingen, 602-702 (1965)

(11) JONES, W.H., FREEMON, J.E., GOSWICK, R.A.: The persistance of loneliness: Self and other determinants. Journal of Personality 49, 1, 27-48 (1981)

(12) MILLER III, I.W., NORMAN, W.H.: Effects of attribution for success on the alleviation of learned helplessness and depression. Journal of Abnormal Psychology 90, 2, 113-124 (1981)

(13) ORPEN, Chr.: Effect of flexible working hours on employee satisfaction and performance: A field experiment. Journal of Applied Psychology 66, 1, 113-115 (1981)

(14) PRYSTAV, G.: Psychologische Copingforschung: Konzeptbildungen, Operationalisierungen und Meßinstrumente. Diagnostica 27, 3, 189-214 (1981)

(15) SATIR, V.: Selbstwert und Kommunikation. München: Pfeiffer (1980)

(16) TYLER, T.R., DEVINITZ, V.: Self-serving bias in the attribution of responsibility. Journal of Experimental Social Psychology 17, 408-416 (1981)

(17) VAGT, G., STAVEMANN, H.H.: Arbeitszeitverkürzung, Freizeitprobleme und Persönlichkeit. Psychologische Beiträge 22, 513-520 (1980)

(18) VINETT, R.A., NEALE, M.S.: Flexible work schedules and family time allocation: assessment of a system change on individual behavior using self-report logs. Journal of Applied Behavior Analysis 14, 39-46 (1981)

STRATEGIES OF RESEARCH ON ECONOMIC INSTABILITY AND HEALTH

Stanislav V. Kasl

Department of Epidemiology and Public Health
Yale University School of Medicine
New Haven, Connecticut, USA

Introduction

Impact research on important and complex social problems is seldom carried out in a setting of unanimity and consensus among the involved members of the research community. The reasons for such disagreements can be manifold; for example: 1) A single, feasible research design cannot encompass all aspects of the phenomenon which need studying and piecemeal studies are the inevitable consequence. 2) Absence of experimental control over possible confounding variables in the real-life field setting precludes clearcut causal interpretations. 3) Opportunistic research which depends on "natural experiments", a sound and cost-effective strategy, yields studies which have unique strengths and unique weaknesses but are difficult to compare. 4) Considerations of cost, manpower, and interdisciplinary expertise lead to varying research design compromises, which inevitably impose limitations on the generalizability and interpretability of the results.

It is not surprising, then, that such impact research frequently generates findings which appear incomplete and inconsistent to the scientist, and of limited usefulness to the policy maker. Furthermore, the above comments suggest that there may be no easy remedy and that in the long run, only a painfully prolonged accumulation of diverse evidence holds the best promise of yielding a reasonably clear picture. Short of that happy end point, it behooves the scientific community to continue evaluating different research strategies which are used (or their use is contemplated) in order to understand their advantages and disadvantages. While it is both undesirable and futile to seek consensus on a single ("best") research strategy to be adopted, it does seem fully appropriate to seek consensus on what are the strengths and limitations of the different designs, and then to bring such consensus to bear on the evaluation and interpretation of findings from specific studies.

All of the above comments are fully applicable to research on economic instability and health: a critical mass of evidence has not been accumulated and a considerable controversy exists about the methods and findings thus far. Specifically, the analysis of the relationship between economic conditions and health at the macro level (that is, using grossly aggregated data, generally at the national level) has dominated the research scene during the last decade. However, it has also attracted an increasing amount of skepticism and criticism and disquietude among scientists and policy makers who are increasingly unwilling to see such important data be based on a single, highly vulnerable methodology (Kasl, 1979b; WHO, 1981).

The present report has three objectives: 1) To summarize the methods and results of a study of the impact of plant closing and job loss in order to illustrate the micro level approach. 2) To use this summary as a taking-off point for a discussion of the strengths and weaknesses of the epidemiologic (micro) level of analysis. 3) To raise a number of general research strategy questions which consider macro and micro approaches and variations on the two.

Methods

The study is a longitudinal investigation of the health and behavioral effects of job loss and of the ensuing unemployment and/or job change experience. It reflects a research strategy of trying to identify significant social events of stressful nature which are predictable and thus can be studied in their natural setting with sufficient scientific rigor.

The design may also be seen as an approach to the study of life events which emphasizes the need to examine a single event in depth, rather than studying superficially an accumulation of diverse events over a span of time, such as might obtain when one uses the Schedule of Recent Experience to monitor periodically events reported by study subjects.

We were able to identify two plants which were going to shut down permanently and where all the employees would lose their jobs. In this way, we were able to accumulate a cohort of men whom we could then follow at regular intervals up to two years as these men went through the stages of anticipation of job loss, plant closing and employment termination, unemployment (for most), probationary re-employment, and stable re-employment.

Our target population were all male blue-collar workers at these two plants who were married, in the age range of 35-60, and who had worked at the company at least 3 years. Of the men eligible for study, 79% agreed to participate.

The men were seen in their homes by public health nurses, with the schedule of visits being as follows:

Phase 1: The first nurse visit took place some 4-7 weeks before scheduled plant closing; the men were still on their old jobs but they were already well aware of the impending shutdown. We have called this the Anticipation Stage.

Phase 2: The second nurse visit took place some 5-7 weeks after plant closing. At this point the men were either unemployed, or they had found a new job but were still in the probationary period of employment.

Phase 3: The nurse visits during this phase took place some 4 to 8 months after plant closing. Some men were seen only once, but for some 60% of the men there were actually two nurse visits during this phase. For these latter men, the average of the two values for each study variable is used in data analysis. During Phase 3, more and more men found new jobs; some were still unemployed, and a few had made another job change.

Phase 4: Here the nurse visits took place one year after plant closing. Most men had achieved a stable re-employment situation, but some were experiencing further job changes and a few remained unemployed.

Phase 5: The last nurse visit took place some 2 years after the original plant closing. A sizeable minority of men had experienced additional job changes and unemployment during the previous year.

In our presentation of results, we refer to these 5 phases as: Anticipation, Termination, 6 Months, 12 Months, and 24 Months, respectively.

During the course of each visit to the man's home, the nurse collected blood and urine specimens, took blood pressure, pulse rate, height and weight, and used a structured interview schedule to collect diverse social-psychological and health data. These included: his current employment situation, his economic circumstances, his subjective evaluation of his job and financial situation, questionnaire measures of mental health and affective reactions, and physical health data. Because there was a great deal of repeated data being collected, two nurse visits were necessary; these two visits came two weeks apart and during this period the men kept a health diary with a daily record of their health.

Most of the data which we collected is based on standardized, explicit (pre-coded) interview schedules and questionnaire measures, developed over a period of some 4 months of pretesting. The public health nurses, all of whom were experienced interviewers, received some additional 2-3 weeks of training in the use of the study's interview schedule and questionnaires. This training was designed primarily to ensure uniformity of interview behavior and strict adherence to the interview schedule, its questions and its built-in probes.

The design of the study also called for the use of controls who were continuously employed men in comparable jobs. They were followed for almost the same length of time and exactly the same assessment procedures were used.

The men who lost their jobs came from two companies. One was a paint manufacturing plant located in a large metropolitan area. The men were largely machine operators, assistants in laboratory, and clerks in shipping departments; the work was relatively light for most of them. The other plant was located in a rural community of some 3,000 people. It manufactured display fixtures used by wholesale and retail concerns, and the men were machine operators, assembly line workers, and a few tool and die workers.

The controls came from four different companies and were quite comparable to the cases on major demographic characteristics, type of work they did, and the rural-urban location of the plant. One was the maintenance department in a large university and the men were largely machinists and carpenters. The second company was a plant manufacturing parts for heavy trucks; it was located in a large metropolitan area and the men were machine operators and assembly line workers. The other two companies were both rural manufacturing concerns where the men again were primarily machine operators and assembly line workers.

Table 1 presents the major socio-demographic characteristics of the terminees -- the men who lost their jobs -- and the controls. The two

Table 1

A Comparison of Terminees and Controls

	Terminees	Controls
Companies involved	1 urban 1 rural	2 urban 2 rural
Number of men in study	100	74
Initial participation rate (% of target population)	82	75
Mean age	48.1	50.1
Mean years of schooling	9.5	10.0
Mean number of children	2.9	3.3
Non-white, %	8	11
Mean years at (original) company	19.4	21.1
Mean hourly wage (initial)	$2.96	$3.58
Mean Duncan code of occupational status	28.2	32.2
Mean employability (combines age, education, nurse's rating of health, and Duncan code of highest previous job held)	2.5($\pm$0.5)	2.6($\pm$0.5)

Terminees and Controls also comparable on:

a) Need for social approval (Crowne-Marlowe scale)
b) Ego resilience (Block)
c) Flexibility-rigidity (California Psychological Inventory)
d) Self-rated health (on initial visit)

groups are quite comparable and none of the differences in Table 1 are significant. It is worth noting that the terminees had worked at the company almost 20 years, on the average. Given their age, this would suggest that the plant closing meant for most of them a separation from the primary place of employment of their adult work career.

The bottom of Table 1 shows that terminees and controls were also comparable on diverse additional variables, such as: a) Crowne and Marlowe's (1964) measure of the Need for Social Approval, useful as an indicator of defensiveness in self-report; b) Block's (1965) Ego Resilience Scale, a measure of general adjustment; c) The CPI Flexibility-Rigidity Scale (Gough, 1957); d) global self-rating of health on the initial visit.

Let us briefly characterize the unemployment experience of the men during the 2 year follow-up period. Overall, the men experienced an average of about 15 weeks of unemployment during the 24 months; for most of them, this was the period between plant closing and the time they started on their new, full-time job. However, 20% of the men were unemployed two or more times. In the urban setting, the experience during the first year was less severe: 25% experienced no unemployment (i.e., they found a new job at once) and another 50% has less than 2 months of unemployment. In the rural setting, the men had a more difficult time finding a job; even some 3-4 months after plant closing, one third of the men were without a job. By the end of the 1st year, the men in the rural setting had experienced an average of 12 weeks of unemployment, in contrast to 7 weeks for the urban one. During the 2nd year, the situation was reversed and more men in the urban than in the rural setting experienced additional periods of unemployment. Thus by the end of the 2 year period, the cumulative experience of the men in the two companies was about the same.

A separate analysis of the social context of the two companies (Gore, 1973) has revealed that in the urban setting, where the men lived scattered throughout the city, the plant itself was an important focus of a sense of community and social support. With the plant closing down, this "community" died (Slote, 1969). But in the rural setting, the small town itself and the people in it were the major source of a sense of community and social support for the men, while the plant had never become fully integrated into the community life. When the plant closed down, the community and its social organization remained largely intact and social interaction with former co-workers who were friends was not so severely disrupted.

These differences in the severity of the unemployment experience and in the social setting of the urban and rural companies have to be kept in mind as the results are presented and discussed. The reader is referred to the NIOSH Technical Report (Cobb and Kasl, 1977) for full details of the study methodology.

Summary of Results and Discussion

This section will highlight some of the major findings which have been obtained from this study. The reader is urged to consult the original publications (Cobb, 1974; Cobb and Kasl, 1977; Kasl, 1979a; Kasl and Cobb, 1970, 1979, 1980; Kasl and Cobb, in press; Kasl and Cobb, and Brooks, 1968; Kasl, Gore, and Cobb, 1975) for much fuller detail regarding the various outcomes.

The first set of findings to be summarized are those which may be thought of as characterizing the <u>total</u> or <u>average</u> impact of the experience. The salient ones were:

1) The men who became unemployed did not blame themselves for this; however, for those who continued being unemployed (6 months or more), self-blame did go up (Cobb and Kasl, 1977).

2) Job satisfaction data for re-employed men, collected one year after plant closing, showed equal or higher job satisfaction on the new jobs, compared to the old ones. Strikingly higher satisfaction with co-workers and supervisers on the new job was particularly suprising, given the 20 years of seniority at the old plant (Cobb and Kasl, 1977).

3) Analysis of intra-person differences between occasions when a man was unemployed and when he was re-employed revealed a clearcut impact of employment status on sense of economic deprivation and specific work-role deprivation dimensions (e.g., "chance to use skills you are best at;" "feelings of security about the future"). However, on diverse indicators of mental health status (e.g., depression, anxiety-tension, psychophysiological symptoms) no significant differences attributable to employment status could be detected (Kasl, 1979a; Kasl and Cobb, 1979). Correlational analyses of the subjective index of economic deprivation with the various indicators of mental health status also failed to establish a link that would be suggestive of an impact (an indirect one via economic deprivation) of the job loss experience on mental health: the correlations were quite weak and no different from those among the controls. Furthermore, phase-to-phase changes in economic deprivation did not correlate with corresponding changes in mental health.

4) Measures based on a 2-week health diary, such as Days Complaint ("did not feel as well as usual") and Days Disability ("did not carry on usual activities"), showed significant fluctuations over time, but not those which could be linked to employment-unemployment status changes (Kasl, Gore, and Cobb, 1975). For example, Days Complaint were elevated at Anticipation Phase, when all men were still working. At Phase 2, when many of the men were unemployed, levels of Days Complaint were significantly below average and this was true irrespective of working status. At Phase 3, the levels were again elevated -- as much for men still unemployed as for those recently re-employed or those who were stabilizing their employment (passed their probationary period).

5) There was a small group of men who were still unemployed at one and/or two-year follow-ups. These men gave every evidence of poor mental and physical health; for example, they had elevated levels of Depression and Days Complaint. However, these men showed stably elevated levels throughout the study, including the Anticipation phase. This tends to rule out the effect of unemployment and suggests, instead, a "reverse causation" interpretation: initially poor health was interfering with their ability (or desire) to find work.

6) Analyses of cardiovascular risk factors (blood pressure, serum cholesterol, cigarette smoking, body weight) did not at any point reveal a level of cardiovascular risk among men losing their jobs exceeding the risk among controls (Kasl and Cobb, 1980). Cigarette smoking was found to be an exceedingly stable habit in our study subjects and essentially no changes could be identified and studied. The other risk factors (especially cholesterol) did prove to be sensitive to the employment status changes experienced by the terminees;

however, this was because of extra low levels during reemployment rather than elevated levels during unemployment. Overall, the findings failed to provide support for the hypothesis, derived from the business cycle and mortality analyses (Brenner, 1971; Brenner and Mooney, in press; Bunn, 1979), that major cardiovascular risk factors will be found elevated at some point during the job loss-unemployment-reemployment experience.

7) The vast majority of the dependent variables in this study (physiological, mental health, and work-role deprivation) showed a similar pattern of dynamic changes: a) Between Phase 1 and Phase 2, they were reliably sensitive to the difference in employment status, that is, going from Anticipation to unemployment vs. to prompt re-employment; b) Between Phase 2 and Phase 3, men continuing to remain unemployed tended to return to "normal" levels similar to the men who were becoming re-employed at that time. This pattern suggests that the men did not maintain a state of arousal, distress, and sense of work role deprivation as long as the unemployment experience lasted; rather, they showed evidence of adaptation so that following an initial period of unemployment those remaining unemployed could not be distinguished from those finding a new job. In short, it appeared that we could demonstrate acute effects of the plant closing and job loss experience but not prolonged or chronic effects.

In general these findings tend to illuminate the process of coping and adaptation to losing one's job, but they do not suggest a strong and lasting average impact of the experience. Thus, for example, it is difficult to interpret the cardiovascular risk factor findings as providing evidence that, with a larger sample and longer follow-up, higher incidence of cardiovascular morbidity or mortality would have been observed. However, it is still possible that even if standard risk factors don't change, morbidity or mortality can go up. (For example, Eliot and Buell (1981) have noted a 50% increase in sudden death rate among men at the Kennedy Space Center during the mid-1960's, even though traditional risk factors showed little.) Furthermore, even transitory, self-limiting, reversible elevations in blood pressure or serum cholesterol could conceivably indicate at least a temporary increase in risk of morbid outcomes, which when aggregated over large units (states, nations) might reveal a detectible increase in actual morbidity and mortality. In short, the findings are not supportive of the business cycle analyses and results, but cannot be interpreted as being definitely contradictory.

The results may also be seen against a background of research on low-skill blue-collar jobs (Kasl, 1974 and 1978). Many workers adapt to dull and monotonous jobs by disengaging and by giving up expectations that work will be a meaningful human activity. Thus, aside from the financial considerations, the adaptive demands of the loss of the work role may be only self-limiting, with a correspondingly limited impact, among such disengaged blue collar workers.

There were additional findings which came out of the study that can best be viewed as _selective_ impact or _interactive_ effects, rather than general impact (Kasl and Cobb, in press).

One powerful source of variability in results obtained had to do with the location of the plant, the large metropolitan area vs. the small rural community. 1) The primary objective index of severity of the job loss experience, number of weeks of unemployment experienced during the first year, showed substantial correlations with a subjective index of job loss "stress," with

Relative Economic Deprivation and with the Work Role Deprivation scales. However, this was only true in the urban setting; in the rural setting, the correlations were nonsignificant and in the opposite direction. Clearly then, to the extent that these subjective variables reflect relevant mediating perceptions and processes, the dynamics of the plant closing-unemployment experience appear to have been quite different in the two settings. 2) Analyses of intra-person differences between occasions when a man was unemployed and when he was re-employed revealed an impact of employment status on the work role deprivation scales primarily in the rural setting and an impact on some of the mental health scales only in the urban setting (Kasl and Cobb, 1979). This is consistent with the notion that there are rural-urban differences in the meaning of work: there is some evidence that small town workers are less alienated from middle-class work norms than are urban workers (Hulin and Blood, 1968; Turner and Lawrence, 1968), and thus there is a greater attachment to the work role in the rural setting.

Another major source of variation in results which we have encountered (Cobb and Kasl, 1977; Kasl and Cobb, in press) was due to differences in Perceived Social Support. The major findings involving this measure provided a fair amount of support for the general proposition that, among men who went through a more severe plant closing-job loss experience, higher levels of perceived social support tended to ameliorate the negative impact of the experience, both for psychological and physiological indicators. For example, social support was found to influence the relationship between length of unemployment and scores on the subjective job loss "stress" index: among men high on social support, length of unemployment had very little influence on job loss "stress", while among those low on social support, a substantial positive association was seen between length of unemployment and job loss "stress".

Level of social support contributed to selective or variable impact of the job loss experience in even more complex ways by interacting with other variables. For example, the role of social support depended sometimes on the stages of adaptation to the experience (Kasl and Cobb, in press). Phase-to phase analysis of changes in anxiety-tension revealed that the benefits of prompt re-employment (i.e., reduction in level of anxiety by Phase 2 among those with new jobs) were seen primarily among those with <u>low</u> social support. However, later phase-to-phase changes (e.g., from Phase 2 to Phase 3) revealed that among those whose employment situation remained uncertain (still unemployed, or further job changes), high levels of social support were associated with reductions in anxiety-tension, and low levels of support, with increases. This pattern of findings suggests that social support as a buffering influence did not come into play until later, i.e., when it appeared that stable re-employment was not easily attained; on the other hand, the combination of prompt re-employment and low social support might have led to a sense of accomplishment and mastery by the unsupported individuals. Similar analyses of changes in the physiological variables (blood pressure, serum uric acid, serum cholesterol) also showed that the buffering effect of social support was phase-specific, i.e., evident at some stages of adaptation to the plant closing experience but not at other stages.

In general, these results on variability of impact of the job loss experience suggest that a) the dynamics of adaptation to the experience and the mechanisms of impact can differ for subgroups of individuals, thus suggesting b) that these individuals are not equally vulnerable to the possible adverse impact of the job loss experience.

Epidemiologic (Micro Level) Research on Economic Instability and Health

In this section, we shall use the research design of the above study as a starting point for a discussion of research strategies involving the epidemiologic or micro level approach to the problem.

Let us begin by clarifying and making explicit some of the research design advantages and disadvantages of utilizing the above "natural experiment" approach.

The prospective study of plant closing has several advantages. One is that there is no plausible self-selection process involved. The job loss experience is faced by all working at the plant (with an average of almost 20 years of seniority) through no fault of their own, and personal characteristics such as poor health or depression are not influential in increasing the person's risk for losing his job. The second advantage is that the cohort of subjects is picked up prior to plant closing and before they go through the experience of job loss. Such baseline data permit a "before-after" analysis within the cohort of men losing their jobs. However, the baseline data are of an admittedly limited usefulness: the men already knew the plant closing was coming and thus the initial data collection was sensitive to the impact of anticipation. A true baseline data collection during a time when a plant closing is not anticipated or even rumored would be difficult to accomplish and would likely be an expensive design.

Simple cross-sectional analysis of data on a community or national sample, in which respondents are classified as employed or unemployed, is almost certain to reveal differences on unhappiness, distress, anomie, and psychiatric disorder (Bradburn, 1969; Campbell, Converse, and Rodgers, 1976; Fried, 1969). However, such differences are suspect because of the severe problem of self-selection as an alternative explanation: a) Subjects with prior distress or unhappiness may be at greater risk for being unemployed. b) Subjects with lower education or fewer job skills may be at greater risk for both distress and unemployment. c) Subjects with prior distress or unhappiness may be at greater risk for a longer episode of unemployment before finding a new job; such a longer episode would then increase their chances of being included in the "unemployed" group in a cross-sectional survey conducted at any one particular time. Retrospective questioning regarding the circumstances of the job loss might identify a sub-group of unemployed respondents for whom self-selection processes are unlikely to have been present. If their level of distress is no different from the others who are unemployed, then this would argue for an impact of unemployment rather than for self-selection. However, the validity of such retrospective questioning may be difficult to establish.

Under certain ideal circumstances, a cross-sectional survey of a community or a well-defined "catchment area" may reveal differences between those employed and those unemployed which suggest an impact rather than self-selection. Suppose our diagnostic interview schedule reveals a prevalence rate of "current depression" of 4% among the employed and 20% among the unemployed. Given the community rate of unemployment of, say, 20% (and assuming representative sampling) we would project a prevalence rate of 7.2% of depression for the total community irrespective of employment status. If we are using an instrument on which population norms indicate that the expected community rate of depression is 5%, then our findings would seem to demonstrate an excess which may be attributable to the unemployment rate. However, we would have to make certain assumptions, such as no biased in- or out-migration from the community. But the most important assumption would be that the population norms of the test are an applicable basis for calculating "expected" rates. On whom was the test normed? If on employed people only, then clearly those are inappropriate norms. If on a national sample, then we must ask if the community we are studying is strictly comparable to the national "average." Perhaps the most convincing basis for such norms would be self-same community data from the recent past -- at which time, incidentally, the unemployment rate was much lower. But then, the issue simply becomes one of interpreting secular change in community prevalence rates by paying attention to one intervening change (in unemployment) and ignoring other possible historical events and changes. In short, this discussion reveals that cross-sectional comparisons of employed and unemployed are likely to remain a problematic methodology.

A non-prospective design which includes longitudinal follow-up appears to hold some promise. Such a study starts out as a cross-sectional survey of the community; those initially unemployed and a representative (or matched) subset of those employed are then followed up. It may be argued that if the unemployed persons started out with higher levels of depression (for example) and that if those who became re-employed showed reductions in depression, then such a pattern of results is more compatible with the impact interpretation and less compatible with the self-selection hypothesis. However, there are limits to such an argument. For example, if there are enduring or chronic effects of the unemployment experience, one would falsely attribute the lack of return to "normal" levels to an initial self-selection process, thereby grossly underestimate the impact of unemployment. Furthermore, only a very close monitoring of the subjects would be able to pin down securely the proper causal interpretation. If, for example, a person is both unemployed and depressed on one occasion and re-employed and of normal affect six months later, the above assumptions would call for the causal interpretation of unemployment influencing depression. However, if the actual sequence of events were recovery from depression at month 2 and re-employment at month 3 (not detected by the actual follow-up schedule), then a "reverse" causal interpretation would seem more appropriate.

Thus far we have discussed research design issues which reveal problems of causal interpretation. These can be summarized by noting that short of being able to impose random assignment of subjects to job loss (vs. continued employment), the best approach seems to be a "natural experiment" in which a whole plant closes down in a deus ex machina fashion (in the specific instance of our study, corporate headquarters a thousand miles away deciding to build a new plant in a different region of the country because of labor costs and unrelated to worker performance or product demands). However, various practical limitations of field research may pose problems: 1) Baseline data from even before the plans to close down become known to employees may be difficult to obtain and anticipation effects may intrude. 2) Comparison companies serving as controls will at best be only approximately comparable. 3) Severity of the experience (such as weeks unemployed or the number of job changes after plant closing) is an additional important independent variable, but it is no longer exempt from the suspicion of "self-selection" bias; a different "natural experiment" would be needed to compare, with minimum self-selection bias, those exposed to brief vs. lengthy unemployment.

It is a common dilemma in quasi-experimental field research (Cook and Campbell, 1979) that a trade-off exists between internal validity (strong causal inferences) and external validity (generalizability). In the case of the plant closing study described earlier, it may be seen that its external validity is rather limited. Generalizability may be seen in terms of who were the subjects who were studied and just what part of the total phenomenon (economic instability) was addressed with that "natural experiment" design.

Some obvious limitations of the generalizability of that study must be noted: 1) Only blue-collar male workers were studied. There is no question that inferences about impact cannot be made regarding women, white collar workers, professionals and scientists, and so on. Low skill blue collar workers have a relatively weak attachment to the work role (Kasl, 1974 and 1978) and possibly to the specific work place (The Company) as well. 2) The selection criteria which defined eligibility for participation in study (e.g., male, age 35-60, married, several years of seniority) further limit the generalizability of the findings. The rationale behind these criteria was to define a homogeneous subgroup, of a sufficiently large number, for whom the impact of job loss might be particularly strong: the primary breadwinner in the family, in an age range where early retirement is unlikely, where work career pattern has been established, and with financial responsibility for one or more dependents. However, such criteria were developed more or less on an intuitive basis and they need not have all operated in the direction of greater impact. For example, increased responsibility due to being married may be more than compensated for by the increased potential for social support. In short, other subjects would need to be studied -- single workers, those with irregular work careers, those who recently entered the labor market -- before we can have a good picture of the impact of a plant closing on different subgroups of workers.

It is likely that the best strategy for a study of the impact of plant closing is at the level of the community (Sklar, 1980). Such a study would thus include other persons who do not themselves go through the job loss experience: wives of the workers and the children; selected members of the business community most likely to be affected by the plant closing; young persons about to enter the labor market; and so on. In addition, data would need to be collected regarding the functioning of various agencies and institutions at the community level in order to paint a better picture of the way the community is responding to and coping with the plant closing.

So far we have discussed limitations on generalizability which relate to who was and was not studied. The other aspect of generalizability is: what aspect of the total phenomenon was studied? 1) There is no question that the plant closing study was carried out at a time when the national and local economic situation was rather benign. Hence, the duration of the unemployment for most was reasonably short and the prospects of reemployment among the job searchers were presumably never desperately bleak. A similar study carried out today in an economically depressed state like Michigan might reveal quite a different impact. Specifically, analyses designed to distinguish acute and prolonged impact might now demonstrate chronic stress effects among those remaining unemployed. 2) As was noted earlier, studying an entire plant where everybody (outside of a few in higher levels of management) lost their jobs through no fault of their own is a "natural experiment" which controls rather well for self-selection biases. However, the trade-off is that only a particular type of job loss experience is being studied. For example, it represented a situation where self-blame was at a minimum; studies from the Depression era (Kasl, 1979a) suggest that self-blame may be an important prelude to other adverse reactions, such as depression and loss of self-esteem. Furthermore, since the entire cohort of workers was going through the experience together, the potential for sharing of the experience among those affected and for the building of community support structures (particularly in the rural setting) could have been greatly enhanced. 3) It may also be noted that a 2 year follow-up period may not be sufficient for detecting long term effects or delayed effects. This comment, of course, is particularly relevant to the study of impact of long episodes of unemployment in a depressed economic market. The issue of delayed effects is difficult to speculate about, with one exception: In our study we noted (Cobb and Kasl, 1972) that irrespective of how rapidly the terminees become re-employed, their situation with respect to retirement benefits was bleak because they had to start de novo with their own and the employer's contributions at the new place of employment. Consequently, at the time of retirement, their private benefits (aside from Social Security payments) will be less than if the plant had not closed and their pension plan liquidated. Thus the post-retirement economic well-being of these men, who suffered relatively short unemployment, would be worth additional study.

The last point above raises a general problem which as yet has not been addressed adequately by available unemployment studies. The issue is how to decompose, conceptually and operationally, the particular experience under study. For example, the experience of losing one's job may be thought of as consisting of three primary components: 1) Those which are purely economic or financial, such as change from certain income due to wages, to 80% of wage income coming from unemployment insurance, to no income when the period of coverage for such insurance runs out. 2) Those which pertain to activities and behaviors associated with going to work: the commuting, the socializing at work, the physical expenditure of energy or the utilization of special skills (as applicable), the structuring of passage of time, and so on. 3) Those which pertain to issues of self-concept or self-identity: for example, one may substitute or replace job activities and insurance may replace lost wages, but the self-identity (and public identity) of "not working", "but of work" "unemployed", persists. Similarly, within the family one may lose the identity of "chief breadwinner" or "head of household."

Clearly, the above ideas are just the beginnings of a theory which would define the necessary components of the unemployment experience and suggest adequate operationalizations for such concepts. However, such a decomposition is necessary since even though the unemployment experience is unitary, remedial actions designed to ameliorate impact are bound to be piecemeal, such as financial help, re-education with respect to leisure activities, or self-help support groups. Furthermore, the differential vulnerability of subgroups of workers cannot be easily understood unless we again decompose the total phenomenon in order to pinpoint specific processes accounting for the differential vulnerability.

While this discussion has centered on studying the impact of job loss on health, there are clearly other aspects of the notion of "economic instability" which are eminently worth studying: indefinite layoffs, temporary layoffs (either scheduled and predictable or unexpected), inability to find employment among those trying to enter the job market for the first time, working reduced hours, being forced to change jobs within a company, and continued employment in a setting of great economic insecurity.

Studies of Economic Instability and Health at the Macro and Micro Levels

Much of the recent research on unemployment has utilized a macroeconomic approach, linking aggregated data on economic change (particularly percent unemployed) to fluctuations in other indicators, also aggregated for a whole state or country (Brenner, 1971, 1973, 1975, 1979; Bunn, 1979). This proliferation of the business cycle studies by its practitioners has taken place in relative isolation from methodological criticism of this whole approach. Some have questioned the interpretation of the associations, but not the basic methodology (Eyer, 1977, 1980); others question it as an approach to detecting the health and mental health costs of unemployment (Kasl, 1979b; Marshall and Funch, 1979; Ratcliff, 1980); and still others have raised broad methodological criticisms of the whole approach of utilizing ecological data (Firebaugh, 1978; Stavraky, 1976). The concern with "ecological fallacy" is, of course, not very new (Robinson, 1950).

The specific analytic techniques applied to the macro level studies of economic change have undergone revisions over the years and certain concerns and criticisms from earlier studies may no longer be applicable. For example, the highly inappropriate detrending practices (e.g., Brenner, 1973) are no longer evident. Furthermore, additional variables have been included in the multiple regression models which thus strengthen these analyses -- for example, per capita cigarette consumption when looking at cardiovascular mortality (Brenner and Mooney, in press). Finally, we are beginning to see re-analyses of data from earlier reports (e.g., Gravelle, Hutchinson, and Stern, 1981) which tend to clarify the issue of robustness (vs. sensitivity) of the results as changes in the analytic methodology are explored.

Clearly, there is much need for additional exploration of the strengths and weaknesses of different methodologies and of different levels of analysis. The recent work of Catalano and Dooley (Catalano and Dooley, 1979a and b; Catalano, Dooley, and Jackson, 1981; Dooley and Catalano, 1979 and 1980) and Sklar (1980) shows promise of clarifying the troublesome issue of generalizations across levels of analysis and establishing strategies of research for studying the health impact of business cycle changes and of the individual experience of unemployment.

Much of the work involving macro analysis of business cycle and mortality data has stagnated at the stage of post-hoc analyses and interpretations (e.g., Brenner, 1979) and has failed to avail itself of the opportunity of proposing and testing a priori hypotheses and predictions. History of science strongly suggests that offering a testable proposition and then collecting (or analyzing) data to see if it is supported, is preferable to allowing oneself total freedom of post-hoc interpretation. This is particularly applicable since the data analyzed are macro level data, but interpretations and suggestions regarding causal dynamics are at the level of individual (e.g., Brenner, 1979).

What testable propositions are possible and would be helpful? Three types of testable propositions would represent modest steps forward. 1) Apply already accomplished analyses to forecast future trends in a particular dependent variable, such as infant mortality. Thus far, there is no evidence of any utility of past analyses for forecasting future trends. For some outcomes, the success of such forecasting is difficult to imagine; for example, the decline in cardiovascular mortality during the past 10-15 years has taken place against a background of considerable economic turmoil in the last decade. 2) Set up analyses to permit cross-validation of results. For example, divide the total period examined (say 1920 to 1980) into 2 periods, so that model parameters based on the first period are used to project trends in mortality for the second period. This is, in effect, forecasting done in retrospect. 3) The third type of testable proposition takes advantage of natural variations in the total, global picture. For example, regional variations in the unemployment picture can be exploited to make differential predictions about changes in the dependent variable, applicable to one or another region. Similarly, different socio-demographic subgroups offer an opportunity for making predictions and carrying out sub-analyses. Thus the impact of the fluctuations in unemployment should be different for those who are retired and on pensions or retirement plans adjusted for inflation, than for middle-aged blue collar workers with limited skills.

The above suggestions for expanding the type of analyses to be carried out represent only a small step toward fully exploring the basic issue: how to achieve a better understanding of the role of different research designs, carried out at different levels of aggregation or on different units of observation, in generating data on the impact of economic instability on health.

At this point it seems useful to close this report with a series of questions which may help us focus on some of the issues ahead. (Some of the following questions are more rhetorical than others).

A. Questions with respect to macro-level analysis:

1) Do we at the present time understand the differences in results which have been obtained across different recent macro level analyses? Do we know what analyses (or what studies) would be needed to reconcile these differences?

2) Would we learn anything useful from additional macro level analyses? What? How should they be different from those already carried out?

3) Since macro level analyses need to examine a reasonably long chunk of the past, can they ever tell us anything meaningful about the present or the near future?

4) Since macro level analyses are very inexpensive (dirt cheap?) to carry out, but potentially devastatingly expensive when providing false leads, do we at present have a methodology for separating useful from useless leads (suggestions, hypotheses)? Is it a macro level methodology?

5) Since macro analyses depend on data collected by others (archival or institutional data), do we at present use any guidelines for evaluating the quality and validity of data and for deciding when to accept or reject a new data source?

6) Can macro level data analysts identify the types of data they would like to have made available to them? Are there some data which are crucial and without which macro level analysis might be deemed inadequate?

7) Since many of the multivariate macro-level regression "models" are already "explaining" close to 100% of the variance in mortality data, what criteria can we set up so that we answer the question: Is the new "model" better than the old one?

8) Are there at present any internal checks on the way the data analysis is being carried out so that technical problems (such as, excessive error variances when working with partial associations among strongly intercorrelated variables) are avoided?

9) Does the macro level accept the notion of "spurious" associations, or are all associations at the macro level "real" and equally valuable (valid)? If associations can be "spurious" at the macro level, are there principles and methodologies for identifying them and removing their influence?

B. Questions with respect to micro-level analysis:

1) Can we identify the major types of research designs that are included here? Do they have a priori strengths and weaknesses, or does that depend on the actual execution of a particular study and the types of questions being asked? Can any be labelled a priori as "useless," "essential," "unrealistic," "too expensive," and so on.

2) Can we identify essential types of information that <u>all</u> studies should be collecting? For example: about the economic climate, about social insurance policies applicable to subjects being studied, about type of experience being studied (financial, career, job change, reduced hours, layoff, etc.), and so on?

3) Since at the micro level we can choose the data we intend to collect, is there any consensus on dependent variables (or impact criteria) that might

lead us to label them "important," "trivial," "unmeasurable at present," etc.? Should we have any priorities? What proxy indicators (e.g., risk factors instead of disease outcomes) are most useful?

4) What are the relative merits of naturalistic experiments on adverse impact vs. controlled studies of benefits of various policies/programs/interventions?

5) Since the issue of generalizability of findings is such an important one -- results appear to be highly specific to occupational subgroups, types of experiences, nature of support systems, etc. -- can we identify research designs and subject populations which offer the greatest promise of generalizable findings?

6) Can we identify major methodological concerns to which all micro-studies, no matter what design, should be sensitive? Certainly, there must be an overwhelming concern with the direction of causality i.e., separating out impact of the experience from self-selection processes (reverse causation). Similarly, there must be some concern with the behavioral or biological validity of impact criteria being assessed. What are the other major concerns?

7) Given such methodological concerns, can we prefer certain research designs; e.g. those which minimize self-selection, those which provide us with some baseline information on our subject from the past, and so on?

8) Since the 2 directions of causality are not mutually exclusive (e.g., those in prior poor health are at greater risk for experiencing some form of economic instability, which, in turn, may accelerate the downward course of their health), can we develop principles of methodology which would enable us to study both? What retrospective accounts do we find useful? How good

must be our initial assessment of physical and mental health status if we study subjects where the self-selection process has already taken place?

9) Is there any consensus on the length of observations needed before the full impact of a particular experience can be described? Do different experiences call for different lengths of observations?

C. Questions with respect to cross-level comparisons:

1) Since the distinction between "micro" and "macro" levels is an oversimplification, what are the levels (units) of observation which are actually available to the investigator: individual, family, social network, organization/institution, community, region, nation. Have they been studied equally dilligently? Should they be?

2) Do these levels of observation call for unique data collection methodologies, or are there fewer unique research designs then levels?

3) Can we identify <u>unique</u> contributions to knowledge which go along with working at a particular level of analysis?

4) Are policy issues and intervention efforts uniquely anchored to specific levels of analysis so that appropriate data collection only at that level must take place?

5) Are there research methodologies which <u>cross</u> levels of analysis? What are their special features?

6) Is any cost/benefit analysis of research at different levels of analysis at all possible? That is, can one assess "usefulness" of knowledge at each level? And costs?

7) Have we identified principles of scientific (causal) reasoning which can guide to us to proper interpretations which <u>go across</u> levels of observations?

8) Are there types of information or data collected which are _tied_ to particular levels of observation so that they cannot be properly used except at that level? Are there other types of information which are of general usefulness so that they can be used at any level of aggregation?

9) Do we understand the consequences of changing units of aggregation -- temporal, geographical, socio-political and so on?

References

Block, J. *The Challenge of Response Sets*. New York: Appleton, 1965.

Bradburn, N. *The Structure of Psychological Well-Being*. Chicago: Aldine Press, 1969.

Brenner, M.H. Economic changes and heart disease mortality. *American Journal of Public Health*, 1971, 61, 606-611.

Brenner, M.H. Fetal, infant, and maternal mortality during periods of economic instability. *International Journal of Health Services*, 1973, 3, 145-159.

Brenner, M.H. Trends in alcohol consumption and associated illnesses: Some effects of economic changes. *American Journal of Public Health*, 1975, 65, 1279-1292.

Brenner, M.H. Mortality and the national economy. A review and the experience of England and Wales, 1936-1976. *Lancet*, 1979, 2, 568-573.

Brenner, M.H., and Mooney, A. Economic change and sex-specific cardiovascular mortality in Britain, 1955-1976. *Soc. Sci. & Med.*, in press.

Bunn, A.R. Ischaemic heart disease mortality and the business cycle in Australia. *American Journal of Public Health*, 1979, 69, 772-781.

Campbell, A., Converse, P.E., and Rodgers, W.L. *The Quality of American Life*. New York: Russell Sage Foundation, 1976.

Catalano, R., and Dooley, D. Does economic change provoke or uncover behavioral disorder? In L.A. Ferman and J.P. Gordus (Eds.) *Mental Health and the Economy*. Kalamazoo: The W.E. Upjohn Institute for Employment Research, 1979(a).

Catalano, R., and Dooley, D. The economy as stressor: A sectoral analysis. *Review of Social Economy*, 1979(b), 37, 175-188.

Catalano, R., Dooley, D., and Jackson, R. Economic predictors of use of mental health facilities in a non-metropolitan community. *J. Health & Soc. Behav.*, 1981, 22, 284-298.

Cobb, S. Physiologic changes in men whose jobs were abolished. *J. Psychosom. Res.*, 1974, 18, 245-258.

Cobb, S. and Kasl, S.V. Some medical aspects of unemployment. In Shatto, G.M. (Ed.) *Employment of the Middle-Aged*. Springfield, Ill.: C.C. Thomas, 1972

Cobb, S., and Kasl, S.V. *Termination: The Consequences of Job Loss*. Cincinnati: DHEW (NIOSH) Publication No. 77-224, 1977.

Cook, T.D., and Campbell, D.T. *Quasi-Experimentation*. Chicago: Rand McNally, 1979.

Crowne, D.P., and Marlowe, D. *The Approval Motive*. New York: Wiley, 1964.

Dooley, D., and Catalano, R. Economic, life and disorder changes: Time-series analyses. American Journal of Community Psychology, 1979, 7, 381-396.

Dooley, D., and Catalano, R. Economic change as a cause of behavioral disorder. Psychological Bulletin, 1980, 87, 450-468.

Eliot, R.S., and Buell, J.C. Environmental and behavioral influences in the major cardiovascular disorders. In Weiss, S.M., Herd, J.A., and Fox, B.H. (Eds.) Perspectives on Behavioral Medicine. New York: Academic Press, 1981.

Eyer, J. Prosperity as a cause of death. International Journal of Health Services, 1977, 7, 125-150.

Eyer, J. Social causes of coronary heart disease. Psychotherapy and Psychosomatics, 1980, 34, 75-87.

Fried, M. Social differences in mental health. In J. Kosa, A. Antonovsky, and I.K. Zola (Eds.), Poverty and Health: A Sociological Analysis. Cambridge: Harvard University Press, 1969.

Firebaugh, G. A rule for inferring individual level relationships from aggregated data. American Sociological Review, 1978, 43, 557-572.

Gore, S. The Influence of Social Support in Ameliorating the Consequences of Job Loss. Philadelphia: Unpublished doctoral dissertation, The University of Pennsylvania, 1973.

Gough, G. The California Psychological Inventory Manual. Palo Alto: Consulting Psychologists Press, 1957.

Gravelle, H.S.E., Hutchinson, G., and Stern, J. Mortality and unemployment: A critique of Brenner's time-series analysis. Lancet, 1981, 2, 675-679.

Hulin, C.L., and Blood, M.R. Job enlargement, individual differences, and worker responses. Psychological Bulletin, 1968, 69, 41-55.

Kasl, S.V. Work and mental health. In J. O'Toole (Ed.), Work and Quality of Life. Cambridge: The MIT Press, 1974.

Kasl, S.V. Epidemiological contributions to the study of work stress. In C.L. Cooper and R. Payne (Eds.), Stress at Work. Chichester: J. Wiley & Sons, Ltc., 1978.

Kasl, S.V. Changes in mental health status associated with job loss and retirement. In J.E. Barrett (Ed.), Stress and Mental Disorder. New York: Raven Press, 1979(a).

Kasl, S.V. Mortality and the business cycle: some questions about research strategies when utilizing macro-social and ecological data. American Journal of Public Health, 1979(b), 69, 784-788.

Kasl, S.V. and Cobb, S. Blood pressure changes in men undergoing job loss: a preliminary report. Psychosom. Med., 1970, 32, 19-38.

Kasl, S.V. and Cobb, S. Some mental health consequences of plant closing and job loss. In L.A. Ferman and J.P. Gordus (Eds.) Mental Health and the Economy. Kalamazoo: The W.E. Upjohn Institute for Employment Research, 1979.

Kasl, S.V. and Cobb, S. The experience of losing a job: Some effects on cardiovascular functioning. Psychotherapy and Psychosomatics, 1980, 34, 88-109.

Kasl, S.V., and Cobb, S. Variability of stress effects among men experiencing job loss. In Goldberger, L., and Breznitz, S. (Eds.) Handbook of Stress. New York: The Free Press, in press.

Kasl, S.V., Cobb, S., and Brooks, G.W. Changes in serum uric acid and cholesterol levels in men undergoing job loss. J. Amer. Med. Assoc., 1968, 206, 1500-1507.

Kasl, S.V., Gore, S., and Cobb, C. The experience of losing a job: Reported changes in health, symptoms, and illness behavior. Psychosomatic Medicine, 1975, 37, 106-122.

Marshall, J.R., and Funch, D.P. Mental illness and the economy: a critique and partial replication. Journal of Health and Social Behavior, 1979, 20, 282-289.

Ratcliff, K.S. On Marshall and Funch's Critique of "Mental Illness and the Economy." Journal of Health and Social Behavior, 1980, 21, 389-391.

Robinson, W.S. Ecological correlations and the behavior of individuals. American Sociological Review, 1950, 15, 351-357.

Sklar, E.D. Community economic structure and individual well-being: A look behind the statistics. International Journal of Health Services, 1980, 10, 563-579.

Slote, A. Termination: The Closing at Baker Plant. Indianapolis: Bobbs-Merrill, 1969.

Stavraky, K. The role of ecological analysis in studies of the etiology of disease: a discussion with reference to large bowel cancer. Journal of Chronic Diseases, 1976, 29, 435-444.

Tiffany, D.W., Cowan, J.R., and Tiffany, P.M. The Unemployed: A Social-Psychological Portrait. Englewood Cliffs, N.J.: Prentice-Hall, 1970.

Turner, A.N., and Lawrence, P.R. Industrial Jobs and the Worker. Cambridge: Harvard University Graduate School of Business Administration, 1968.

WHO: Study on the influence of economic development on health. Report on a WHO Planning Meeting, Nov. 11-13, 1980, Copenhagen. WHO: 1981.

METHODOLOGICAL PROBLEMS IN THE MEASUREMENT OF HEALTH CONSEQUENCES OF UNEMPLOYMENT IN SAMPLE SURVEYS

Klaus Preiser

Forschungsgruppe Arbeit und Gesundheit GmbH
Dortmund, Federal Republic of Germany

0. Introduction

The author's interest in work with this theme dates from years of empirical work on the relationship between job characteristics and their influence on the health of employees. Through secondary analysis it was tried to demonstrate or to reject a relationship (cp. B. HAMACHER, K. PREISER, 1977; N. GARRETT-BLEEK u.a., 1976; INFRATEST SOZIALFORSCHUNG und FORSCHUNGSGRUPPE ARBEIT UND GESUNDHEIT, 1979; R. MÜLLER u.a., 1979). Much too often this work has been overshadowed by irritations about the various kinds of methodological dilettantism in the analyses so far done.

This may be a consequence of the low stage of development of the epidemiologic and social-medical research in the Federal Republic of Germany. The reasons and causes for this are not to be followed here. It is not surprising, then, that a majority in this country support the thesis: "Unemployment makes sick".

This paper is intended to draw attention in short form on the methodological traps and weakness which pose themselves in this connexion. We deal with the exclusive question of the empirical clarification of the problem in sample surveys. After having read the paper the reader might ask himself whether it is possible at all to proof health consequences of unemployment. The author cannot give a final judgement on that question.

1. Terms

<u>Methodological problems</u> are meant to comprise the whole research design, proceeding from the context of findings (hypothesis), its transformation in empirical procedures and instruments (measurement), including the empirical survey and finally the evaluation of the results. Our focus here is on making the research concepts operational.

<u>Sample survey</u> means interviewing a subpopulation, selected from a total population, through a mainly standardized questionnaire in a personal contact or by mail.

As <u>unemployed</u> we mean to be understood persons, which at a given moment or a reference period have no gainful employment, but seeking work.

<u>Health</u> should be a "condition of complete physical, psychological and social well-being" (WHO-definition). Unemployment is said to have effects on the well-being, if the state of health varies as a result of this event.

2. Theoretical concepts to construe the relationship between unemployment and health

A homogeneous theoretical concept to describe this relationship is not available. "It is the lack of theory, which makes the research results look so fragmentary" (D. FRÖHLICH, 1979, 36). FRÖHLICH traces this back to a missing theory of work susceptable to empirical proof. The following concepts can be seperated:

1. The stress concept

First stress is a normal biological reaction of man to a lot of stimuli from the environment. The physiological result of stress is the release of energy ready to be spent in muscular exertion. The effects of stress on health depends on its intensity and the possibilities of muscular exertion. Normally no health risks are given. If however the strength and the length of a stress are continously high or long, then health risks result. Often reported symptoms are e.g. weariness, headache, constipation or diarrhoea; it can cause an ulcer of the stomach or duodenum (cp. W. MÜLLER-LIMM-ROTH, 1977). Alcoholism, criminal behavior and susceptibility to drugs are more likely to occur (ib.). It is taken for granted, that the event of unemployment and its length have qualities of stress.

2. The psychosomatic concept

According to the psychosomatic concept the roots of the illness-releasing conflict is to be looked for in early childhood. Through the unemployment (as a loss of the object) the conflict which lies dormant deep inside is actualized. This loss of object can be expressed in wishes of dependence, resistence to aggression, reduced introspection, a feeling of emptiness compensated by depressive moods, limitation of perception and a look of the ability to bear conflicts (cp. M. BAUER, 1976, 140).

WACKER (1976, 67) said about this concept, that "the loss of the job should not thinned to the release of personal crisis." THOMANN (1978, 203) is correct in saying, that with this concept "the central role of work in human life" is discredited.

In default of a conclusive theoretical concept the following procedure is usually applied: Some functions, inherent in the work, like earning money, orientation in time, self-esteem, social contacts etc. are defined. The effects of the loss of any of these functions are then observed in a measurable form and explained through the suppression of the functions (cp. D. FRÖHLICH, 1979, 37). FRESE and MOHR (1978, 285) noted, that not only the degree of variety of the dependent and independent variables are not satisfactory but it is not sufficiently clarified which variables are causes and which are effects. Normally intervening variables are missing.

Summarily, we can say at this point, that in most research of the effects of unemployment on wellbeing there is a lack of homogeneous theory and of well founded hypotheses (cp. the summary paper of M. FRESE, G. MOHR (1978) and K.-D. THOMANN (1978)). This has the effect, that as the result of the analysis there are detected significant single relationships, but that a closed and complete system of dependent, independent and intervened variables has not been tested.

3. Measurement of unemployment and other independent variables

Unemployment was broadly defined above as job-seeking coincident with a loss or lack of a job. It can be arguable, whether 'job-seeking' is a significant criterion of definition. There are good reasons to assume that the wish of work is a criterion. E.g. a house-wife ought to be counted as unemployed in her own account, if she wishes to work, but because it is hopeless to be assigned a job she is not registered as unemployed.

A precise definition of the term unemployment is necessary for the definition of the universe. The sample surveys in this country have usually started from a definition of unemployment in terms of social security regulations: a job-searching person is assumed unemployed, if he/she
"a) is not disabled for work or
 b) is not or only insignificant by working (...) as employee, home worker, family worker or self-employed worker and
 c) does not want only insignificant work (...) or work for a particular firm or work as home worker (excluding those receiving unemployment benefit) or not only look for an employment up to 3 months" (cit. from M. FRESE, G. MOHR, 1978, 282).

In this definition are absent:
- disabled (because of sickness) unemployed persons (absence-rate about 5 - 6 %);
- persons in re-training and further education;
- job-searching women and young people, who have not registered as unemployed because they are not entitled to unemployment benefit;

- job-searching permanently disabled persons (with invalidity pension);
- part-time workers, which look for a full-time job.

About the size of these groups there are only unreliable estimations. The total number of these persons could be within several 100.000, using cautious estimations.

Moreover, it should be noticed, that part of the receivers of unemployment benefit are not genuine unemployed persons (e.g. so-called "children's allowance unemployed", "unemployed in transition stage"). This group can be estimated at about 10 % (cp. INFRATEST SOZIALFORSCHUNG et. al., 1978, 101-102). Another part of the registered unemployed receive subsidiary income from incidental work - about 10 % of the unemployed (cp. INFRATEST SOZIALFORSCHUNG et. al., 1978). With these groups the loss of the job cannot have significant consequences on health.

A sample survey of unemployed drawn from the data base of the labour offices, therefore, is always a group, defined by the social security regulations, which deals with the problem of unemployment only in a restricted sense. For research by social scientists this approach to the problem has to be considered inadequate.

Another problem comes up when drawing the sample on a fixed reference day by a single sample survey. About the "persons affected" by unemployment one can only make restricted statements. Within one year a total of about 3 million persons will be unemployed. On any fixed day only about 1 million of these will be covered. This 1 million is not a random sample either. On any reference day short-term unemployed are under-represented and long-term unemployed overrepresented with all correlates that go along (age, qualification, health) (cp. F. EGLE, W. KARR, 1977). Now it may well be argued, whether a fixed day or a period are better used to describe the total population. We demand, that this question can be clarified only on the background of a theory rsp. hypotheses.

Unemployment is not the only independent variable, which can explain well-being. Here, too, one misses an acknowledged set of other social indicators. Normally a basis for comparison is missing.

Other psychological stresses (besides unemployment) are taken into consideration most comprehensively in the concepts of the 'life event approach'. The basic hypothesis of this approach is, that above average stress precedes illness (cp. for this and the following H. KASCHNIG, 1980). A list of events is presented to the interviewed person (e.g. wife's death, birth of a child in the family, job change, loss of job, trouble with superior). The interviewed person has to state for a period, whether the event has happened or not. Such events can may elicit adaptive response. More precise information is not yet known (cp. H. KASCHNIG, 1980, 22). Other important points of criticism are:
- Rather global measures are used in indifferentiated and vague designs, expecially in the 'schedule of recent experiences' (cp. H. KASCH-

NIG, 1980, 24-25). The particular events are aggregated additively - without any proof - to sumscores, mainly to make comparisons between groups.
- In the 'life-event-schedule' it is up to the interviewer to standardize the life-event within one field. Only after the interview the answers will be coded.

In spite of all criticism of the concepts of life-event-research there are clearly some merits: Unemployment can be examined along with other changing conditions and the dimension of time is included in the concept. But here again is true, that still the main problems (after about 15 years of research) lie in reliable and precise measurement, that is in quality and not in quantity. Add to this, that intervening variables, as especially individual coping and individual ability to cope with life-events, can account for different results of incidence of illness on the background of the same life-events. They have not been considered up to now (cp. H. KASCHNIG, 1980, 84-85).

4. Measurement of the health consequences

Here problems of measurement of health variables in questionnaires will be described. Medical and psychological anamnestic schedules, which can only by applied through qualified personal, are excluded.

In a model of variables representing the relationship between unemployment and health, the health variables are the dependent variables. It is necessary at first to define the aim of the research in this area, in order to set a base for the definitions. It is not sufficient for this purpose to measure the effects of unemployment on health alone. It is better at this point to state the aim of proving the need of a specific supply for therapy for a given study group. Without a specification of the aim health effects cannot be measured in a meaningful way. In German language research such precise specifications of the aim are not usually given.

Most often psycho-social consequences will include the following dimensions (cp. D. FRÖHLICH, 1979, pp. 71; C. BRINKMANN, 1976, 406-407).
- the experience of time or the decline of the chronological order;
- self-confidence or the feeling of worthlessness;
- the development of social contacts or social relationships (isolation);
- the disturbing of the work role, boredom, uncertanity about the future, fatalism, depression.

In all studies these dimensions are measured in a different manner. BRINKMANN (1976, 406) is right, if he states, that "a homogeneous and operational concept for the measurement of these social and psychological stresses and their causes (...) are not available up to now". There is no basis for comparisons. Therefore, the results vary. Whether these differences are "complementary points of view" (A. WACKER, 1976, 109) may be doubted.

In addition, single variables will usually be summarized to stress-indices. Validity and reliability are not or only superficially examined.

Psychological schedules of questions for diagnosis of psychical disorders, of which there are a lot of tested instruments, are too extensive for a questionnaire in a sample survey. It is necessary to do further research to develop a short and valid instrument for such surveys. Any such instrument should take notice of the duration of the disorder (vgl. H. KASCHNIG, 1980, 14), because many psycho-social disorders can disappear and recur in time.

To cover the state of health poses other difficulties. To begin with there are several global health indicators, of the form: Would you say you are in good, medium or bad physical condition? Such questions can give a first impression on the subjective state of health, but they have faults too. Information, derived from this question alone, is not a sufficient base for taking action. The answer depends on a number of influences (age, risk-factors, qualification, former work-stress, etc.), which have nothing to do with unemployment.

Finally such questions don't allow statements about the course of well-being over time, especially as a function of unemployment.

We shall comment shortly three other concepts, which measure the state of health: lists of complaints rsp. illnesses, absence-days and of activity scales. A vast amount of literature may be consulted on these three topics. We confine ourselves to comment on a few important points.

Lists of complaints rsp. illnesses in Germany were used e.g. in the unemployment-study of INFRATEST SOZIALFORSCHUNG et al. (1978). With some illnesses rsp. complaints it is not quite clear, whether the respondents understand the terms. One may surely expect a class bias here in the sense, that the upper and middle classes have more knowledge and are more capable to articulate themselves than the lower class. Some illnesses (e.g. high blood-pressure) will only be articulated, if there are detected, usually by a doctor. With high blood-pressure in particular, the recognition depends on the use of medical services.

When looking at the numer of sickness days of unemployed, special regard must be given to social security regulations. Sickness days postpone the termination of unemployment benefit. Hence a great number of sickness days may be an artefact of social security regulations.

In the anglo-american epidemiology we find frequent use of activity scales to measure the state of health. Activities are physical and social actions, e.g. running rapidly, going upstairs, but also washing the hands and dressing. The behaviour of a researched population is observed by competent judges (cp. W. E. POLLARD et al., 1976; D. L. PATRICK, 1973).

For the use in sample surveys such scales with over 200 items are too lengthy. Medical action cannot be derived from them (cp. S. BIEFANG, H. POHLMEIER, 1979, 26). With these instruments one can measure the state of health on a fixed day; studies predicting the change in health over a period of time have not been undertaken.

These health indicators need also be regarded over a period of time. Simply because too low a number of complaints, illnesses and activities occurs on a fixed day, a reference period is preferable. To the question, which reference period should be taken, there is no definite answer. By taking too long a period (e.g. one year) one must take into account considerable errors of recall. So the Statistische Bundesamt (internal working paper) has found in the sixties, that the number of accidents (a rather hard event), was reduced about a half, if recalled for a period which dated back 2 months. Expecially minor accidents were forgotten or were remembered as having occurred at some other time.

5. Methodological design

Research on the relationship between unemployment and health in the German-speaking countries is designed as retrospective studies. Here there are problems with the recall of health variables. If changes in the state of health are to be measured, this method is an inadequate solution to the problem. Secondly it will be demanded, that such studies are always carried out with control groups (cp. M. SCHÄR, 1975, 444). In default of proper control groups controle can be produced afterwards through paired sampling. Here particular attention must be paid to sampling.

There is no need to go into the effects of interviewing or the response rates in written mailed interview. They concerned for all interviews likewise. The response rate is lower for questions on health and risk-factors (consumtion of cigarettes and alcohol) are underestimated.

In retrospective studies, if psycho-social effects are to be measured, the choice of the date of the survey is of great importance. KASL et. al. (1975) have pointed out, that the anticipation or fear of an event may cause just as much stress as the event itself. It is fairly common that someone will know or apprehend some weeks or months before that he is likely to become unemployed. Why should his first way to the labour office change his state of health? This more rhetorical question puts the problem very distinctly.

The questions which were posed suggested, that the problems can only be resolved with a longitudinal study and not with a cross-sectional study. The same group of persons will be interviewed at several times. It is even better to reach the unemployed persons for the first time before unemployment starts. Only in this way causal effects can be ascribed to the factor of unemployment.

We may here refer to the 'National Longitudinal Survey' in the United Staates, where unemployed persons are included (questions on the state of health are scarce) and the studies of KASL (cp. f.e. 1975). The first German representative longitudinal survey of unemployed persons was carried out by INFRATEST (cp. for the health questions INFRATEST SOZIALFORSCHUNG und FORSCHUNGSGRUPPE ARBEIT UND GESUNDHEIT, 1979).

Problems have turned up particularly in the data analysis. The various and complex factors which influence the state of health can only be handled by complex statistical procedures. However, one soon is restricted by the limits of too small a number of persons, even with a sample of about 1000 unemployed persons. A change of the state of health is a rare event and happens in both directions. Persons with a better and a worse state of health entered into the average and therefore they are neutralized. Quite apart from the fact that for the analysis of longitudinal surveys no fully developed statistical procedures are available.

The analysis of this longitudinal survey illustrated, that an often practised method is incorrect. From a comparison in retrospective surveys of the state of health of long-term unemployed with short-term unemployed persons it has been concluded that a narrow relationship between the duration of unemployment and the state of health exists. "The more long-term the unemployment is the more negative is the state of health" (D. FRÖHLICH, 1979, 138). As a result of the social, physical, occupational and other factors, these are two completly different groups, so that a comparison is not possible in this manner.

Part 3

FURTHER RESEARCH:

PROPOSALS AND STRATEGY

UNEMPLOYMENT, THE UNEMPLOYED, AND HEALTH
An analysis of the Dutch situation

Ingeborg P. Spruit

Instituut Voor Sociale Geneeskunde
Rijksuniversiteit Te Leiden
Netherlands

In this paper the main attention will be given to the subjective experience of being unemployed. This experience is influenced by a number of social factors and is also related to (health) effects of unemployment, which can be devided into physical and psychosocial effects. The Hypothesis can be drawn from the published research results, and on this basis we shall explore various possibilities for the formulation of problems that might be investigated.

Subjective experience of unemployment

Few studies have dealt with the health of today's unemployed, especially if we wish to exclude the categories of those drawing disability benefits or opting for early retirement. Data on the effects of unemployment, not only in the Netherlands but also other countries, have been provided by highly divergent investigations. Many of those done in the Netherlands were performed to provide a basis for policy-making of the re-incorporation of the unemployed into the labour process or were concerned with the management of social provisions. Findings on the subjective experience of unemployment in these studies are usually obtained coincidentally, or from secondary sources or secondary analyses. A few studies have been primarily concerned with the experience of unemployment and its consequences as experienced by the individual. The heterogeneity of the studies impedes comparison of the results. This report does not represent more than an inventory of the accumulated information, and analysis indicates little more than occasional cases of some degree of agreement. It is, however, striking that in almost all of the studies problems arose in connection with the reaction to unemployment. This probably indicates the severity and penetration of the problems encountered by some of the unemployed.

In 1976, a broadcasting group (K.R.O.) in the Netherlands commissioned Intromarkt[1] to make a survey for their television program called Brandpunt. This survey covered 200 general practitioners considered to be representative of a population of more than 5000 general practitioners. Of this sample, 66 % thought that the economic situation influenced the number of patients and/or the nature of the complaints, 24 % thought there was no such influence, and 10 % had no opinion. Houben[2] found that the reaction to unemployment is always negative to very negative, although it is not considered the worst thing that can happen to a person. The negative feeling about joblessness and (negative) effects of joblessness are closely related. In a study done in the USA at the end of the 1960', Kasl et al.[3] found that the reaction to unemployment was related to ill health. Ex-unemployed who said they had undergone their recent unemployment as a very severe experience had more health complaints during the period of unemployment and a slightly less adequate recovery after re-employment. Since this was a prospective study in which determinations were made at various times, the results may be considered reliable. The research has also shown the negative reaction not only affects and influences the effects of unemployment but in addition that there are certain factors that have a reinforcing influence on the reaction. The processes and parts of processes which have been studied can be represented as follows:

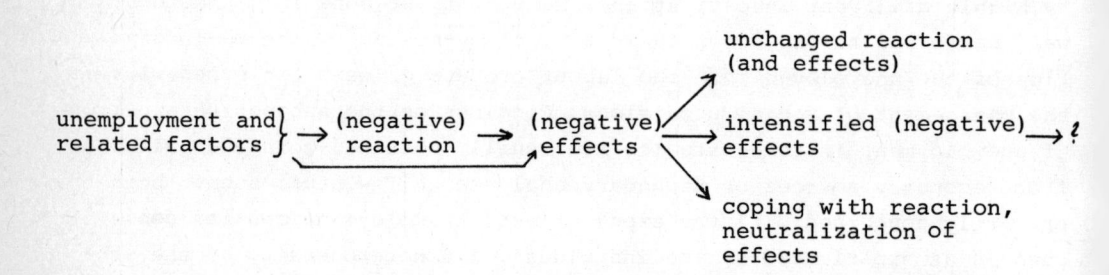

```
                                                  unchanged reaction
                                                  (and effects)
                                                ↗
unemployment and ⎫  → (negative) → (negative) → intensified (negative) → ?
related factors  ⎭     reaction      effects    effects
                                                ↘
                                                  coping with reaction,
                                                  neutralization of
                                                  effects
```

Fig. 1: Schematic representation of researched unemployment processes

The following discussion concerns the factors with an influence on the reaction to and effects of unemployment, and reference will be made to the reinforcing processes, where found.

Work ethic and aspects of work

According to the Science Council for Government Policy[4], work and a sense of duty are still central in the lives of most citizens of the Netherlands. But the data on which this conclusion is based are on the whole crude and rather unspecific, being based on general-attitude surveys performed in divergent categories of respondents. The relative importance of labour is decreasing slightly, but work is still seen mainly as a right and a duty. The idea that an individual can develop himself by work is considered very important. The work ethic is adhered to only slightly more strongly by older people than by younger people. Few things are considered more important than work, and all of them lie in the personal zone and concern, for instance, health, family, and home. The unemployed put a higher value on work than the employed do. It has been postulated that the consciousness of the importance of work increases strongly after the loss of work. The Science Council thinks that this assignment of a central place to work may be ascribed to such work-derivative factors as income, property, and status, and to the fact that there are no other good alternatives for constructive participation in social life.

In a memorandum on the young unemployed, prepared by The Netherlands Social and Cultural Planning Bureau[5], to the difference in work ethic between the young and the older groups is assigned more importance than in the report submitted by the Science Council, but here too a few general-attitude surveys provide the main basis. Reference is made to: "... some cultural changes ... indicating that the attitude of the young to work is changing." This is said to concern a generation-dependent difference in the evaluation of work and leisure, a somewhat weaker work-orientation, and a less strict sense of duty with respect to work. But at the same time it is remarked that a really radical rejection of the social system, to the extent that young people avoid employment in industry as much as possible or do not seek any work at all, cannot be said to be prevalent in the Netherlands and is at most found in a few small sub-cultural groups of young people. Kagan[6] pointed out correctly that although attitudes to work (and the jobless) have proven to be extremely important, little is known about them. This holds particularly for various categories in society. Although research on attitudes is done frequently, it is always difficult to interpret the results. Relationships between attitudes and behaviour and the meaning of various attitudes for the individual are poorly understood. Concerning the 'more liberal views' of the young (compared with the older age groups) the Planning Bureau rightly remarks: 'It is not clear whether this means that after finishing school young people prefer to postpone starting to work for a time or, once they have started to work, accept a period of unemployment more easily.'

Therefore, support for general findings that is provided by studies on the unemployed is of great importance. In four Dutch studies[7-10], a British study[11] and an American study[12] it was found that the reaction to being unemployed is coloured by the work ethic, by the opinions on what the previous work was like or could have been, and on both the material and immaterial benefits of that work. Van Wezel[7] pointed to the relation between the experience of mental and physical stress and the work ethic. He also found that the work ethic and the degree of belief in it vary in a society and are highly individual. The degree to which the work ethic prevails in social groups is impossible to define, and he suspects that it is strongly dependent on personal factors and circumstances. Gravelotte et al.[10] give a more specific definition of the influence of the work ethic on the reaction to unemployment. In a study done in unemployed young people they found that a 'Calvinistic work ethic' has a strong influence on attempts to maintain a normal day-rhythm and to get through the day as well as on boredom and feelings of inferiority.

A strong work ethic implies a rather negative attitude toward the jobless. These views too influence the reaction to unemployment. Van Wezel found that many unemployed individuals themselves share this negative social evaluation of unemployment, and that this leads to negative opinions about oneself as well as other jobless people. Many of the unemployed are extremely conscious of how others see them. The average Dutch citizen sees participation in the labour process as a condition for being a useful and equal member of society and tends to regard the failure to satisfy this condition as, at least partially, a personal failure on the part of the jobless.

In sum, it may be said that the homogeneity of the research findings indicating that the work ethic has an important influence on the reaction to unemployment is rather strong. At the same time, it has been found that this factor exerts its influence in various ways. There is a strong effect of the inability to participate in a positive experience: participation in work as a means of self-realization and then as a condition for being accepted as a worthy member of society, as a means to acquire status, prestige, and income. Not only is the possibility of a more positive reaction absent, but the individual is given an explicitly negative status, both the individual and those around him at the very least questioning whether a personal failure is involved. Among the indicated effects are physical and mental stress, feelings of inferiority, and problems with getting through the day!

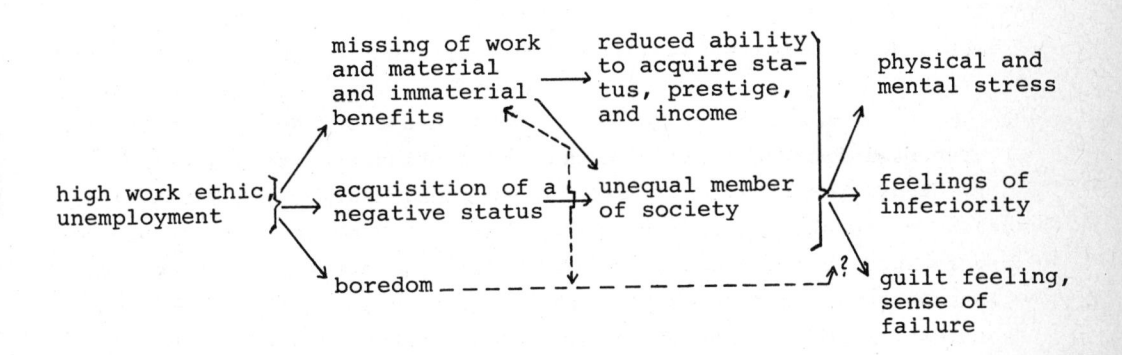

Fig. 2: Work ethic and unemployment

Conditions coinciding with unemployment

In view of the central place of work in life, it is hardly surprising that the conditions under which work is lost play a large part in the experience of the loss of work. Among these conditions the reason for the dismissal is a very important factor for both older and younger workers (Gravelotte et al.)[10]. Marsden and Duff[11] found in England that the mechanism concerned a feeling of guilt accompanied by a sense of powerlessness. Although in most cases the loss of work is involuntary, many unemployed people feel that they bear a share of the guilt involved in the breaking of the contract: had they worked harder they might not have been one of those who were fired. This personal judgement can haunt the jobless individual. In seven studies done in the Netherlands[2, 8, 10, 11, 14, 16] similar findings were made concerning the relation between the conditions of dismissal and joblessness and the reaction to the latter. The feeling of personal guilt and failure is mentioned here not so much as the crucial mechanism, but merely the estimation of the chances of re-employment. The divergent objectives of these studies hamper summarization of the findings, and all of them cannot be indicated.

Both Houben[2] and Hamaker[13] found a relation between ideas of personal failure in the job, estimation of the chance of re-employment, reasons for being fired, and 'job-hunting behaviour'. Houben concluded that the estimation of the chance of finding a new job had more influence on the intensity and negativity of the experience of being jobless than, for example, the duration of the unemployment. On the other hand, the duration of unemployment itself has an influence on the estimation of the chance of finding a new job. Heinen and Vissers[14] found, among other things, that it is difficult to re-employ unemployed who had been jobless frequently or for long periods and rate their chances more negatively. One complicating factor in the evaluation of such research results is that the job-hunting behaviour has often taken a more central position in the problems associated with the investigation than the reaction to unemployment with all its facets. The latter aspects have been identified and described by the investigators, but the analysis of the reaction was orientated toward the interaction with the job-hunting behaviour and not with health. Furthermore, the authors used different models, and it is not clear at which point the negative reaction to unemployment is the strongest for the individual:

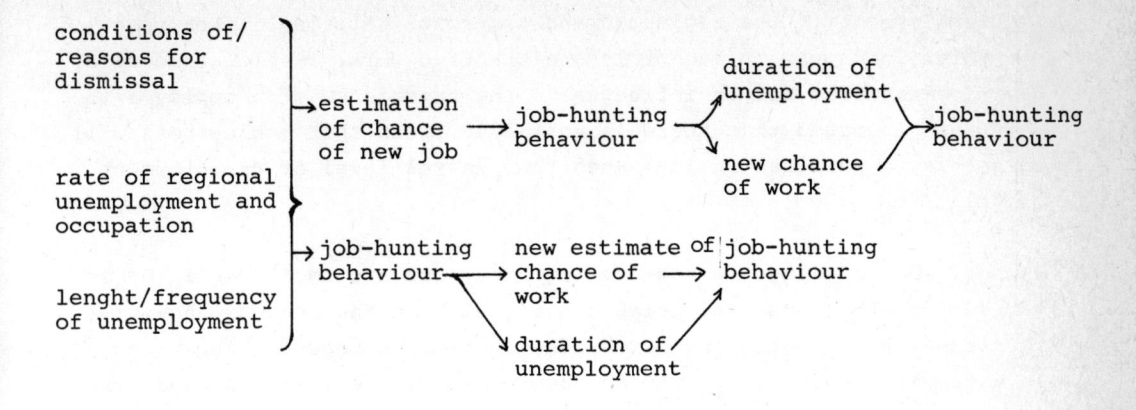

```
conditions of/
reasons for
dismissal                                          duration of
              ⎫   →estimation      job-hunting    unemployment    job-hunting
              ⎪    of chance   →   behaviour   →⟨              →  behaviour
              ⎪    of new job                     new chance
rate of regional ⎬                                of work
unemployment and ⎪
occupation    ⎪
              ⎪   →job-hunting    new estimate of  job-hunting
              ⎪    behaviour  →   chance of     →  behaviour
lenght/frequency ⎪                work            ↗
of unemployment ⎭                ↘ duration of
                                   unemployment
```

Fig. 3:   Schematic representation of research on unemployment and re-employment

These studies do, however, provide important information, because the findings run parallel to those of other investigators who are explicitly concerned with health or other emotional effects. The health effects were most clearly dealt with in a study done by Kesteloo[15] on the effects of planned closure of a large business plant. Judged from the number of health complaints registered by the occupational medical service, these occurred most frequently among: 1. those with a poor chance of re-employment, 2. employees performing relatively specialized work, 3. those who would be difficult to replace and/or 4. were in poorer health, 5. had more disability, and 6. were older. All of these categories can be expected to have difficulty in finding new work. Nievaard[16] too mentions the severe problems of those who, '... because of advanced age or poor health', estimate their chance of finding another job negatively. According to Houben, it is particularly those who have worked for the same company for a long time and the formerly self-employed who have problems in coping with unemployment and a higher risk of poor health. He thinks that this holds expecially in the initial period after dismissal or the liquidation of a company. When the unemployment lasts a long time, these groups lose the desire to work.
This probably does not hold for 'the' unemployed as a category, since other authors have found that prolonged unemployment and/or a high level

of unemployment in the region (or occupational category) often means
a greater readiness to accept less attractive work. The local level of
unemployment also has an influence on the experience of unemployment.
Koopmans[8] reported that there is more likelihood that joblessness will
be seen as a personal failure when the general level of unemployment
is less high.

In sum, when findings on job-hunting behaviour are not taken into consideration, there is appreciable uniformity in the results showing
that the reasons for being fired, the conditions under which an individual becomes jobless, and, to a lesser degree, the frequency and duration of unemployment have an influence on how unemployment is experienced
as well as on the occurrence of health complaints. Two important mechanism here are the estimation of the chance of re-employment and
(under the influence of the unemployment rate) the feeling that personal failure was partially responsible for the loss of work. The findings overlap to some extent, but more often are supplementary:

```
                         reason for discharge ――――→ estimation of chance
                                                    of new employment
┌──────────────┐
│ higher age   │
│              │
│ specialized  │
│ work/trade   │
│              │
│ difficult to │
│ re-employ    │
│              │     negative conditions
│ less healthy/│ ――→ associated with       ――――――→ negative estimation of
│ more disabled│     dismissal                     chance of new work
│              │
│ duration of  │
│ employment   │
│              │
│ self-employed│
│ (ex)         │
└──────────────┘

┌──────────────┐
│ frequent and/or│
│ prolonged      │ ――→ negative unemployment ――――→ negative estimation of
│ unemployment   │     history                     chance of new work
└──────────────┘
```

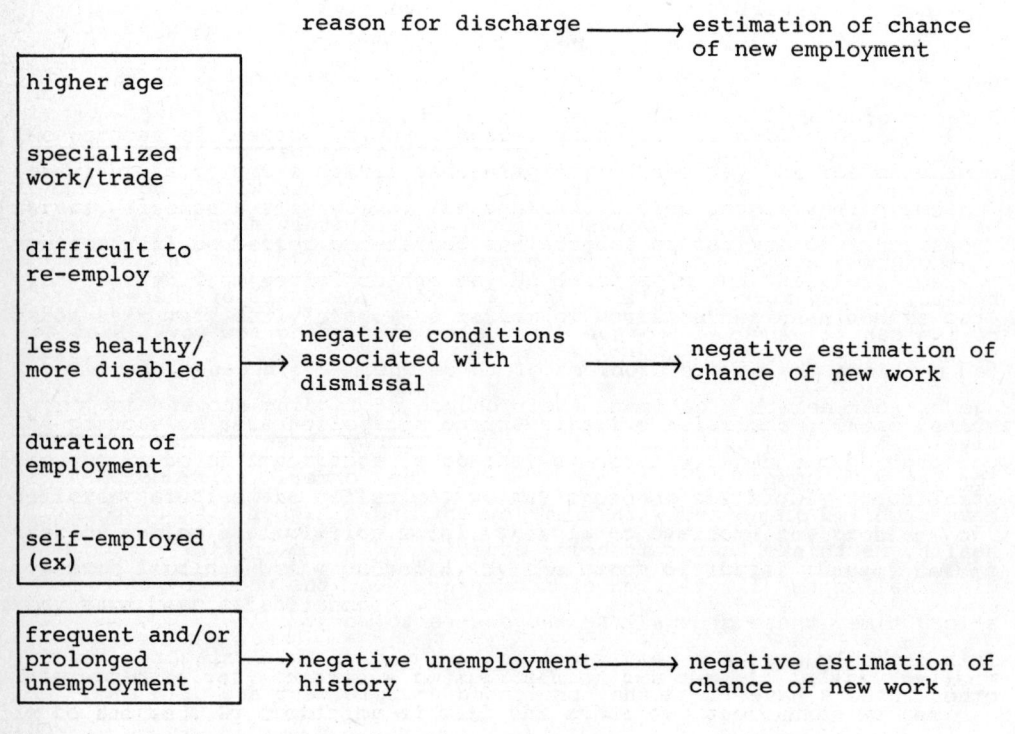

Fig. 4: Factors influencing the experience of unemployment

Various investigators have found factors which lead to a negative estimation of the chance of re-employment. Studies on the influence of these factors on job-hunting behaviour and on the subjective aspects of health problems have led to the conclusion that such factors have a negative influence on both the emotional experience and on the number of health complaints. Furthermore, a low unemployment rate enhances the feeling of personal failure. A high unemployment rate coupled with long duration of unemployment increases the willingness to do lower-status work. The effect which this in turn has on the reaction aspects is not known (see Fig. 5).

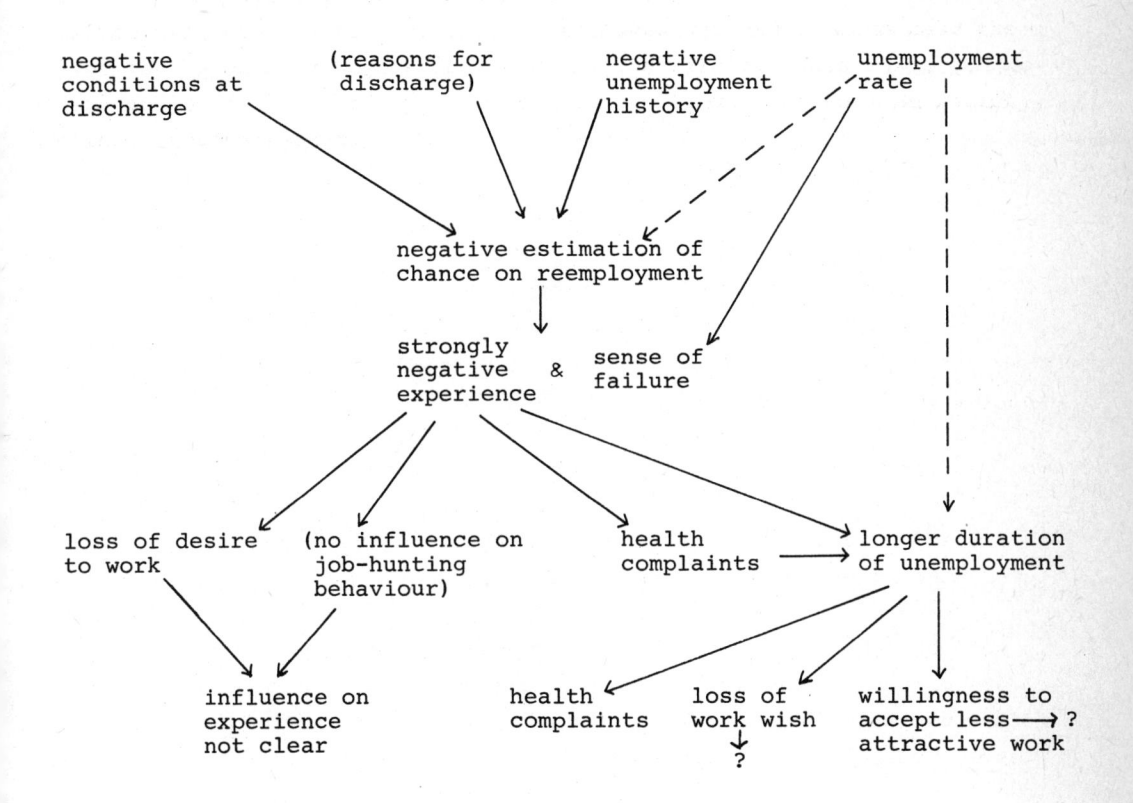

Fig. 5: Hypothetical Process of negative emotional experience of unemployment and health complaints

Frequency and duration of unemployment

The frequency of unemployment can be seen as a condition (in the past) that plays a part in (the reaction on) dismissal, but this is not the case for the duration of unemployment. However, since both factors influence the estimation of the chance of re-employment and therefore the reaction on unemployment, this aspect has already been touched on. Some investigators have provided supplementary information about the how, why, and magnitude of the influence of pessimism as part of the reaction to unemployment. Not only Kesteloo[15] in the Netherlands but also Kasl et al.[3] in the USA have investigated the health situation in this context. Kesteloo did not take the unemployment history into account. Kasl et al. found more health problems among those who had changed jobs frequently and those who had to look for a new job more than once during the study.

In the Netherlands, several authors have reported a loss of self confidence and self respect due to unemployment, which in some of the jobless never disappears entirely. Van Buchem[17] reported that the experience of having a poor chance of re-employment led to an increasingly negative attitude in 70 % of a group who had been unemployed for more than six months. According to Houben[2], the reaction is most intense in the initial period after dismissal, and reoccurs each time application is made for a new job as well as in contacts with employment agencies and welfare personnel, and also when the amount of the unemployment benefit decreases (due to a change in category). Some other authors have found a negative to very negative attitude toward contacts with such authorities (e. g. Barense et al.[18], Smoor[19]) among both younger and older groups (Gravelotte et al.[10]). The influence of financial loss is mentioned by some investigators. Van Wezel[7] found that this was mentioned more often by younger people and this has, according to Gravelotte et al., to do with the more restricted possibilities for use of leisure time. The majority of the investigators found that those in the lower occupational groups mention the financial disadvantage more often, but a minority of the authors report this to be more frequent in those in the higher occupational groups. In England, Marsden and Duff[11] noted that views on the (level of) welfare benefits were related to views on where the responsibility for the dismissal lay and the work ethic. This point has not been considered in Dutch studies.

In sum, negative effects of the frequency of unemployment seem to result mainly from the negative estimation of the chance of re-employment and loss of self respect and self confidence. Negative influences of the duration of unemployment seem to lie not only in these factors but also in the painfullness of being rejected when applying for new work and in applying itself, in a negative experience in contact with mediating and disbursing authorities, and an increasing financial disadvantage. The increasingly negative attitude is already measurable after only six months of unemployment.

Some demographic factors

Evaluation of demographic factors has become obligatory in investigations related to the social sciences. It is not always clear, however, how strong and how independent the relation between such factors and the process under study actually is, or why these factors can be of importance, and for which categories which delimination is relevant. The demographic factors yield the most heterogeneous **research** results.

Van Buchem[17] reported that the willingness to work is greater among those who support others than in those who do not, but this does not mean it is low among the latter. Hamaker[13] found that the degree to which the family and the surroundings exert pressure on the breadwinner is not correlated with the latter's reaction to the situation, job-hunting behaviour, or willingness to accept hardship. Authors usually assume that the feeling of responsibility for the family influences the reaction (and willingness to work). This factor has, however, received little attention, and therefore little is known about it. The findings on education, social position, and salary level before discharge are not in agreement. For example, Heinen and Vissers[14] found that those with a higher educational level are the most positive about working, and Koopmans[8] that they have a more intrinsic work orientation (pleasure in working for the sake of working, immaterial subjective aspects of work). However, the same holds here as was found by the Planning Bureau with respect to the work orientation of younger people: it does not necessarily mean that they take unemployment less seriously. It could also mean that they have developed more coping mechanisms and, for example, can find more satisfaction in volunteer work (for lack of something better). Nevertheless Houben[2] refers to those with more education in the same breath as the groups whose negative estimate of their re-employment chances gives them a higher risk of poor health. According to Van Wezel[7], however, young people and the more educated are among those who most often mention advantages as well as disadvantages of unemployment. His study does not indicate how they weigh against each other, but he reports that advantages were cited particularly by young people with more education who had lost rather uninteresting work. This might mean that a too homogeneous variable was included in the measurement of either the educational level or higher income, or the like, and that the duration of the last employment, the nature of that work, and social status (as interrelated factors) would be more influential variables. In theory, however, unemployment might have such a strong influence that demographic factors of this kind play no role at all.

On the factor of age there is much more agreement between the results. This is also expressed in the conditions of the dismissal, because age is strongly related to the estimation of the chance of finding another job. Only the Dutch Ministry of Social Affairs[21] is of the opinion that age (like sex) is not a factor that impedes the finding of a job but rather that other factors operate via age. These factors are, according to the memorandum of the Ministry: a. older individuals think that they are more difficult to place; b. the employment agencies think that they are more difficult to place and therefore insufficient effort is made to find them another job; and c. their income was higher before the loss of the job. The Ministry seems to be alone in holding this view, however, and the unemployment figures show that the older groups have a very high percentage of prolonged unemployment. In Kesteloo's[15] study the main problem-group was that of the 50- to 55-year-olds, who together with the married women had the most ill health. Van Buchem[17] too put the age limit at 50 years. Older people find it more difficult to obtain a new job because there is a general expectation that their production level will be lower and their absenteeism higher: "Anyone who is older than 50 years and is unemployed is doomed to remain unemployed." He points to the frustrations this situation will induce, because in connection with their welfare benefits these people must continue to try to enter the labour market although they are repeatedly reminded that they have less chance than ever of finding a job. Oveson[20] points out that the normal learning process is violated by not being given the opportunity to learn from experience and having to do the opposite of what experience has taught.

Very little is known about the way in which women undergo unemployment. A study done by van der Linden[22] suggests that for them, too, the negative aspects predominate, but the scale of the investigation was too small to permit far-reaching conclusions.

In sum, the factor of age may be regarded without ambivalence as a 'risk factor'. All studies have indicated that the older group of jobless have more problems caused by lack of work and run a higher risk of ill health. As factors education and/or social status have led to divergent results, and sex and married/breadwinner status have received insufficient attention. No research at all has been done on ethnic minorities.

Reaction of the immediate social surroundings

Earlier experiences, other stressful events coinciding with unemployment, and the presence or absence of social support in the surroundings, can be important for the reaction to unemployment. According to Kesteloo[15], psycho-social problems in the family reduce resistance more strongly than do factors originating from the work environment, and they weigh more heavily in the situation. This study, however, used a form of selection in that the subjects were employees who consulted the occupational medical service. Among this group complaints increased in severity when there were also problems at home. These problems could be independent of unemployment or a result of impending loss of work. Boucher[9] found that some of the long-term unemployed fail to work through negative experiences, particularly with respect to family problems and poor health. This, however, concerned problems induced or aggravated by unemployment. Besides these studies little attention has been given to this subject in the Netherlands and this has left an information gap.

In the United States, Kasl et al.[3] found that social support has more influence on the reaction to unemployment than earlier stressfull experiences. Gore[23] too reported that social support in the family or from significant others can prevent or reduce the negative effects of unemployment to a great extent. These findings seem sufficiently important to warrant further study. So far, this is the only mechanism that has been found to have a positive or curative effect. In this light it is important to include family tensions as a cause as well as an effect of inability to cope with the problem of unemployment and the increased number of unemployment related health complaints.

Only one researcher refers to early experiences of unemployed individuals (an unemployed father, or the influence of the father's unemployment, on growing or job-hunting children), but there are no research results on these points. Tiffany[12] points out in general that the dealing with unemployment (negative or positive) can grow into an institutionalized reaction and be expressed in values, norms, attitudes, and rules of behaviour when population categories are confronted with recurrent unemployment.

In sum, with respect to reactions of those in the immediate social surroundings of the unemployed it may be said in particular that family problems (arising both before and after unemployment) seem to reduce the ability of the unemployed to solve problems and that social support from within the family and from significant others seems to increase this ability.

Conclusion

Every investigator has encountered the negative reaction of the unemployed to their situation. There is a relationship between the intensity of this reaction and health problems. The reaction to unemployment is influenced by a number of factors. Factors with a negative influence have to do with the estimation of the chances of re-employment, the sense of having failed, and the work ethic. Conditions which influence the chance of obtaining a new job include age, employment history, health status, and unemployment history. These processes with a negative effect are shown in Fig. 5, where arrows indicate possible interrelations. Family problems could be included here as a negative element, but have an influence not via the estimation of the employment chances but rather directly on the reaction to unemployment. However, family problems can also arise from the unemployment itself, or be so greatly exacerbated by it that they become part of the negative reaction. A factor with a positive influence on the ability to solve problems or which can diminish the negative reaction is the presence of social support in the family or from significant others. The factors which alone or together form conditions with a negative influence on the reaction to unemployment can be seen as an indication that older groups run a higher risk, because these people haven often done long service with the same company, have a (slightly) stronger work ethic, are often less healthy, have specialized work and somewhat higher wages, and are more difficult to re-employ.

Less research has been done on the reaction of younger age-groups and women, and none at all on that of ethnic minorities. Those who have retired early or have some form of disability are not taken into account here.

Effects of unemployment

'Unemployment in its present form, i. e., large-scale and permanent, is a catastrophe which has struck virtually all of the countries in the world. It is as it were a disease of modern society and as such deserves the attention of the medical profession. Although the investigation of the causes and the planning of attempts to cure society lie outside their competence, they can help to increase insight into the suffering of the victims, the unemployed, and their families.' This citation from a thesis written by Folpmers[24] in 1937 could easily be taken for a recent statement. In the 1930s a number of studies were done on the effects of unemployment, and these are still used as a source of information on the subject. When the economic crisis had passed, some thought that recurrence was impossible and scientific interest in the topic disappeared almost entirely.

At present, unemployment does not have the same radical effects on the individual and the family as was the case in the Thirties. Welfare provisions have improved considerably since then and no one need go hungry, and housing problems are less severe (although far from solved), cold is less of a threat, and medical provisions and sanitation have also been greatly improved. In the Thirties, many investigators attributed the physical, psychic, and social effects of unemployment to the poverty it caused. But a number of these effects are found today despite the relatively lower degree of poverty. This could mean that unemployment itself has effects. Although it would be wrong to underestimate the financial problems (especially when unemployment is prolonged) and the associated material difficulties[43], a number of effects of unemployment appear in an early stage. This has led investigators to distinguish between poverty and unemployment, although this will not always be possible in reality. This distinction has not been worked out very far, however. It has often been reported that the jobless have financial problems due to their unemployment, but there are no data on the effects.

Physical reactions to unemployment or impending unemployment

In the Thirties all investigators reported physical reactions. In the Netherlands most of the research was done on the health of schoolchildren, which Folpmers[24] also investigated. He found mainly nutritional deficiencies which: '... can be mainly attributed to the effects of improverishment, which affects all of the jobless despite the dole.' Furthermore, the children of the unemployed did not seem able to concentrate well at school. With respect to the better off, he says: '... the suffering of the unemployed intellectual(s) is probably mainly if not entirely psychic in nature.'

In Germany, a number of investigators thought that unemployment influenced the incidence of tuberculosis, but consensus was not reached. In England Marsh[25] reported in 1938 that there was correlation between unemployment, blood pressure, and cardiovascular diseases; but in this study cause and effect cannot be distinghuished with certainty.

Few studies have been done on the physical reaction to subsequent periods of unemployment. In England, Mathew[26] thought in 1961 that the cardio-respiratory functions decline and that excessive inactivity leads to atrophy. The physical deterioration accelerates with increasing age of the unemployed. Mathew calls unemployment a causer of disease, just as dust, bacilli, and air pollution are. In the Netherlands in 1975, Barendse et al.[18] reported a lecture given by an internist on the negative effect of unemployment on the physical condition. To stay in condition, at least 30 % of the top capacity must be used; otherwise, the chance of developing a cardiovascular disease increases. He also mentioned stiffening of the motor apparatus and a deterioration of metabolism. It is not clear, however, which observations concern which populations, and one wonders what the situation is with respect to the condition of employed individuals with sedentary work.

There are also four reports[2, 9, 11, 17] on physical reactions described by unemployed individuals themselves. Indications were obtained that there can be a physical reaction to unemployment, equivalent to reactions to severe problems or (heavy) stress. The complaints included sleeplessness at night and fatigue during the day, headaches, lack of appetite, indigestion, stomach complaints, general feeling of being sick and not looking well, indecision and worrying, irritability, crying, yelling, being overwrought, gastric bleeding, heart infarction, and emotional collapse. These complaints were found among both the short-term and long-term unemployed, and in both the jobless men and their wives. The magnitude of the problem is not indicated by these studies. Boucher et al.[9] reported that 30 of the 85 long-term unemployed they studied mentioned physical complaints, in eight so severe that they could no longer seek work. Zanders[27] found that after re-employment there were just as many persons with increasing complaints as persons with declining complaints. A striking finding in this study was the deterioration in the younger age-groups. On the basis of these studies it can only be said that there are individuals who react to unemployment with physical complaints, but that there is considerable difference between individuals and that the magnitude is still unknown.

Two studies have been done on the effects of closure of a company on health, one of them by Kasl et al. in the USA and the other that of Kesteloo[14] in the Netherlands. The latter determined the changes in complaints after the impending closure became known to the employees. As occupational physician he had data on sickness-absenteeism before the closure and could therefore detect changes in the pattern. He divided the complaints into the diagnostic categories applied in occupational medicine, and found the strongest effects of the impending closure in "group 5", i. e., psychic anomalies. Like Zanders, he reported that the younger age-groups were more susceptible to stress than the older age-groups. He also found a slight rise in the incidence of short sickness-absences and of diseases of the circulatory system and motoric organs. No increase was found for diseases of the digestive system or for accidents.

Much more detailed research has been done by Kasl et al.[3, 28-30]. They performed a prospective comparative study in employees of two plants which closed and a control group of workers who still had a job. The unemployed were interviewed and visited by a public health nurse at various times during the period of unemployment, after re-employment, and just before job loss. This concerned mainly short-term unemployment, i. e., 'health problems at the work/no work boundary'[28]. This study permitted a number of conclusions, summarized in Fig. 6.

Specific diseases observed in this study included a rather large number of cases of hypertension and gastric ulcers (the latter especially in the wives) and a higher incidence of colds and flu. Swollen joints and other symptoms of arthritis were seen more often in former employees of the closed company in the city but not in those of the one in the country, where the social networks had remained intact. Differences influenced by age were also found only in the urban situation. Young people reacted more strongly in the first phase (usually people with young children, and not the younger group), but they also recovered better after re-employment. This tendency was found to only a small extent among those with more education. Disability did not show a distinct pattern over the various phases. There was a highly consistent correlation between number of days of disability and the subjective evaluation of the seriousness of the unemployment. Those who remained without work or had had several unsuccesful trail periods showed a significantly higher score.

Persons who took unemployment more seriously showed a slow but steady increase in the number of days of sickness, whereas those who took it less seriously showed a decrease with time in this respect.

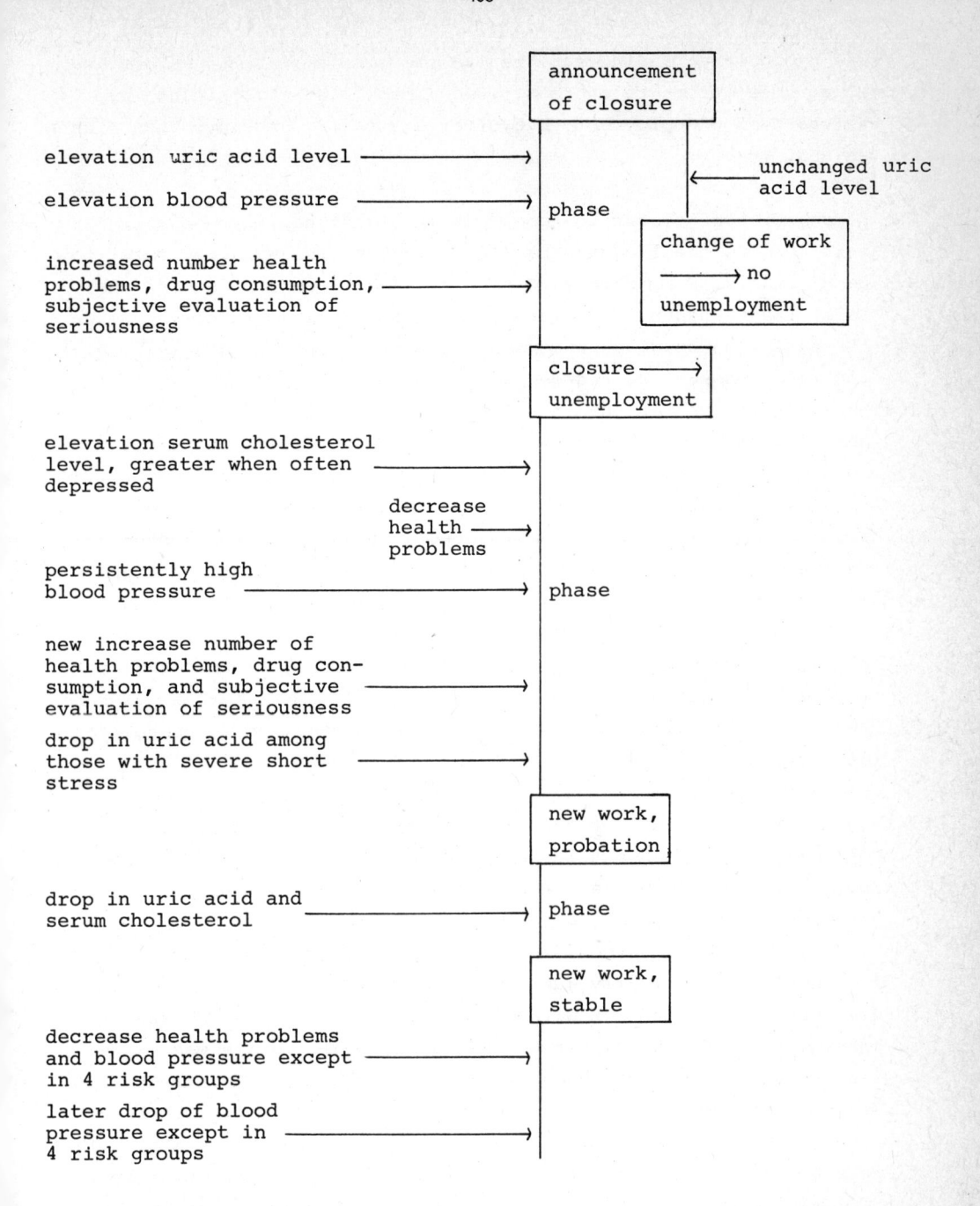

```
elevation uric acid level ─────────→  ┌──────────────┐
                                       │ announcement │
                                       │ of closure   │
                                       └──────┬───────┘
                                              │       ←── unchanged uric
elevation blood pressure ─────────→  phase    │           acid level
                                              ├───────┐
                                              │ change of work
                                              │ ─────→ no
increased number health                       │ unemployment
problems, drug consumption,  ─────→           └───────┘
subjective evaluation of
seriousness
                                       ┌──────────────┐
                                       │ closure ────→│
                                       │ unemployment │
                                       └──────┬───────┘
elevation serum cholesterol
level, greater when often    ─────→
depressed
                          decrease
                          health   ─→
                          problems
persistently high
blood pressure               ─────→  phase

new increase number of
health problems, drug con-
sumption, and subjective     ─────→
evaluation of seriousness

drop in uric acid among
those with severe short      ─────→
stress
                                       ┌──────────────┐
                                       │ new work,    │
                                       │ probation    │
                                       └──────┬───────┘
drop in uric acid and        ─────→  phase
serum cholesterol
                                       ┌──────────────┐
                                       │ new work,    │
                                       │ stable       │
                                       └──────┬───────┘
decrease health problems
and blood pressure except    ─────→
in 4 risk groups

later drop of blood
pressure except in           ─────→
4 risk groups
```

Fig. 6: Findings of Kasl et al. on physical reactions on unemployment (U.S.A.) (ref. 3)

Another noteworthy finding was that people with a higher than average number of life events to overcome, had a much higher complaint level at the start of unemployment, but often had fewer compaints than others at the end.

Kagan[6] and Oveson[20] refer to some Scandinavian studies on health indicators. Due to the language barrier only the findings they refer to can be discussed. For example, Grönqvist (1977) found in Sweden that the sale of anti-hypertensive drugs rose with rising unemployment. In two other Swedish studies on company closures, mention is only made of psychic reaction such as reduced self-confidence and self-respect and loss of identity. After the shutdown of a Danish company, psychological symptoms were also seen among those who were thrown out of work. Joint pains were, however, milder in the unemployed or more severe in the new work situation. Kagan did not consider these studies to be convincing methodologically. Oveson reports a study done by Jacobsen in 1972 in Denmark. He analysed a number of cases of sickness in a group of employees before they knew about the closure, after they had been informed, and during unemployment. Jacobsen found a significantly increased number of first consults of the general practitioner in the month after the announcement and a peak in the month after the closure. In a second study Jacobsen found more sickness the more stressful the social situation.

In sum, it may be said that the only large-scale study on physical reactions and health problems in relation to unemployment is that published by Kasl et al. in the USA.
Since this study only dealt with short-term unemployment it is, however, not clear if the processes that are found are merely due to social change or specifically due to unemployment. The results of Dutch studies are not in conflict with these findings, but are too scanty to provide support. It is noteworthy that younger people were found by Kasl et al. and in two Dutch studies to react more strongly to stress but the age classification was not entirely similar. In this young group Kasl et al. found a greater capacity for recuperation. This point was not considered by the Dutch investigators. Another striking finding was the recuperative capacity of individuals with an above-average number of life events, which suggests the existence of a kind

of training effect. Here, as for the factors influencing the estimation of the seriousness of the situation, social support was found to have a positive effect.

Psychic and social reactions to unemployment

With respect to psychic reactions there is an obvious similarity between the findings of studies done in the Thirties and recently. They all show the same tendency as that found by Houtman[31] in a study on collective discharge: 'it is a great disaster, dominated by feelings of powerlessness and insecurity.' This general finding of a tendency does not mean that the results were very similar and reasonably conclusive. Concepts are applied very differently, quantification is very difficult and also rather divergent, and the same holds for the way in which feelings are described and operationalized. This is related to the degree of difficulty involved in such research. Folpmers was explicit on this point in 1937: 'The suffering due to unemployment differs widely between individuals: in describing their feelings some use such expressions as total demoralization, never happy again, being desperate; whereas others say only that they are very disappointed ...', and: 'some of the jobless who because of their character ascribe their difficulties to hostile surroundings, become suspicious.' Now, too, various investigators seem to use many words to describe what is probably the same thing. It is, however, particularly difficult to measure and compare the severity of psychic and social effects, as well as to determine patterns and differences in time, but even more difficult to distinguish what is a result of unemployment and what is due to other factors.

The findings of Eisenberg and Lazarsfeld[32] serve to illustrate the research done in the Thirties. In 1938, they found as the predominant psychic reactions emotional instability, anxiety feelings, lower morale, feelings of inferiority, and introversion. In English[11] and American[3,23,33] studies roughly the same conclusions have been reached on current unemployment. Use is made of such terms as depression, loss of morale, identity loss, difficulty in concentrating, apathy, powerlessness, relational problems, inferiority feelings, loss of self respect, alienation, and the feeling of having been expelled from society. The Braginskys[33] add that the unemployed incur permanent scars, and Oveson[20] too underlines the fact that many will never again function at the same level as before. Dutch researchers use fewer of such terms than their English-speaking colleagues. They have a tendency to restrict themselves to functional descriptions or to use rather neutral terms such as: the predominance of negative feelings, working-through problems, and so on. Moreover, their studies were not specifically concerned with the detection of psychic problems or done with a psychological approach. There is also no question of the detection of processes or patterns, but rather of the registration of feelings reported by the jobless. This 'registration' can be distinguished in the rather universal findings and findings about which there is little agreement. Almost all of the authors mention a feeling of being rejected and of lacking value, boredom, and difficulty in filling up the day. Most of them are also of the opinion that there are phases in the reaction to unemployment, but a general pattern cannot be deduced from the literature. Various authors mention that (government-stimulated) creation of contacts with other unemployed are not generally seen as positive, and there are objections to the uselessness and pointlessness of the leisure activities. Leisure and creative development only make sense in relation to a work situation and not when the filling of a (frequently empty) day is concerned. When the work situation disappears, and especially when there are other identity problems as well, leisure occupations are rather futile. Oveson[20] says literally: 'An unemployed individual has no free time, because there is nothing that he has time off from.'

Relatively little attention has been given to problems encountered by the jobless in dealing with officials who dispense assistance and money. The few reports are rather negative: the unemployed speak of a stirring up of the guilt feeling and the descent to a split personality. If the futility of applying for work is experienced often and over a long period, there is a tendency to reconsider the situation and attempt to live without work. At least in the Netherlands, those who make the benefit payments are obligated by law to make certain that the unemployed really seek work. If too few or no applications are made, the amount paid will be reduced radically. The underlying frustration is, in the words of one jobless man, 'being punished materially for attempting to survive psychically by learning to accept your new identity'. This can lead to intense rage and feelings of powerlessness. The comments about financial disadvantages and shortages found in many structured interviews might mask this problem partially. It is only reported by those who used open interviews. An occasional investigator mentions that at the very beginning the reaction to unemployment can be a sense of relief, a liberation from a mental and physical load that had become (too) heavy. But with longer unemployment these feelings disappear. Boucher et al.[9] put forward a theory in which they distinguish the following types of problems among the jobless: problems with making a choice ('I don't know what I want any more, what I should do, or how I should go about it') problems in dealing with negative reactions (especially when they lead to identity and/or family problems), alienation, and social isolation. This 'theory' does not comprise a clearly demarcated and described problem classification but is merely a restatement of the emergence of problems brought up by the jobless themselves. Especially problems in dealing with the experience and (to a smaller extent) problems of choice in the sense of the ability to reorientate one's life, were found by these authors. On a number of phenomena, lastly, the findings are rather divergent. Such findings include shame about being without work and the importance of the loss of contacts with fellow workers, on both of which the divergence is particularly strong. This also holds for the presence or absence of an increase in the intensity of the negative reactions to continued unemployment. Far too few studies have been done in this area as well.

The family situation has received even less attention than the psychic problems. The scanty data suggest, however, that it is unlikely that serious problems of the husband have no influence on the family and, vice versa, that family problems have no influence on the reaction to unemployment. In this field the classic study done by Lazarsfeld-Jahoda and Zeisl[34] in 1933 has not been equalled. Their participant study was done in the Austrian village of Mariental, which was totally unemployed. They found four distinct family attitudes: 1. resignation; without hope and without plans, life goes on reasonably well, people make the best of things; 2. unbroken; the future still exists and efforts are still made to find work; 3. despair; one attempts to keep going but feels depressive and useless. In these three types the family life remains orderly and attention is given to the children, but this is not the case for the fourth type: apathy. These individuals are broken and have given up totally. In 1938, Eisenberg and Lazarsfeld[32] found that the children of the unemployed achieved less at school, showed (and internalized) the same emotional instability as their parents, and had many conflicts with the parents. In studies on the unemployment of the current recession, family problems are seldom the main subject and an attempt is usually made to detect a single tendency in family reactions. The results of course differ. In fact, the conclusion drawn by Lazarsfeld-Jahoda and Zeisl still seems the most acceptable: essentially good relations between husband and wife become stronger and better, essentially bad relations become worse. Possible effects of the father's unemployment on the children are mentioned only by Lente[35]. When young people became unemployed, Gravelotte et al.[10] found the same pattern as Lazarsfeld-Jahoda and Zeisl found for families with unemployed parents, i. e., that the relationships in the home are reinforced by unemployment, in the sense that good relations are improved and bad ones deteriorate further.

All studies mentioned here were restricted to the unemployed and no control group was used for comparison. Only Ormel[42], who investigated the relation between (social) conditions, mental stress, and lack of well-being, studied a mixed population as far as employment was concerned. As indication of lack of well-being he took pleasant and unpleasant feelings, physical and psychic complaints, and social discomfort. One of his striking findings is that most of those with the strongest lack of well-being did not belong to the 'usual' categories such as women, residents of large cities, or the aged, but were found especially among the 'non-active' (unemployed, disabled) and the lowest social class.

Suicide

There are reasonably reliable indications that suicide is correlated with unemployment. Most of the information comes from studies on the occupational status of the population of suicides and attempted suicides. The proportion of unemployed in this population can be remarkably high, expecially in large cities, ranging from 50 to 65 %[36, 37]. Cobb and Kasl[28] found a high percentage of suicides among their jobless population. Rushing[37] wanted to know whether income is an intervening factor, and found (for the USA) that unemployment is more often correlated with suicide in the low and intermediate income groups and that less suicide occurred in the higher income groups. This correlation with income is stronger when the general unemployment level is low than when it is high. For the low and intermediate income groups Rushing refers to the predominance of fatal suicide as defined by Durkheim.

In sum, in most of the studies done in the Netherlands and other countries, reactions to unemployment were often found to be severe and to lead to long-term problems. It seems obvious that unemployment has psychic effects, but too few studies have gone into this point in any depth, and little is known about the nature and severity of these problems. Even less research has been done on the family and family relations in this respect. Studies done in the Thirties make it likely that families react in different ways, perhaps in dependence on the family situation and relations before the loss of work.
The existence of correlation between suicide and unemployment has seldom been disputed.

Discussion and summary

Generally, it is suggested that the problem of the relationship between unemployment and health is as shown in Fig. 7a.

Fig. 7a:

changes in supply and ⟶ unemployed ⟶ poor health
demand on the labour   people
market
|_____| |_____| |_____|
         cause   problem   result

This problem can be solved as shown in Fig. 7b.

Fig. 7b:

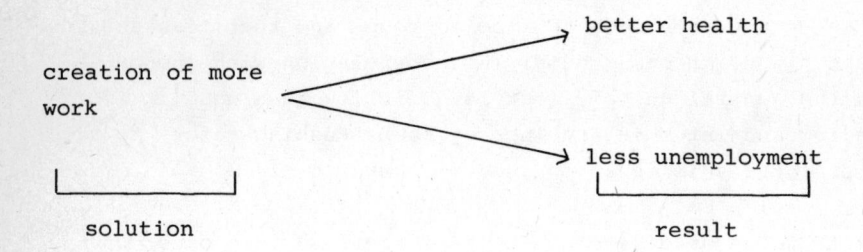

```
                              → better health
creation of more
work           ───────<
                              → less unemployment
|_____|              |_____|
  solution                      result
```

This is the solution aimed at by the Dutch Ministry of Social Affairs[38]. A policy-related formulation leads to Fig. 8a.

Fig. 8a:

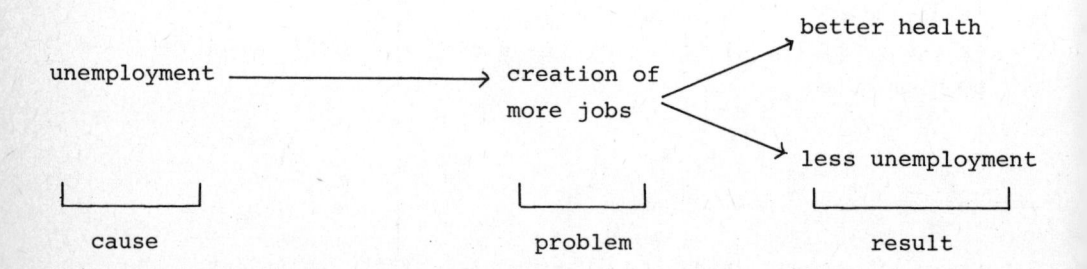

```
                                              → better health
unemployment ─────────→ creation of    ──<
                        more jobs
                                              → less unemployment
|_____|           |_____|          |_____|
   cause                  problem                   result
```

Despite its simplicity and apparent logic this formulation of the problem does not give us much help. There are two reasons for this:
1. Poor health is not the only possible consequence of unemployment. Other effects have already led to the Dutch government to decide to stimulate employment. Apart from political opinions on the degree and success of these efforts, information on health in relation to unemployment would not lead to changes in programs. The solution is evident before the data become available and 2. a vicious circle is inherent in this formulation of the problem, as shown in Fig. 8b:

Fig. 8b:

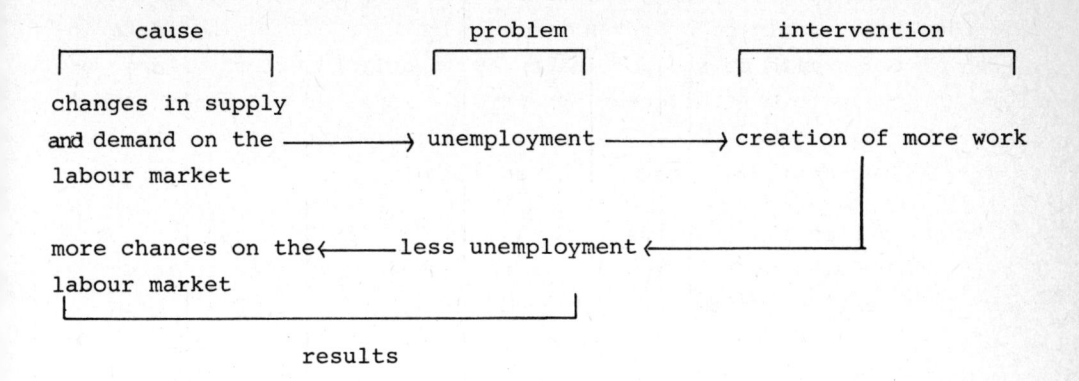

```
      cause                    problem                 intervention
┌──────────────┐           ┌──────────────┐       ┌──────────────────┐
changes in supply
and demand on the ─────→ unemployment ─────→ creation of more work
labour market                                              │
                                                           │
more chances on the ←───── less unemployment ←─────────────┘
labour market
└──────────────────────────────────────────┘
                      results
```

So this way of identifying the problem is fallacious; the true problem is how more work is to be created. The first, apparently simple, formulation thus leads us away from the question of whether there is a relation between unemployment and health and the possible consequences. If we start from a socio-medical formulation of the problem, we find considerably complexity, as can be seen from Fig. 9.

Fig. 9:

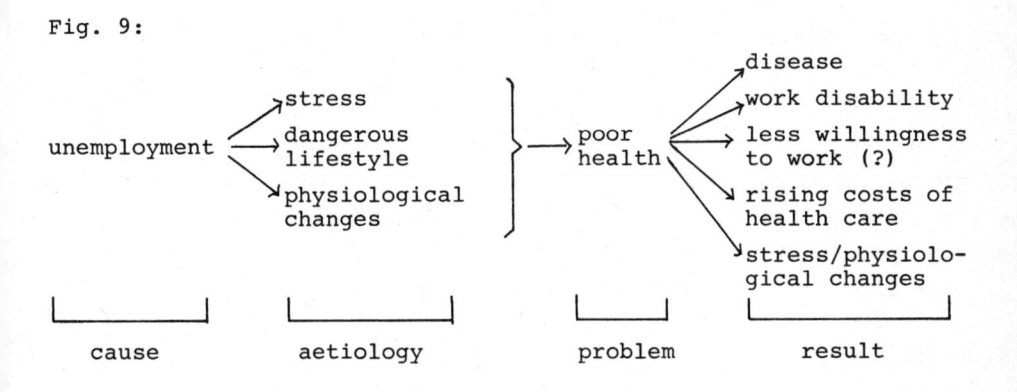

```
                    ↗ stress                              ↗ disease
                   /                                     ↗ work disability
                  /   dangerous          ↘  poor       /
unemployment ────→    lifestyle    }  ─→    health  ←───→ less willingness
                  \                                       to work (?)
                   \  physiological                     ↘
                    ↘ changes                            ↘ rising costs of
                                                           health care
                                                         ↘
                                                          stress/physiolo-
                                                          gical changes
└──────────┘      └──────────────┘     └────────┘      └──────────────┘
   cause             aetiology           problem           result
```

This problem definition helps us in the formulation of assumptions and questions that could lead to intervention possibilities. If we accept the hypothetical relations in this figure:

1. The solution arising out of the first (economic), problem definition i. e., the creation of more jobs, is less obvious and complete. This solution would mainly be a preventive measure to avoid further deterioration of the health of the population. This only requires research on the question as to whether unemployment is a cause of bad health. Then the 'cause' has to be removed, according to logic, so it is implicity assumed that unemployment can be solved and gives no alternative.

2. A greater number of persons with (partial) disability for work could arise, persons who may 'disappear' in the category "difficult to mediate for" or in the category of the 'difficult to re-employ', both rather at random registered. One category is included in the national unemployment rate, the other is not.
These people are involuntarily jobless but not unemployed in the sense that they could be re-employed if more jobs became available. In the first place, this complicates the relation between supply and demand on the labour market, and in the second place such 'hidden reduction' of unemployment cannot be seen as a socially desirable situation.

3. The question as to whether and, if so, to what extent diseases and disability induced by unemployment can be cured, as well as the problem of the degree of possible recurrence, or the occurrence of other diseases of disabilities, all depend on a number of (partially) unknown factors. These concern the following questions: 1. Which disease(s) or complaints can be induced by unemployment; 2. To what extent can these cause invalidity; 3. What relation exists between unemployment (cause) and possible disease aetiology? 4. Is intervention in this relationship possible? 5. When are disease-predisposing processes irreversible? 6. Can intervention in aetiological factors lead to a reduced chance of poor health or does the factor of unemployment (cause) as such bear more risk than the (aetiological) processes it leads to?

The studies done so far and discussed here are mainly social-science investigations with a social-science definition of the problem. Some of the available results derive from studies on the reaction to unemployment and the results of being unemployed as experienced by the individual who has lost his job. Another part of the information was obtained by chance or from subsidiary points. Taken together, all these results attempt to answer the question which is shown schematically in Fig. 10.

Fig. 10:

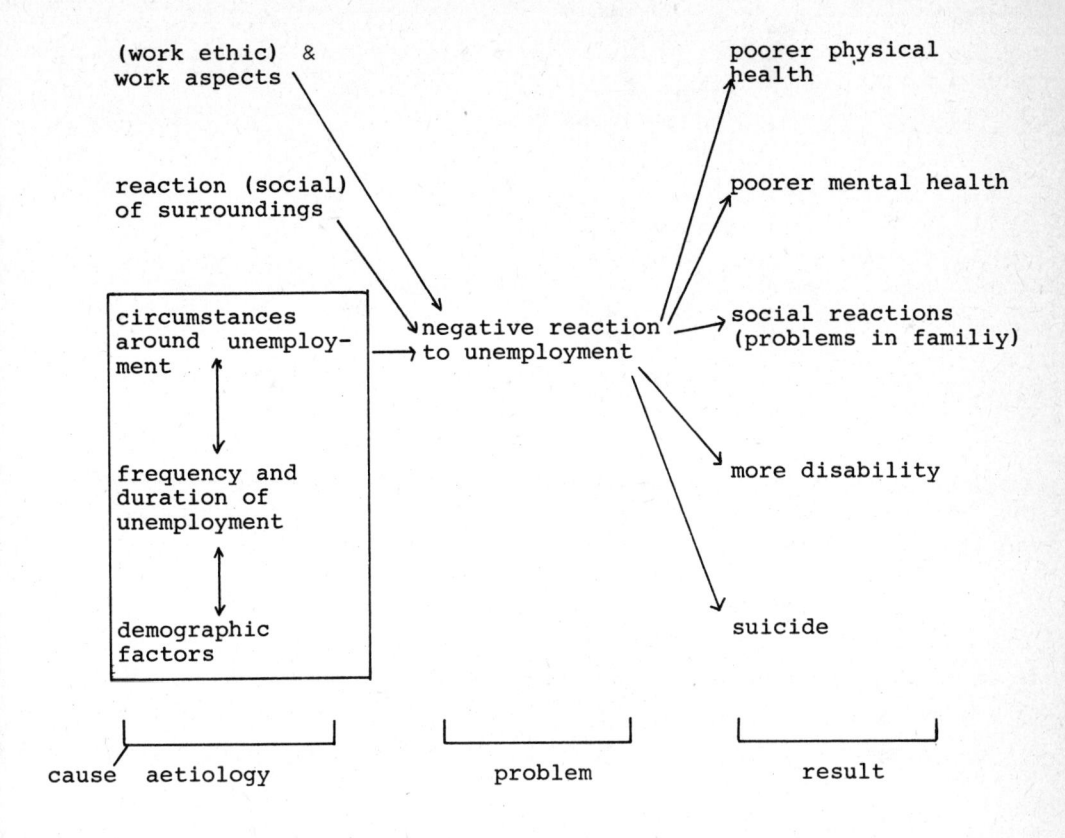

```
                                                    poorer physical
   (work ethic) &                                   health
   work aspects  \
                  \
   reaction (social)                                poorer mental health
   of surroundings \
                    \
   ┌─────────────┐   ↘ negative reaction  ──→ social reactions
   │circumstances│  → to unemployment         (problems in familiy)
   │around unemploy-│
   │ment    ↑    │          ↘
   │        ↓    │            more disability
   │frequency and│
   │duration of  │              ↘
   │unemployment │                suicide
   │     ↑       │
   │     ↓       │
   │demographic  │
   │factors      │
   └─────────────┘
   └──────┬──────┘     └───┬───┘        └───┬───┘
   cause  aetiology      problem           result
```

At the same time, these studies show that the consequences found in this way can start to act as 'causes' for intensified negative reaction (e.g apathy) and thus can generate a self-amplifying negative process (except in cases of suicide, which is an end). Deteriorating health is, therefore, not the end of the possible consequences. Consequently, we can easily link these two formulations as shown in Fig. 11.

Fig. 11:

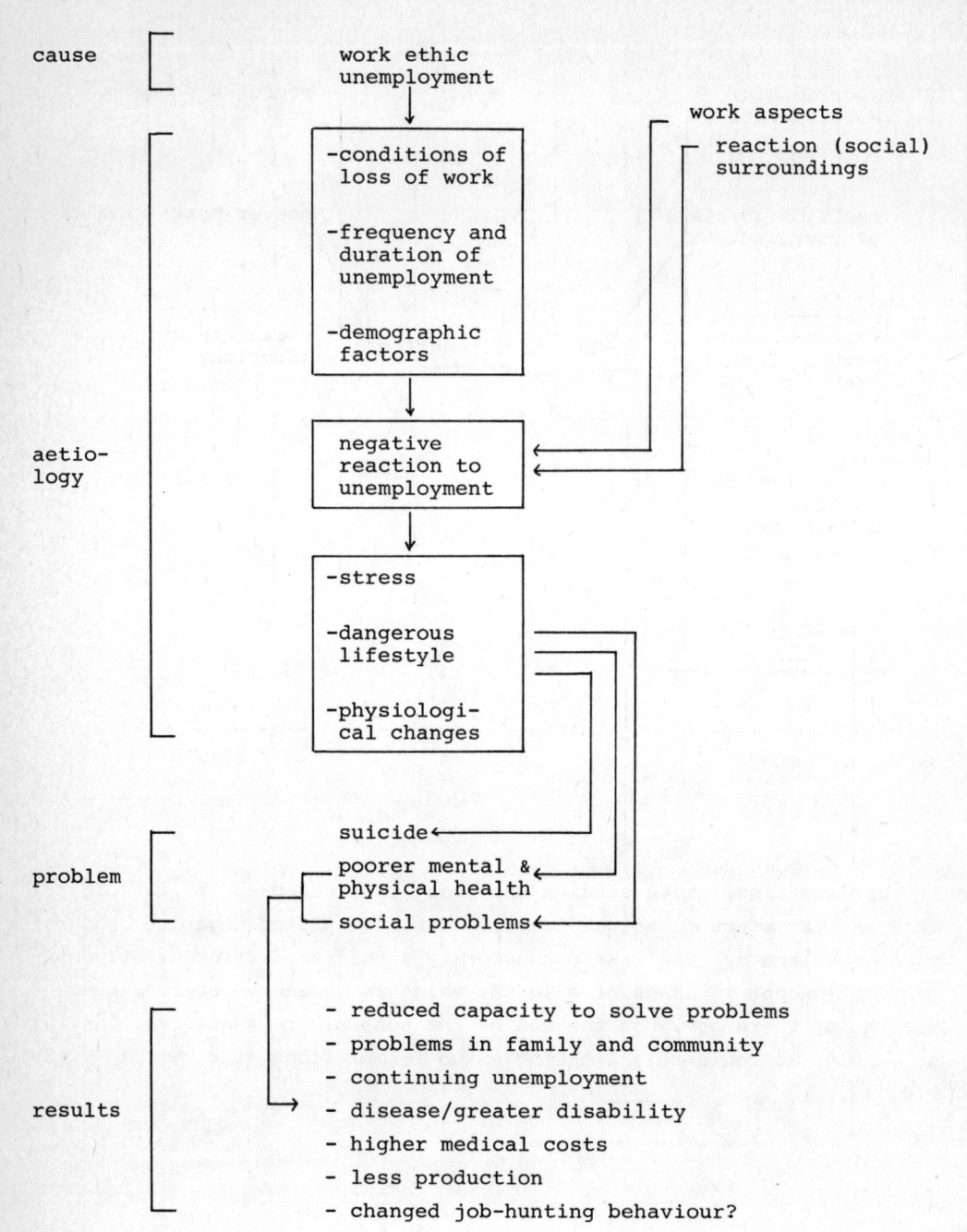

```
cause ⎡                  work ethic
      ⎣                  unemployment
                              ↓
          ⎡        ┌─────────────────┐                    work aspects
          ⎢        │ -conditions of  │
          ⎢        │  loss of work   │               ⎡ reaction (social)
          ⎢        │                 │                 surroundings
          ⎢        │ -frequency and  │
          ⎢        │  duration of    │
          ⎢        │  unemployment   │
aetio-    ⎢        │                 │
logy      ⎢        │ -demographic    │
          ⎢        │  factors        │
          ⎢        └─────────────────┘
          ⎢                 ↓
          ⎢        ┌─────────────────┐
          ⎢        │ negative        │ ←──────┐
          ⎢        │ reaction to     │ ←──────┤
          ⎢        │ unemployment    │
          ⎢        └─────────────────┘
          ⎢                 ↓
          ⎢        ┌─────────────────┐
          ⎢        │ -stress         │
          ⎢        │                 │
          ⎢        │ -dangerous      │
          ⎢        │  lifestyle      │
          ⎢        │                 │
          ⎢        │ -physiologi-    │
          ⎣        │  cal changes    │
                   └─────────────────┘

          ⎡             suicide ←
problem   ⎢             poorer mental & ←
          ⎢             physical health
          ⎣             social problems ←

          ⎡        - reduced capacity to solve problems
          ⎢        - problems in family and community
          ⎢        - continuing unemployment
results   ⎢  →     - disease/greater disability
          ⎢        - higher medical costs
          ⎢        - less production
          ⎣        - changed job-hunting behaviour?
```

In this scheme the most important research findings are classified in order of possible relationships. A causal-analytical approach of this kind, which is used in the field of medicine, lends itself to several formulations (Armstrong)[39]. Such a formulation can be dependent on the institution that must solve what it feels to be the main problem. If, for instance, we trace a curative medical approach, the possible relations would appear as in Fig. 12.

Fig. 12:

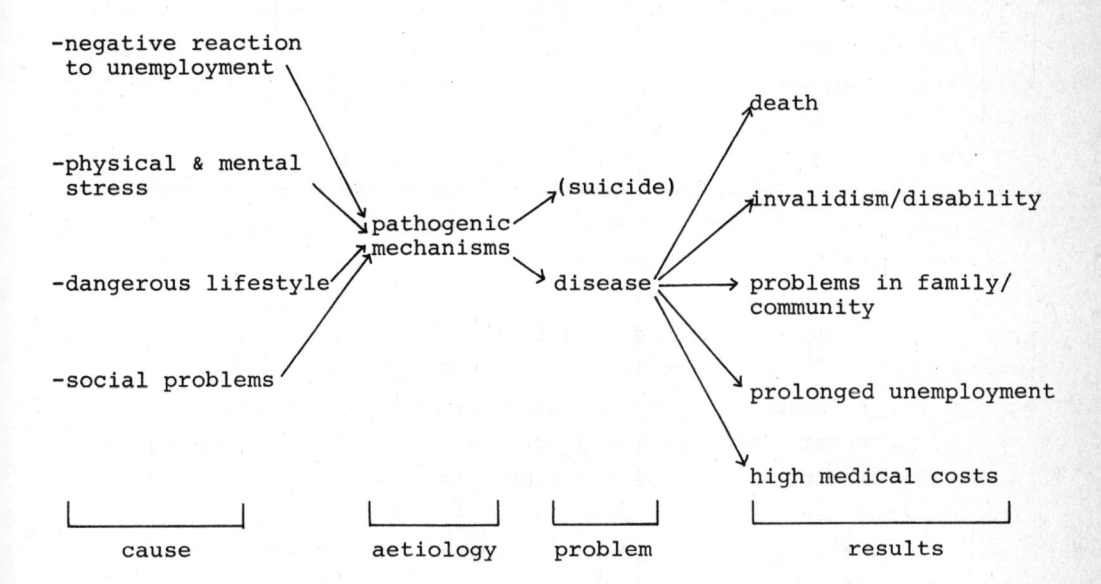

```
-negative reaction
 to unemployment  \                                  → death
                   \
-physical & mental  \                               → invalidism/disability
 stress              ↘                    ↗(suicide)
                      pathogenic
                      mechanisms    → disease      → problems in family/
-dangerous lifestyle ↗                                community
                    /
                   /
-social problems  /                                  ↘ prolonged unemployment

                                                     ↓ high medical costs

└────────┘      └──────────┘  └───────┘   └──────────────────┘
  cause          aetiology     problem          results
```

To detect differentiated processes situated between the social situation (e.g., unemployment) and disease, Kagan[6] formulated a number of hypothetical relationships which can be depicted as in Fig. 13.

Fig. 13:

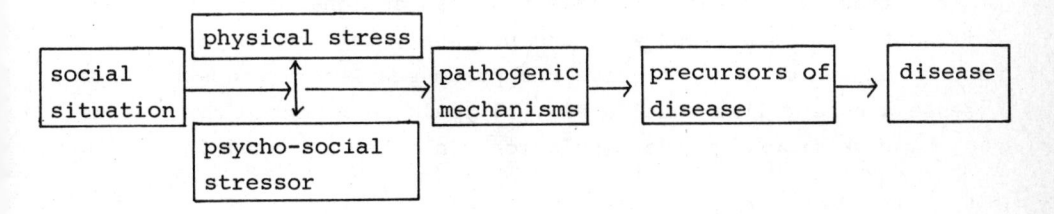

```
                ┌─────────────────┐
                │ physical stress │
┌──────────┐    └─────────────────┘   ┌─────────────┐   ┌──────────────┐   ┌─────────┐
│ social   │          ↑              →│ pathogenic  │ → │ precursors of│ → │ disease │
│ situation│→  ⇒ ─ ─ ↓ ─ ─ ─ ─ ─ ─→   │ mechanisms  │   │ disease      │   │         │
└──────────┘    ┌─────────────────┐   └─────────────┘   └──────────────┘   └─────────┘
                │ psycho-social   │
                │ stressor        │
                └─────────────────┘
```

In this scheme, too, the arrows show possible consequences. If we apply this to unemployment, such a process could be:
a) a social situation (e.g. prolonged unemployment) may lead to:
b) physical stress, due to poorer quality of food, housing etc. and
c) psycho-social stressors like a perceived threat of losing identity, reduction of self-confidence and the like, according to the individual and the presence of such phenomena;
d) pathogenic mechanisms may/can develop, like anxiety and depressions.

These may result in:
e) precursors of disease, which again will be dependent on the individual, his/her social surroundings and the phenomena (a - d) present. Examples of such precursors of disease are apathy, dangerous life-style, raised blood pressure etc. At the end:
f) disease might arise from the cumulative effect of these processes, if all processes occurred and the circumstances (individual characteristics, reaction social surroundings)were negative. This may be cardiovascular diseases, arthritis, addiction, etc.

Schemes 11 - 13 show a reductionistic way of thinking that is necessary for a causal-analytical method used to detect processes leading to disease (Spruit)[40]. The main attention is always given to negative effects. The population in which accumulation of effects stops, is not taken into account from that moment on, because it may be assumed that the process leading to disease has been arrested by then.

After all, not every negative reaction will lead to the loss of self-respect (or one of the other processes mentioned), and not every loss of self-respect will lead to health problems, just as not every case of fatalism will lead to suicide or every elevated cholesterol level to a cardiovascular disease. Which questions can we answer with the different formulations? The processes sought with the aid of scheme 13 would seem to lead to the detection of possible risk factors, but only extensive research will show how great a chance (and which one) of injury to health or disease they entail. In this scheme the social situation is a rather diffuse factor and no place has been assigned to findings on the circumstances coinciding with unemployment, the unemployment history, and so on, which can influence the processes leading to stress. In this sense a scheme like that in Fig. 11 would be suitable for the detection of risk groups in the population. In schemes 11 and 12, however, factors such as a 'negative reaction to unemployment' and 'poorer health' are vague and poorly defined variables. A definition of health (and sickness) is still lacking, and research has usually been concerned with complaints and provided no conclusions about the severity and health-endangered character of those complaints. In view of the limited amout of research done and the degree of difficulty of the prolems, this is hardly surprising. Hypotheses are, however, indispensable. For instance, Daeter[41] concludes that it has been proven that unemployment can lead to disease, and he assigns the most frequently mentioned reactions, psychic and physical phenomena, and complaints, to either a category called psychosomatic-disease or a category called psychosomatic complaints.

The criteria applied in this connection are obscure, the classification vague and arbitrary. Kesteloo[15] uses diagnostic groups, as applied in occupational medicine, but the category 'psychosocial complaints' is a vague one used collectively for anything that cannot be classified elsewhere (wastebasket).

If we want to use the above schemes as a basis for research, the expansion of the social situation (as in Fig. 11) allows in particular for the detection of risk groups, and expansion of the negative reaction (as in Fig. 13) allows for the detection of processes (risk factors). In both cases, longitudinal studies will be required in a population for which a number of prior characteristics (before unemployment) are known and thus can be followed in the process of unemployment and compared with a population of employed individuals.

If we start from a more holistic, descriptive socio-scientific approach, the correlations and results found so far can be represented (hypothetically) as in Fig. 14.

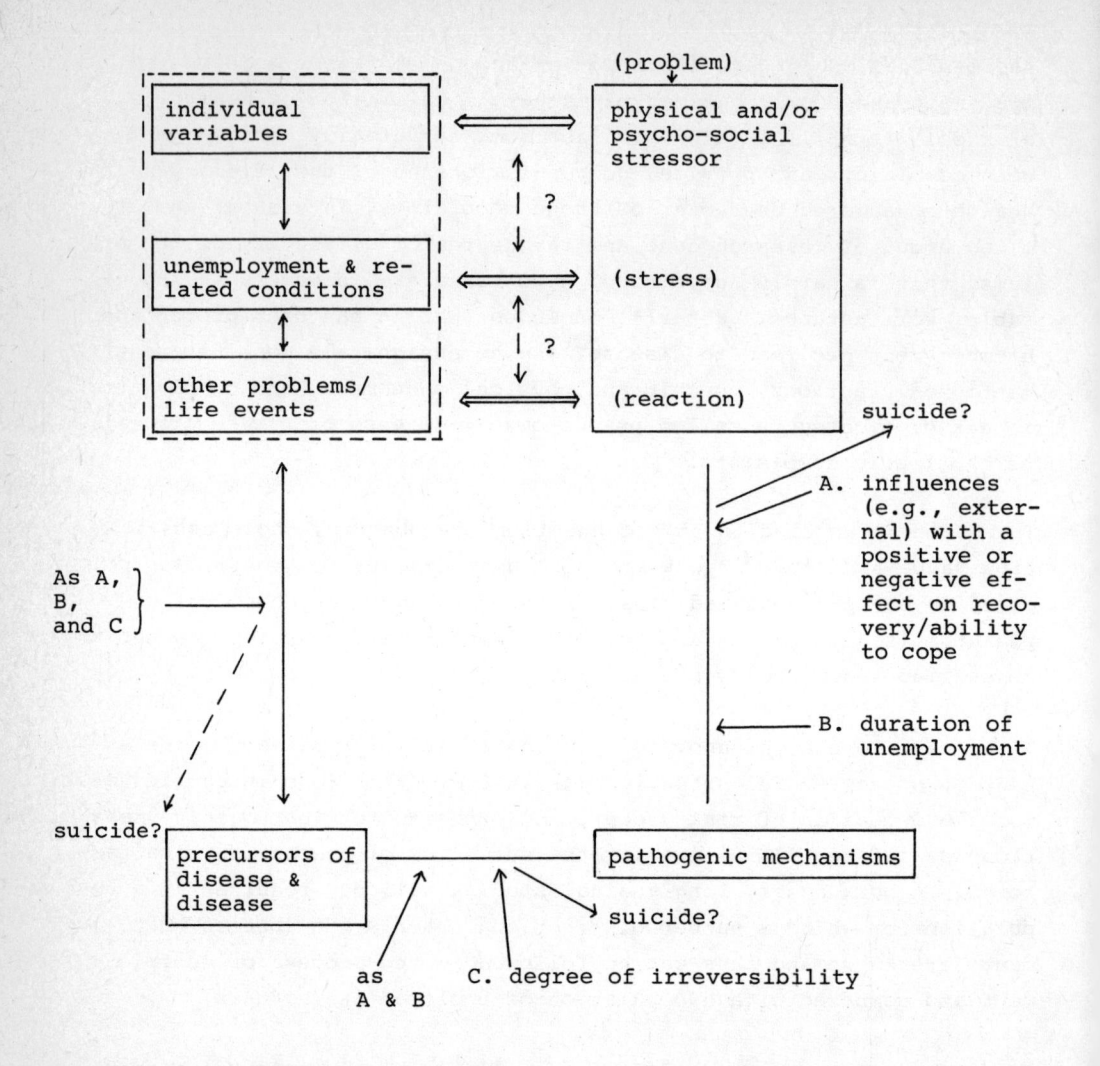

Fig. 14: The experience of unemployment and disease

In this scheme, the 'self-intensifying effect' of various processes introduced more explicitly, as are the possible inter-relationships between a number of factors and influences that (might) promote or retard the process leading to disease:

a. The basis taken was the strong relationship found between unemployment and a negative reaction. This is, according to Kagan's hypotheses, interpreted as a factor that yields stressors (and possibly direct stress), in view of Kasl et al.'s findings that the severity of the reaction is related to the severity of the health problems.

b. Both unemployment and the social conditions coinciding with it are social factors that influence the reaction just as other problems and individual variables do. These are, however, (also) interrelated, although it is not clear just how. There are, nevertheless, a few indications. For instance, it has been found that (more advanced) age often coincides with conditions influencing the reaction to unemployment negatively. It is also possible that there are groups with 'double deprivation': those who, for instance, have a relatively low educational level and belong to a lower social class have a higher health risk as well as more chance of becoming unemployed (and having poor health).

c. The emotional reaction, stressors, pathogenic mechanisms, and disease can influence both the individual variables (e.g., the degree of ability to work) and unemployment (longer duration) and other problems (which can be enhanced by the cumulative effect or an effect on the ability to cope with problems). Thus, a vicious circle of self-intensifying processes can arise. For instance, an older unemployed man with a specialized skill who sees his chance of re-employment as small and possibly already has a poorer physical condition, will in all probability experience his unemployment as something very serious. As a result, health complaints can develop and/or recovery be poorer, which will lead to a very negative reaction and a longer duration of unemployment, which in turn will activate (irreversible) pathogenic mechanisms.

d. Research has revealed positive and negative influences on the reactive and possibly disease-inducing process. Positive elements (in the sense of preventing or reducing complaints) include intact social networks and the presence of social support, possibly via a good family relationship. It has also been shown for instance, that young people may have more ability to recover (although they react more strongly to stress) and that there is a possible training effect of having experienced a higher than average number of life events. Negative elements (in the sense of enhancement of complaints) can be such factors as a strong work ethic, long duration of unemployment, contacts with welfare authorities, and experiences associated with applications for work.

e. The phase in which suicide is most frequent is not known. The same holds for (the genesis of) a dangerous lifestyle.
Use of a scheme like that in Fig. 14 as a basis for research could yield hypotheses for retrospective cross-sectional studies making use of comparable population categories. Such studies would probably reveal correlations of various strengths, but causal interpretation would be impossible. Extrapolation from the degree of correlation to social situations is also far from simple, but the finding of unequivocal causal relations via analytical socio-medical problem definition will not be easy either, because the investigator will be confronted with processes of many kinds that have not been incorporated into the schemes. This will make it extremely difficult to isolate mechanisms leading to disease.
In addition to the formulation of hypothetical schemes based on correlations and factors reported in the literature, it is also possible to indicate aspects which have not received sufficient attention from investigators. For instance, it is remarkable that so little consideration has been given to the implications of a dangerous lifestyle. There are indications of a correlation between the unemployment rate on the one hand and reduction of the quality of food and increased alcohol consumption on the other, but little attention has been given to a possible correlation with the use of such drugs as tranquilizers or other medicaments and no attention at all to possible relations with the use of drugs and tobacco. Kesteloo's findings suggest that occupation is a contributory factor. No research has been done to compare groups with different occupations, and the same holds for comparative studies dealing with different countries. Little is known about who becomes unemployed, except in terms of a few demographic factors, and nothing is known about who is unemployed frequently or for long periods. With respect to this last point, we know only that the age factor exerts an influence. There is also a remarkable lack of data of unemployed ex-self-employed individuals and, for instance, single women with children, or about the influence of unemployment on the partner or the family.

We may conclude that up to now, research has yielded as many questions as answers, but that there is every reason to take the health implications of unemployment seriously and to recommend that much more research be undertaken in this field.

REFERENCES:

(1) BRANDPUNT / K.R.O.: Onderzoek uitgevoerd door bureau Intromarkt. News Item, Survey performed by Intromarkt. Persbericht (1976)

(2) HOUBEN, P.P.J.: Ervaringen en oriëntaties van werklozen. Experiences and orientations of the unemployed. Mens en Onderneming 26, 284-394 (1972)

(3) KASL, S.V., GORE, S., COBB, S.: The experience of losing a job. Reported changes in health, symptoms and illness behavior. Psychosomatic Medicine 37, 2, 106-122 (1975)

(4) WETENSCHAPPELIJKE RAAD VOOR HET REGERINGSBELEID: Verdeling en Waardering van Arbeid. Division and evaluation of labour. Tilburg: I.V.A. (1976)

(5) SOCIAAL EN CULTUREEL PLANBUREAU: Jeugdwerkloosheid; achtergronden en mogelijke ontwikkelingen. Unemployment among the youngs; background and possible developments. Rijswijk: S.C.P. -cahier no. 20 (1980)

(6) KAGAN, A.R.: The evidence for a relationship between unemployment and ill health and lack of well being. (Unpublished manuscript) Stockholm (1980)

(7) WEZEL van, J.: Beleving van werkloosheid. Experience of unemployment. Gedrag, T.v. Psych. 2, 63-79 (1974)

(8) KOOPMANS, E.: Onderzoek onder werklozen I en II. Study on the unemployed, I and II. Tilburg: I.V.A. (1977)

(9) BOUCHER, Ph.W.G., ROBERTUS, T., SYTSTRA, H., WIERSUM, T.M.K, WIJN, M.A.M.: Onderzoek langdurige werkloosheid. Evaluatie van een project in Overijssel en een beeld van de problematiek 1976. Study on long-term unemployment; evaluation of a project in Overijssel and a picture of the problem in 1976. Groningen: Groningse Stichting voor Personeelsbeleid (1976)

(10) GRAVELOTTE, R., HATENBOER, A., KOSTER, A.: Jeugdwerkloosheid in Leiden, II. De belevingsaspecten nader onderzocht. Unemployment of young people in Leiden, II Further investigation of reactive aspects. Leiden: Vakgroep Klinische Psychologie, R.U. Leiden (1975)

(11) MARSDEN, J., DUFF, E.: Workless, some unemployed men and their family. Harmondsworth: Penguin (1975)

(12) TIFFANY, D.W., COWAN, J.R., TIFFANY, Ph.M.: The unemployed. A social-psychological portrait. N.Y.: Englewood Cliffs (1970)

(13) HAMAKER, H.G.: Het arbeidmarktgedrag van werklozen. Behavior of the jobless on the labourmarket. Mens en Onderneming 26, 295-308 (1972)

(14) HEINEN, T., VISSERS, A.: De houding tegenover werken/niet werken. Attitude to working/not working. Tilburg: I.V.A. (1978)

(15) KESTELOO, A.: Bedrijfsgeneeskundige aspecten van een dreigende bedrijfssluiting I en II. Occupational medical aspects of an

intended factory-closure. T.S.G. 53, 472-277 and 516-520 (1975)

(16) NIEVAARD, A.C.: Beleving van werkloosheid; bévindingen uit een onderzoek. Reaction to unemployment; findings made in a study. Intermediair 13, 21, 29-35 (1977)

(17) BUCHEM van, A.L.J.: Effecten van het voortduren der werkloosheid; een secundaire analyse van gegevens uit een onderzoek onder werklozen. Effects of continued unemployment; a secondary analysis of data from a study done in unemployed persons. Tilburg: I.V.A. (1975)

(18) BARENDSE, K., BUIJZE, Q, CAPEL, C.: DOORNEBAL, F., OLDE DAALHUIS, A., STEGINGK, M.: Werkloosheid en gezin. Unemployment and the family. Wageningen: De Uitbuyt (1976)

(19) SMOOR, B.L.: G.S.D.-Kliënten en hun belevingswereld; deelrapport in het kader van het onderzoek gemeentelijke sociale dienst. Clients and their emotional world; interim report of a study on municipal social services. Tilburg: I.V.A. (1978)

(20) OVESON, E.E.: Werkloosheid, een inzicht in de psychische en maatschappelijke gevolgen van werkloosheid. Unemployment, a view of the psychic and social consequences of being jobless. (Vertaald uit het Deens). (Translated form Danisch) Rotterdam: Kooyker (1977)

(21) MINISTERIE VAN SOCIALE ZAKEN: Nota Langdurig Werklozen. Memorandum on long-term unemployment. Weergave en beoordeling van een aantal onderzoeksresultaten met het oog op de beleidsvoering. Verslage en Rapporten Ministerie Soc. Zaken, jrg. 1976-5. Den Haag: Staatsuitgeverij (1976)

(22) LINDE v.d., S.A.G.: Werkloosheid als vrouwenprobleem. Unemployment as a problem of women. Groningen: Soc. Inst., University of Groningen (1979)

(23) GORE, S.: The effect of social support in moderating the health consequences of unemployment. Journal of Health and Social Behavior 19, 157-165 (1978)

(24) FOLPMERS, G.J.: Over de gevolgen van werkloosheid in Nederland. On the consequences of unemployment in The Netherlands. Utrecht: Thesis (1937)

(25) MARSH, L.C.: Health and unemployment; some studies of their relationships. Oxford: Oxford Univ. Press (1938)

(26) MATHEW, G.G.: Unemployment and health. J. Industr. Nurses 314-319 (1961)

(27) ZANDERS, H.: Omschakeling ex-mijnwerkers. Retraining of ex-miners. Tilburg: I.V.A. (1971)

(28) COBB, S., KASL, S.V.: Some medical aspects of unemployment. Industr.Geront. 8, 8-15 (1972)

(29) KASL, S.V., COBB, S., BROOKS, S.W.: Changes in serum uric acid and cholesterol levels in men undergoing job loss. Journal of American Medicine Association 206, 1500-1507 (1968)

(30) KASL, S.V., COBB, S.: Blood pressure changes in men undergoing job loss a preliminary report. Psychosomatic Medicine 32, 19-37 (1970)

(31) HOUTMAN, J.: Collectief ontslag. Collective discharge. Leiden: Thesis (1978)

(32) EISENBERG, PH., LAZARSFELD, P.F.: The psychological effects of unemployment. Psychological Bulletin 35, 358-390 (1938)

(33) BRAGINSKY, D.D., BRAGINSKY, B.M.: Surplus People. Psych. Today, p. 69-71 (1975)

(34) LAZARSFELD-JAHODA, M., ZEISL, H.: Die Arbeitslosen von Marienthal. Ein Soziographischer Versuch über die Wirkungen langdauernder Arbeitslosigkeit. Leipzig: Hirzel (1933)

(35) LENTE van, A.C.: Werkloosheid en vervroegde pensionering. Unemployment and early retierement. Evangelie en Maatschappij, p. 339-348 (1969)

(36) SMITH, J.C.: Changes in the patterns of admission for attempted suicide in Newcastle upon Tyne during 1960's. British Medical Journal 4, 4, 412-415 (1971)

(37) RUSHING, W.A.: Income, unemployment and suicide: an occupational study. Sociological Quarterly 9, 493-503 (1968)

(38) MINISTERIE VAN SOCIALE ZAKEN: Jaarverslag Arbeidsmarkt 1980. Report Labour Market. Den Haag (1981)

(39) ARMSTRONG, D.: An Outline of Sociology, as applied to Medicine. Bristol: Wright & Co. (1980)

(40) SPRUIT, I.P.: The applicability of medical anthropological research results to medicine. (In press)

(41) DAETER, H.G.M.: Ziekte en werkgelegenheid. De rol van de medische sociologie. Disease and unemployment; the role of medical sociology. Med. Cont. 35, 49, 1519-1524 (1980)

(42) ORMEL, H.: Moeite met leven of een moeilijk leven. Difficulties with living or a difficult life. Groningen: Thesis (1980)

(43) BELJON, J.A.S.: Consumptieve bestedingsmogelijkheden bij werkloosheid. Consumption spending possibilities of unemployed. Sociaal bestek 35, 405-422 (1975)

PREVALENCE OF UNEMPLOYMENT AMONGST THOSE BECOMING ILL

C.A. Birt

Stockport Area Health Authority

and

Department of Community Medicine
Manchester University Medical School

Great Britain

The aim of this project is to explore the relationship between longer-term unemployment and certain health indicators as observed in certain groups of individuals becoming ill in Stockport. Expressed in terms of a null hypothesis, the hypothesis to be tested is that the incidence of the conditions to be studied in Stockport does not differ significantly between the employed and unemployed parts of the population within each sex and age group.

Background to the Study

The previous seminar held in Copenhagen, and presumably this one also, held in Munich, can, at least to a certain extent, be described as debates carried on in the shadow of the soul of Professor Harvey Brenner. He must indeed be given the credit for awakening interest in the inter-relationships between the health of a national economy and the physical and mental health of its inhabitants, by providing a hypothesis concerning this issue which can be discussed. Many of his original findings, in the USA, and in particular in New York State, as well as in the United Kingdom and Australia, are well known. He found associations between changing rates of employment and deaths from coronary heart disease, cerebrovascular disease, malignant conditions, cirrhosis, homicide and suicide, as well as with infant deaths. He also noted relationships between changing levels of employment and prison and mental hospital admission rates.

The study of associations between one group of variables and another always presents great problems and dangers. Even if there can be shown to be a causal relationship between two variables, how does this operate, and which way round? One hypothesis suggests that the physical and mental health of a population varies in a cyclical manner, and the health of the economy gains and suffers accordingly. It has even been suggested that there may be an association between cyclical variations in human health and the sunspot cycle!

However, particularly when associations between the functioning of the economy, and the behaviour of communities and individuals are being studied on the one hand, and meanwhile other associations between behavioural variables within communities and health indices are also being studied on the other hand, the number of possible variables and associations between variables is almost uncountable. It is obvious that unemployment and becoming unemployed are likely to be associated with altered behaviour, and behaviour which is different to that observed in the employed population. Relationships in the home will become affected, as will relationships with work colleages. Altered patterns of behaviour will follow these changed relationships and also will be brought about by changed economic circumstances, which will impinge upon many aspects of day-to-day life and recreation. Meanwhile, the recession associated with unemployment will also have reduced the bargaining power of the labour force, with the result that working conditions themselves are likely to have become less favourable. The same recession may well have brought about a deterioration in the level of social service provision, upon which many of the poorer members of society may depend for their welfare. Many of the resultant aspects of altered behaviour may be associated with various health expectations, but any causal relationships are difficult to ascertain.

If increasing unemployment and deteriorating community health are associated, this may merely be on account of an association between poverty and ill health, and increasing poverty in the community following reduction in family income. Associations between poverty and ill health are no recent revelation, and have been clearly identified in the United Kingdom since the last century, when Rowntree identified such associations in York. More recently, the last Secretary of State for Social Services, David Ennals, set up a working party under the chairmanship of Sir Douglas Black, the President of the Royal College of Physicians of London, to identify relationships between social inequalities in the United Kingdom and health expectations. The resultant report shows that, not only do health expectations vary very considerably between social classes within the United Kingdom, but that these differences indeed appear to have increased during recent decades.

Harvey Brenner himself, however, has tended to suggest that unemployment is associated with deterioration in health on account of increased stress suffered by those who become unemployed. Unfortunately, stress remains a subjective term, which remains to be adequately defined. Be that as it may, whatever definition is applied to stress, there is good reason and some evidence to attribute stress both to those who are overworked as well as to those who are unemployed. As regards the latter group, the work of Leonard Fagin has taught us much, as indeed we are learning here at the seminar in Munich. He has certainly shown some ways in which stress is manifested within families where one member becomes unemployed. But if such stress is to be a mediator of ill health, what evidence is there to support such a hypothesis? It has been shown by various workers that, following the death of one partner of a marriage there is considerably increased risk of death of the other partner within the subsequent year. Other workers have shown similar findings in respect of those who retire as compared with those of the same age who remain in work. As regards coronary heart disease deaths following death of a spouse, the peak incidence occurs six months after the initial death. Yet Brenner suggests that there is a two-year delay between a peak of unemployment and a maximum incidence of coronary heart disease deaths. This anomaly may perhaps be explained by the fact that people become unemployed, as a rule, at a different stage of life to that at which marriage partners frequently die. The latter event is likely to occur later in life, by which time the early stages of coronary heart disease may have had the opportunity of already developing further.

Assuming that an association between rising unemployment and subsequent increasing ill health within a community can be shown to obtain, various questions remain. Is the increased incidence of disease to be found amongst those who have themselves become unemployed, or, is the increasing level of unemployment associated with other factors within the community which results in other people within that community becoming ill? Moreover, if the functioning of the economy can be shown to be clearly associated with the health of the people, what are the time-relationships? Is increasing ill health clearly related to increasing unemployment, or is it more related to the subsequent economic upturn, as has been suggested by some workers? As regard an answer to the first question, the work of Kasl, Cobb and Brooks possibly provides at least a hint of an answer. They followed a cohort of workers employed in a plant where a closure was announced, a closure took place, and the workers became unemployed. Subsequently, most of them obtained new jobs. These workers were able to show that various physiological variables became altered during this period. When the plant closure was announced, they noted that serum uric acid and diastolic blood pressure began to rise. Following plant closure, serum cholesterol was shown to rise. Serum cholesterol and uric acid began to fall following re-employment, and the raised diastolic blood pressure fell back to normal after workers had been re-employed for some months. At least some of these physiological variables may be regarded as possible coronary heart disease risk factors. But risk factors for disease are not the same thing as the disease itself. The question therefore remains, is the incidence of illness increased in those who become unemployed? If so, after what time interval does this become evident? These are the principal questions which this study aims to investigate.

Methodology of the Proposed Study

This study will attempt to investigate the incidence of certain conditions as between employed and unemployed populations. Unemployment itself is a vague concept, which has developed over various decades. In economic and philosopical terms, an unemployed person, will, for the purposes of this study, be regarded as one who has attempted to sell his labour on the labour market, and who has been unable to find a buyer. For practical purposes, this will require, because of the age limits being imposed, that an unemployed worker was previously constructively employed, that at some time he lost his job, and that subsequent to this he has been unable to obtain another one. Thus, housewives would not be considered to be unemployed, and nor would   self-employed people who might regularly expect periods of idleness of a few weeks or months.

The conditions to be studied are acute myocardial infarction (ICD 410), cerebro-vascular disease (ICD 430-437), poisoning ICD 965 (poisoning by analgesics, antipyretics and antirheumatics), ICD 967 (poisoning by sedatives and hypnotics), ICD 969 (poisoning by psychotropic agents), and ICD 980 (toxic effects of alcohol)), and malignant tumours (ICD 140-208). The subjects to be studied will be all men and women aged between 25 and 64 admitted to Stepping Hill Hospital, Stockport, on account of one of the conditions being studied, and who are resident within agreed geographical limits, plus all those who, in the same age group and resident within the same geographical limits, die of one of the same conditions outside Stepping Hill Hospital.

The Department of Employment has agreed to provide full details, every three months, in respect of each of its unemployment office areas, of the numbers of people, broken down by sex and age group, who are registered as unemployed for up to one month, for over one month, for over two months, for over three months, etc., up to a maximum of over thirty-six months. It is therefore necessary to define the area of the study taking account both of the hospital catchment area, and of the geographical limits of the areas served by each of the Department of Employment's local offices. Unemployed people do not, in the United Kingdom, have to register at their local office, but information supplied by the Department of Employment suggests that the overwhelming majority do register at their own local offices, so that, in practice, it is not difficult to define employment office area boundaries with a fair degree of precision, and the Department of Employment is doing this. Similarly, patients have absolute freedom as regards which hospital they are admitted to (and general practitioners are free to admit their patients to the hospital of their own choice), but, once again, the overwhelming majority of patients are admitted to local hospitals. In this case, the situation can be monitored with greater precision, as every admission to hospital within the United Kingdom (or to be precise, every discharge from hospital) is recorded on the computerised Hospital Activity Analysis system. Besides much other information, this records the home address of every patient. Thus, using this system, it is possible to define the catchment area of Stepping Hill Hospital, for the purposes of this study, as being that area from which 90% of patients admitted to hospital on account of their suffering from the conditions being studied are admitted to Stepping Hill Hospital. The employment office areas, as already defined, are then

superimposed upon the hospital catchment area, and the outer limits of the
hospital catchment area are excluded from the area to be studied, until the
boundaries of the employment office areas and the remainder of the hospital
catchment area are coterminus. This, then, will mark the boundary of the
area within which patients will be studied.

A questionnaire has been devised which will be used by research workers working
on this study. They will interview each patient, or a close relative (in the
case of a death, it will naturally be a close relative), using this questionnaire.
It is designed to ensure the recording of personal information, information
concerning the admission to hospital (if any), social information (including
information regarding the employment status of any spouse), diagnostic
information, and information regarding the employment or unemployment status
of the individual. This employment information will include a detailed
employment history for each preceding month of the preceding total of thirty-
six months. Thus, it will be possible to detect the nature and extent of any
period of unemployment during the thirty-six months prior to the onset of
disease. The diagnostic information will record other information in addition
to that pertaining to the immediate illness, so that patients with long-standing
recurrent illness or with any type of chronic sickness can be excluded from the
study.

In respect of patients admitted to hospital, the interviews will have to be
carried out following the making of an initial diagnosis by the doctor responsible
for the case. It will therefore be necessary for the final diagnosis of all
patients admitted to Stepping Hill to be checked prior to their discharge.
This will enable patients whose final diagnoses are inappropriate to the study
to be excluded, and will also ensure the detection of patients whose final
diagnoses reveal that they should have been admitted to the study, but who
were missed at the initial diagnostic stage. These patients, or their relatives,
can then be interviewed, either in hospital, or subsequently at home.

For the purposes of this study, the employed population will be defined as the total
population between the ages of 25 and 64 (25 and 59 for women) which is not unemployed.
On the basis of the information supplied by the Department of Employment, and obtained
from the study of patients with disease, it will then be possible to calculate
an incidence of each condition being studied in the employed population, the
incidence of each condition in those unemployed for one year or more, the
incidence of each condition in those unemployed for two years or more, and
the incidence of each condition in those unemployed for three years or more.
The expected number of interviews per year is 1,500 (1,150 following admission
to Stepping Hill Hospital, and 350 following death not taking place in Stepping
Hill Hospital). It is intended that the study should last for two years,
and it is therefore likely that the total number of interviews will be
approximately 3,000. The anticipated cost of this study is £25,000, or
DM 115,000.

If the null hypothesis is correct, and the incidence of these conditions is the
same in both the unemployed and the employed population, it is to be expected that
only approximately 60 of the patients entered to the study each year will have been
unemployed for more than one year. If the incidence of disease in the unemployed
is higher than in the employed population, then this expected number of 60 will
be exceeded.

There have been considerable difficulties in arranging the necessary finance to support this study. The National Health Service does enjoy its own arrangements for the funding of research, but such research is normally concerned with the medical and natural sciences. It would appear to be more difficult to obtain finance within the National Health Service to fund studies which include a social science perspective, however limited. However, other opportunities do exist, and it seems likely that this study can be financed directly by one of the British Government's own schemes, which is administered through the Department of Employment itself, known as the Community Enterprise Programme.

Finally, it should be added that, in addition to the study described, workers in Stockport and Manchester are considering and discussing the protocol of another research proposal. This would consist of a case control study between patients admitted to hospital with coronary heart disease and other patients admitted on account of their requiring acute abdominal surgery. Coronary heart disease patients, admitted to hospital following acute myccardial infarction, would be matched according to various characteristics, including age, sex, social class, health behaviour (e.g., tobacco and alcohol behaviour), etc., with patients admitted for acute abdominal surgery. The unemployment rate (and the length and period in time of unemployment) would then be investigated in both groups of patients, to detect whether or not there is an increased prevalance of a history of unemployment in the acute myocardial infarction patients as compared with those patients undergoing acute abdominal surgery.

REFERENCES:

1. Titmuss, R.M.: "Birth, Poverty and Wealth: A Study of Infant Mortality", Hamish Hamilton, London, 1953.

2. Townsend, P.: "Inequality and the Health Service", Lancet 1974, I, 1179-1184.

3. Morris, J.N.: "Social Inequalities Undiminished", Lancet, 1979, I, 87-90.

4. "Inequalities in Health", Report of a research working group (Chairman: Sir Douglas Black), DHSS, London, 1980.

5. Brenner, M.H. : "Economic Changes and Heart Disease Mortality", American Journal of Public Health, 1971, 61, 606-611.

6. Brenner, M.H. : "Fetal, Infant and Maternity Mortality During Periods of Economic Instability", International Journal of Health Services, 1973, 3, 145-159.

7. Brenner, M.H.: "Trends in Alcohol Consumption and Associated Illnesses : Some Effects of Economic Changes", American Journal of Public Health, 1975, 65, 1279-1292.

8. Brenner, M.H.: "Time Series Analysis of Relationships Between Selected Economic and Social Indicators", U.S. National Technical Information Service, Springfield, Virginia, 1971.

9. Brenner, M.H.: "Mortality and the National Economy : A Review, and the Experiences of England and Wales, 1936-76", Lancet 1972, II, 568-573.

10. Kasl, S.V., Cobb, S. Gore, S.: "Changes in Reported Illness and Illness Behaviour Related to Termination of Employment: a Preliminary Report", International Journal of Epidemiology, 1972, 1, 111-118.

11. Kasl, S.V., Cobb, S.: "Blood Pressure Changes in Men Undergoing Job Loss: A Preliminary Report", Psychosomatic Medicine, Vol. XXXII, No. 1, 1970.

12. Kasl, S.V., Cobb, S., Brooks, G.W.: "Changes in Serum Uric Acid and Cholesterol Levels in Men Undergoing Job Loss", JAMA, November 11th, 1968, Vol. 206, No. 7.

13. Rabkin, J.G., Struening, E.L.: "Life Events, Sress, and Illness", Science, Vol. 194, 3rd December, 1976.

PROPOSED RESEARCH ON THE
EFFECTS OF UNEMPLOYMENT ON HEALTH IN SCUNTHORPE

Gill Westcott

Nuffield Centre for Health Services Studies
University of Leeds
Great Britain

Background

Because of the difficulties with large scale statistical analysis of the relationship between unemployment and health (explored in the WHO seminar on this subject in Copenhagen last year), and because so far there are few contemporary case studies in Britain, there has been felt a need for further case control studies to show how far, in the present circumstances, unemployment does influence health. A second aim of the proposed research project is therefore to find out, if health changes do result from unemployment, what aspects of this situation are most crucial and which factors directly cause the health changes.

In this type of enterprise one cannot expect that unemployed workers in different regions will be precisely the same. Some of Brenner's work suggests that the response of overall mortality rates to a rise in unemployment level is greater in a town like Liverpool with long standing unemployment, than in a relatively prosperous town such as Nottingham. Local history, the character of local industry and of the workforce all condition how people respond to becoming unemployed.

The proposed study described here is one of several being carried out in different regions of the UK which attempt to gauge the effects of unemployment on health in their locality.

Location

Scunthorpe has long been a town with expectations of prosperity. Jobs for school-leavers have been ensured until recently by the presence of British Steel, the largest employer in the area. This has changed dramatically in the last few years, with the closing of one of the two steel plants and the pruning of the other. There were 1000 redundancies in late 1979 and 1980, and a further 4,100 jobs will have gone by the end of 1981. Several other factories are about to close or lay off large numbers of workers.

Scunthorpe is therefore a more extreme example of a situation typical of many areas in the UK, i.e. of a recent, acute unemployment problem in a location where workers have not previously experienced much instability in the job market.

The fact that there will be such a large number of redundancies in certain occupations mean that differences in responses to unemployment resulting from factors such as social support, age, etc. should be readily determined. The study was originally requested by the local branch of MIND, the National Association for Mental Health. The support and interest of local voluntary organizations and agreement of those involved in dealing with the redundancies at British Steel and elsewhere also make this a very suitable location for research and one where the findings might have potential applications.

This is not to imply that there can be a "solution" to the problem of unemployment by providing services, voluntary and statutory, and helping the unemployed to "cope" better with their situation. Nor can the problem be removed by a Keynesian deus ex machina, as the call for a return to full employment policies implies. In view of the present world economic climate, and the continuing technological change affecting the structure of employment opportunities, the problem seems virtually certain to continue for some time to come, without a great deal more democratic control over the amount and type of employment opportunities available.

When we discover the reasons for the health effects of unemployment, a great deal of light will also have been thrown on the sickening effects of employment, for the unhealthy features of being jobless - poverty, boredom, aimlessness, ingestion of harmful substances - are also present in varying degree in the work situation.

This being so, the involvement of a great many more of the people whose lives and work are affected by unemployment in understanding and acting must be an essential ingredient in any long term constructive measures.

It is therefore planned to feed back to the community as far as possible the results of the research as they become available and to aid and stimulate where possible seminars and programmes based on the problems revealed.

Study design

The hypotheses to be tested are, therefore: that

i) indicators of mental and physical health will deteriorate following unemployment and will remain low as long as unemployment lasts. (Two alternate hypotheses are that health may improve; or that a temporary deteroriation is followed by a readjustment);
ii) health indicators for the families of the unemployed will also be adversely affected;
iii) behaviourial changes will occur, such as the taking of drugs, alcohol and tobacco consumption, changes in diet, utilization of health services;
iv) weight gain will occur; and
v) that the adverse effects upon the unemployed will be reduced if the following factors are present:
 - age below 40
 - previous experience of changing jobs and skills
 - spouse's employment
 - social support
 - material support (including the scale of redundancy payments)
 - finding meaningful life activity *)
 - redundancy was, on balance, desired by the respondent.

Sample

A stratified sample of 500 unemployed workers will be drawn from among those who previously worked with British Steel, another factory which is closing in Scunthorpe, and if possible through the local job centre.

---

*) a preliminary definition of meaningful life activity is: those activities which the respondent feels to be worthwhile and proper to him or her, rather than being undertaken primarily to pass the time.

This size of sample will be required to determine adequately any differences in health status associated with different situations represented in the sample. A smaller sample will be drawn from this group for more extensive interviews, about a year after redundancy.

A control sample of employed workers will also be drawn to allow a comparision between the health of the employed and unemployed. This will be much smaller than the main sample, as it is not planned to study differences within it. It would be desirable to find a matched group of workers still employed. Similar data will be collected for the control group as for the main sample except for the in depth interviews. The samples will be contacted by post. Those agreeing to participate will be visited at home.

Data collection

Two visits, a fortnight apart, will be made at four-monthly intervals for a period of at least a year, if possible two years.
On the first visit the following information will be collected
    General Health Questionnaire (Appendix I)
    Initial Family Health and Employment Questionnaire.
On the second visit, a fortnight later
    Health Diaries for Family (Appendix II)
will be collected. On subsequent rounds, at the first of the two fortnightly visits the Life Activities Questionnaire would be carried out in place of the Initial Family Health Questionnaire. In addition, at whatever time is appropriate a
    First Year Assessment Questionnaire
will be administered to a subsample of the families in the unemployed sample.

Measures of Health

It was originally intended to use two self-administered health questionnaires, one to identify a tendency to mental health problems and one to measure problems of physical health.

1. For mental health, it is intended to use the General Health Questionnaire (GHQ) developed by Goldberg to detect psychiatric disorders among subjects in a community setting (3). The GHQ has been validated on groups in a London general practice, and has been found

to discriminate extremely well between people who are likely to be found suffering from a mental illness of a 'neurotic' kind by psychiatric interview and those who are not. The GHQ has the advantage of having been used also in studies of the unemployed (e.g. of the mental health of unemployed teenagers in Sheffield (4).

To measure physical health it was felt that clinical measures such as blood pressure, would require clinical expertise beyond the resources of this particular study. Hence it was decided to consider the Nottingham Health Profile(NHP), a measure of physical health status. This profile has been tested on a group of elderly patients (5) and is in the process of being validated on a more diverse group. Initial results suggest that the measures obtained agree well with the judgment of physicians.

However, the NHP as it stands contains a number of statements which are of specific relevance to the elderly and infirm, such as "I have trouble getting up and down stairs or steps". These are of minor relevance to the proposed sample, and yet when they are removed, the remaining questions in the NHP (dealing with such things as sleep, energy, social isolation, emotional reactions) resemble very closely the GHQ questions. Other health profiles for mental health (the Foulds/Bedford Personality Disturbance Inventory (6), the adapted version of the Cornell Medical Index (CMI) used by Fagin (7), and the Middlesex Hospital Questionnaire (8)), include again a fairly similar range of questions.

It would appear that the same sort of questions can be used to distinguish those suffering from mental and physical health problems!

It was decided, therefore, to use only one questionnaire. The GHQ has been well tested, and would provide comparability to other studies. However, certain criticisms have been made of its use:

i)   The questions are asked in the form "have you recently....." experienced certain feelings or symptoms. Although it reflects <u>changes</u> in health, it would seem that those who have adjusted to a situation in which they are unhappy or unwell will answer these questions with "no more than usual". This possibility was considered by Goldberg in the validation studies but, he states that "only a small minority of patients with chronic disorders are misclassified because they have responded "same as usual". Most of them seemed to sustain a notion of their "usual selves" as people who are free from symptoms, even after illnesses that have lasted many years"(9).

ii) The GHQ also misses patients with dementia, chronic schizophrenia and hypomania. These are, however, a small proportion of the mentally ill. It also misses defensive people. Goldberg also avers these are a small proportion.

iii) There may be some disagreement as to whether psychiatrists actually do denote something meaningful by assigning the label "mental illness". There may be less disagreement that whatever it is that is recognised entails distress for the person involved.

The Cornell Medical Index health questionnaire, in contrast to the GHQ, refers to a state of health at a point of time regardless of past experience. It is criticised for not distinguishing traits and symptoms, for being loaded with hypochondriacal items and being subject to 'yea-saying' bias (unlike the GHQ). However, if it reflects, as Fagin states (10), 'sick role tendency' this does not invalidate the rule of the questionnaire to explore the extent of sick-role behaviour.

A small pilot study was carried out, consisting of 23 interviews with employed and unemployed people of different ages. They were contacted through a drop-in centre for young unemployed people and through personal links. The unemployed and employed groups were matched as far as possible for age, sex and social class. Each person was asked to complete a questionnaire including the 20 item GHQ, followed by an additional 10 questions to cover most of the items in the CMI as used by Fagin which were not covered at all in the GHQ. The Family Health and Employment Questionnaire was also given.

The numbers in the pilot study are too small for reliable statistical analysis. Nevertheless the interviews threw some light on the points made above. A woman whose agrophobia was apparently worsened by her husband's unemployment gave low scores on the CMI questions and, especially on the GHQ. A measure which detects <u>changes</u> in health status is what is required for the present study, especially in the early phases; but it must be borne in mind in the analysis that a decline in the GHQ may not in fact be associated with a health improvement. There is a need for another measure of the <u>state</u> of health, which the CMI or the Health Diary could do better.

For what they are worth, there was a correlation of 0.673 between the scores on the GHQ and CMI in related questions. The CMI questions pick up a greater number of physical symptoms. The divergence between the two measures may be augmented by the fact that the majority of the pilot study were young (11 were under 25) and some moved in circles where it was acceptable to express malaise in ways other than adoption of a sick role. Six of the young people were known to have been involved in crime while they were unemployed, and another three while they were employed or still at school. One might test the hypothesis that the high GHQ scores indicate not only a tendency to health problems but also in these cases reflect involvement in crime and expectations of trouble with the police.

The danger that a defensive attitude would prevent the expression of malaise through the GHQ may not matter if this attitude is associated with a rarity of illness. Stoicism is a virtue highly valued in Yorkshiremen. However of the 8 highest GHQ scores 7 were men (6 were unemployed). Of the 6 who showed higher CMI-related scores than the GHQ would seem to warrant, 5 were women.

2. <u>The Health Diary</u> (11) is a fortnightly record of perceived health experience (see Appendix II) and can be kept for the whole family. It was used by Kasl and Cobb in their two year study of job loss, when the number of 'Days Complaint' was found to be a sensitive measure of health status and responsive to the perceived stressfulness of experience. (Similar associations with perceived stress were found for serum uric acid, blood pressure levels and serum cholesterol) (12). From the diary, Days Disability and the use of health facilities and pharmaceutical products may also be gauged, though the numbers over a fortnight were rather small for statistical analysis.

Thus with the periodic use of both the GHQ and the Health Diary adequate indicators of perceived health will be obtained, indicators which have been shown to be related to psychiatrists' judgements in the one case, and physical and psychological indicators of stress in the other.

Related information

A family health and employment questionnaire will be used to collect the basic demographic data and employment history of the respondent and spouse (13). It also covers aspects which will be regularly updated through the Life Activities questionnaire in later visits: housing, financial situation, smoking, drinking, socializing and other life activity. Some results of the pilot study with the questionnaire are given in Appendix III.

In the final analysis, two sorts of comparisons will be possible:

i) between the employed and unemployed samples for the present time, and between different groups of the unemployed with respect to the variables mentioned above. Path analysis could be used to elucidate the chains of causation.

ii) between the employed and unemployed situation at present and their own past experience.

In this way one could distinguish changes over time relating to the whole population including the effects of recession, from the effects of unemployment at present.

Implications of Unemployment for the Social Services

Data available from official sources and voluntary agencies will be used to complement the findings of the survey. Changes in health on a city-wide basis will also be apparent. Information on the pattern of utilization of social services and any changes in this pattern (e.g. the demands made on social workers, might also yield insights on the health-related factors which might be affected by unemployment. A study of this kind, together with the findings from the sample survey, could enable the build-up of a coherent picture of likely trends in mental illness and of potential channels for intervention and preventive work.

APPENDIX I

HEALTH QUESTIONNAIRE

Please read this carefully:

We should like to know if you have had any medical complaints, and how your health has been in general, over the past few weeks. Please answer ALL the questions on the following pages simply by underlining the answer which you think most nearly applies to you. Remember that we want to know about present and recent complaints, not those that you had in the past.

It is important that you try to answer ALL the questions.

Thank you very much for your co-operation.

HAVE YOU RECENTLY:

1. been able to concentrate on whatever you are doing?	Better than usual	Same as usual	Less than usual	Much less than usual
2. lost much sleep over worry?	Not at all	No more than usual	Rather more than usual	Much more than usual
3. been managing to keep yourself busy and occupied?	More so than usual	Same as usual	Rather less than usual	Much less than usual
4. been getting out of the house as much as normal	More than usual	Same as usual	Less than usual	Much less than usual
5. felt on the whole you were doing things well?	Better than usual	About the same	Less well than usual	Much less well
6. been satisfied with the way you've carried out your task?	More satisfied	About same as usual	Less satisfied than usual	Much less satisfied
7. felt that you are playing a useful part in things?	More so than usual	Same as usual	Less useful than usual	Much less useful
8. felt capable of making decisions about things?	More so than usual	Same as usual	Less so than usual	Much less capable
9. felt constantly under strain?	Not at all	No more than usual	Rather more than usual	Much more than usual
10. felt you couldn't overcome your difficulties?	Not at all	No more than usual	Rather more than usual	Much more than usual

11.	been able to enjoy your normal day-to-day activities?	More so than usual	Same as usual	Less so than usual	More less than usual
12.	been taking things hard?	Not at all	No more than usual	Rather more than usual	Much more than usual
13.	been able to face up to your problems?	More so than usual	Same as usual	Less able than usual	Much less able
14.	found everything getting on top of you?	Not at all	No more than usual	Rather more than usual	Much more than usual
15.	been feeling unhappy and depressed?	Not at all	No more than usual	Rather more than usual	Much more than usual
16.	been losing confidence in yourself?	Not at all	No more than usual	Rather more than usual	Much more than usual
17.	been thinking of yourself as a worthless person?	Not at all	No more than usual	Rather more than usual	Much more than usual
18.	been feeling reasonably happy, all things considered?	More so than usual	About same as usual	Less so than usual	Much less than usual
19.	been feeling nervous and strung-up all the time?	Not at all	No more than usual	Rather more than usual	Much more than usual
20.	found at times you couldn't do anything because your nerves were too bad?	Not at all	No more than usual	Rather more than usual	Much more than usual
21.	been having pain in my back?	Not at all	Rarely	Sometimes	Often
22.	been having bad headaches?	Not at all	Rarely	Sometimes	Often
23.	been suffering from indigestion or an upset stomach?	Not at all	Rarely	Sometimes	Often
24.	been breathless or had a pounding of your heart?	Not at all	Rarely	Sometimes	Often
25.	been feeling tired most of the time?	Not at all	Rarely	Sometimes	All the time
26.	found that people annoy and irritate you?	Not at all	No more than usual	Rather more than usual	Much more than usual

27.	been waking up in the early hours in the morning ?	Not at all	No more than usual	Rather more than usual	Much more than usual
28.	been feeling there is nobody you are close to ?	Not at all	No more than usual	More than usual	Much more than usual
29.	been frightened of going out alone or meeting people ?	Not at all	Rarely	Sometimes	Often
30.	been having feelings of panic, for no good reason ?	Not at all	Rarely	Sometimes	Often

APPENDIX II

DAILY HEALTH RECORD   FOR:

Week beginning:

EACH DAY, mark (X) any of these three columns which apply			EACH DAY, mark (X) the columns below which apply:					EACH DAY, mark (X) in these columns if:		EACH DAY, if any columns except 3 and 9 have been marked, describe what the trouble was:
			Didn't carry on usual activities - had to:			Carried on usual activities				
Was sick, had an ailment or did not feel as well as usual	Had an accident or injury or felt effects of previous accident or injury	Felt as well as usual	Stay in hospital	Stay in bed at home	Stay in the house but not in bed	But not able to do as well as usual	As well as usual	Any drugs or medicines or pills were used	A doctor was seen or contacted	—for each sickness, write in what was wrong. If a doctor was seen, put what he said the trouble was: —for each accident or injury, make sure you put what parts of the body were hurt, how each part was hurt, & how & where the accident happened. —If any medicines or pills were taken put what they were, and what they were taken for. If any illness stays the same for more than one day, write in "Same". (Use back of sheet if more room needed)
(1)	(2)	(3)	(4)	(5)	(6)	(7)	(8)	(9)	(10)	(11)
DAY										

If in hospital as a patient this week, give name and address of hospital:

Give the name and address of any doctor seen during this week:

APPENDIX III

Report on a Pilot Study with the Family Health and Employment Questionnaire

The pilot study was used to identify difficulties arising in the process of interviewing, in the questionnaires, and in the coding and analysis of information collected. Some 'findings' are discussed briefly here, in order to illustrate the hypotheses which can be tested with a larger sample.

Respondents appeared to find both questionnaires acceptable, and all those asked agreed to have the interview recorded.

For 6 pairs of respondents matched for age, sex and social class, the average GHQ's of the unemployed group (10.6) indicated a poorer state of health than those in the employed group (6.9). In only 2 of the 6 pairs was the unemployed member more healthy as measured by the GHQ. The unemployed group had double the average rate of illnesses reported over a period of time compared with the employed group, illnesses which also tended to be more severe and long lasting.

The CMI-related questions indicated a much smaller difference between the employed und unemployed group (indices of 5.6 and 5.9 respectively).

A large proportion of the sample, when describing what illnesses they had had over the last 2 years, were able to attribute or link them with events or changes in their lives, such as moving to new accomodation, family changes and separations, etc. Although no questions were asked about diet, two people stated that they got digestive problems resulting from irregular diet when unemployed, and two others lost weight.

Backache was the major complaint originating from work. But 2 respondents indicated that they had had considerable health problems while working which had disappeared when they became unemployed. In both cases the ill effects were related to their unsuitedness to the work rather than to occupational hazards as such.

The interviews bore out the point that health consequences were the result of a multiplicity of causes, usually involving a preexisting situation, some of which were worsened by unemployment. For example, Laurie, a plumber, experienced bouts of severe scariasis since working in a rubber factory 8 years before. He developed ulcer-like symptoms when under great stress and a bad cough most winters. Unemployment compounded problems in his marriage, whereupon the scariasis worsened, he had stomach pains and vomiting, though no ulcer was found, and the chest problem was diagnosed as being akin to TB and treated as such.

It appeared that involvement with child care, whether in men or women, and the responses which quite young children would on occasion give to their parents, ameliorated the depression and boredom which were visible particularly in the younger and more socially isolated unemployed.

The two women with children interviewed both felt frustrated by their inability to find a job which would use their skills. Yet their education also helped them to use their time constructively at home; so did their involvement with their children provide full time occupation at home, though both would have accepted full time employment had it been available. Neither were registered as unemployed.

There might be problems in interviewing in a family situation when attempting to discover the attitudes of one partner, particularly women. All the interviews in the pilot study were conducted with one person at a time, although this may not be practical in the main study. It remains to be seen whether there is any point in aiming for solo interviews with one partner on some occasions.

The use of state agencies (including social services, housing department, social workers, probation officers and community health services) was more than twice the level of the employed group in the unemployed. The changes in smoking and drinking brought about by unemployment were more ambiguous. Some cut down, others increased their consumption, particularly among young single people of lower social class. 5 respondents had definitely cut down their drinking when unemployed, while only 2 increased it notable, but these had become very heavy drinkers. (Perhaps this is connected with the finding that in recession, beer consumption falls, while that of spirits increases.)

Close relationships appeared to be adversely affected by unemployment, and so in some cases was social support. In the 30's age group however, a few had developed good support structures for themselves, both material and social: a food co-operative was flourishing in one area, together with arrangements for reciprocal child care and borrowing of money, cars etc. in a group of whom several parents were unemployed. It was a mother in this group, living on an income of £65 for two adults and three children, who said that she did not miss at all the racier life she had lived as a teacher now that both parents were unemployed. This couple were well educated and their unemployment was partly the result of an effort to achieve more balance in child care and external roles. Both did part time voluntary work, and though they struggled financially, they found unorthodox holidays and enjoyed much material and social support on a reciprocal basis. They were highly unusual.

REFERENCES:

(1) SCHWEFEL, D., BRENNER, H.(Rapport.): Study on the influence of economic development on health. Report on the WHO Planning Meeting, Copenhagen, 11.-13.11.1980. In this volome.

(2) WORLD IN ACTION: The reckoning. Granada Television (9.1.1979)

(3) GOLDBERG, D.: Detection of psychiatric illness by questionnaire. London: Oxford University Press (1972)

(4) STAFFORD, E.M., JACKSON, P.R., BANKS, M.H.: Employment, work involvement and mental health in less qualified young people. Journal of Occupational Psychology 53, 291-304 (1980)

(5) HUNT, S.M., et al.: A quantitative approach to perceived health status: a validation study. Journal of Epidemiology and Community Health 34, 281-286 (1980)

(6) BEDFORD, A., FOULDS, G.A., SHEFFIELD, B.F.: A new personal disturbance scale (DSSI/sAD) British Journal of Social and Clinical Psychology 15, 387-394 (1976)

(7) FAGIN, L.: Unemployment and health in families: Case studies based on family interviews - A pilot study. London: Dept. of Health and Social Security (1981)

(8) CROWN, S., CRISP, A.H.:Manual of the Middlesex Hospital Questionnaire (MHQ). Barnstable: Psychological Test Publications

(9) GOLDBERG, D.: op.cit., p.99

(10) FAGIN, L.: op.cit., p.12

(11) KASL, S.V., COBB, S., GORE, S.: Changes in reported illness and illness behaviour related to termination of employment: a preliminary report. International Journal of Epidemiology 1, 2, 111-118 (1972)

(12) ibid., p.114-115

(13) I am indebted to Dr. I.M. STANLEY for help with this questionnaire.

OUTLINE OF A STUDY ON THE IMMEDIATE AND LONGTERM ILL-EFFECTS
OF A PLANT SHUTDOWN IN A RURAL COMMUNITY

Heikki Salovaara[1]
Occupational Health Centre
Olofström, Sweden

The setting of the research project:

- Olofström, a community in Southern Sweden with 15.400 inhabitants, of these 10.000 in the township of Olofström.
- In this community there are 7.500 salaried workers, of them 4.000 employed at the local VOLVO factory not included in the study.
- There are some 430 unemployed = approx. 5 % at the present, and a comparable level of unemployment in the region giving a total of over 2.000 unemployed competing for presently available 12 jobs within a community distance of 30 miles from Olofström.
- The big multinational telecommunications company LM Ericscon has a plant at Olofström employing about 550 persons (85 % women) 1976, but only 250 (80 % women) 1981. During a period of relative uncertainty 1976-81 300 have left their jobs.
- The company decided to shut down the plant in question: 100 must leave by April 1st, 1982. The other 150 by December 31st, 1982.
- The employees included in this study have been extensively studied by the Occupational Health Centre with a lot of base-line data available from the years 1972-81.
- It is possible to find a group of 250 matched controls not experiencing job loss and with the same kind of base line data as the LM-group. These could be picked out from the collective of 2.700 employees served by the Centre.
- Another control group could be found from an array of joblosers in the neighbouring and entirely comparable communities

---

1) with the cooperation of the WHO Institute of Psychosocial Medicine / Prof. Lennart Levi, Stockholm

in plants not served by the Centre. They could be used as controls for intervention effects.
- A parallel study should be made of the 300 who left the plant in question 1976-81.

The study could consist of 3 different parts on the time schedule:

- A retrospective study covering the prospering phase 1972-76 and the phase of insecurity 1976-81.
- A short-term follow-up of the transition stage from employment to unemployment Oct. 1981 - Dec. 1982.
- A long-term follow-up of the unemployment period (up to 10 - 12 years).

Variables that I plan to study:

- economic
- psychosocial
- stress-physiological
- medical

Questions I would like to be able to answer:

- What ill-effects on health can be found retrospectively from the period of uncertainty 1976-81?
- What ill-effects on health can be observed in the transition period since the announcement of plant shut-down?
- What ill-effects on health can be observed in the long-term follow-up of the unemployed in a situation without choice?
- What methods of intervention: social, physical, educational activities, can be of help to alleviate the observed ill-effects on health?
- What ill-effects on health can be observed in the spouses and children of the employees losing their jobs?
- What are the practical implications of the ill-effects on health of losing job? How should a plant shut-down actually be managed to minimize the damage to the effected individuals, their families and the community as a whole?
- What are the actual total costs of a plant shut-down of this size - affecting directly 3 % of the total number of employees in the community - taking in account the costs for both individuals and the community affected? Could these costs be reduced by a different management policy of economically inevitable needs of restructuring?

SOME SUGGESTIONS FOR FUTURE RESEARCH
ON ECONOMIC INSTABILITY AND HEALTH

Aubrey Kagan

Laboratory for Clinical Stress Research
Stockholm, Sweden

The problem and our present position

The questions most of us wish to answer are:
- What aspect or correlate of economic change predisposes what kind of person through what kind of mechanism to what kind of disease?
- What kind of interventions will protect against such ill effects?

An appreciation of the papers so far presented does not take us much further than the position based on a review of the literature 2 years ago. My conclusions now as then, are that there is some support for the notion that something connected with economic change has an effect on ill health and lack of well-being and that this may act through psychosocial as well as physical stressors. Before we can recommend to those concerned actions to prevent ill effects and retain the good effects of economic change we need more understanding. But the demand for action is strongly felt and is increasing.

The purpose of this paper is to suggest a strategy of research likely to be both efficacious and efficient in improving our understanding at the time as it helps people concerned to find practical solutions to their own 'burning' problems of the present and near future.

Reasons for past inadequacy

In the early 1960's as a cardio-vascular epidemiologist I had good reason to ask 'Why is the epidemiological method so ineffective?'. This was twenty years after World War II. Billions of dollars had been spent on research, a large and intelligent body of epidemiologists and others had applied themselves full time to the task. The practical results were zero. By comparing successful and unsuccessful epidemiological investigations I came to the conclusion that it was not a problem specific to cardio-vascular disease. The difference between success and failure was essentially that the former hypotheses of cause and effect were tested and the latter were not.

This was not confined to epidemiology. Sociologists were singularly ineffective in contributing to the health and well-being of mankind and singularly reluctant to test hypotheses of cause and effect. Looking at the contributions of other disciplines it seemed at that time, and still does, that pharmacology had made steady contributions of a high magnitude not only to health and well-being but also to biological understanding. In the latter cellular and subcellular biology had made big contributions. Both these disciplines are characterized by hypotheses testing, and pharmacology by its rigid adherence to evaluation of applications for efficiency, safety and cost.

Of course in these cases of social/health problems there were real difficulties in testing hypotheses and evaluating health or social actions. But there were reasonable hypotheses to test. My conclusion was that we must overcome the difficulties. We must search for situations, methods and ideas that will enable hypotheses to be tested. We must avoid the temptation of wandering away from the target in directions that will produce papers for publication but which will never conclude anything other than more work needs to be done before we can draw any conclusions that will be of any practical use.

Difficulties in testing hypotheses and evaluating interventions in groups of people

The technical difficulties in testing hypotheses and evaluating health actions are known and can be overcome sometimes. The ethical constraints can be complied with usually. We must bring into conjunction the demand, the situation; the appropriate study design and methods.

As a general rule the situations we are concerned with are characterized by
1) the need to show cause and effect
2) the need to evaluate interventions
3) a probability of multiple causation
4) a certainty of many powerful interacting variables
5) a number of suspected factors that can be measured and will be; a number of such factors that can be measured but won't for reasons of cost or convenience; a number of such factors which can be measured; a number of important but unsuspected factors that won't be measured
6) the effects to be estimated will neither be very rare nor very frequent

7) some causes may take a long time to have an effect
8) the change in frequency of effects due to "treatment" will seldom be greater than 50%.

Tactics to meet the difficulties

These characteristics will restrict and to some extent decide what tactics we can or cannot use. Thus:
- Since we are aiming to test hypotheses of cause and effect we must put forward suitable hypotheses, (1) above;
- Since we are proposing to evaluate interventions we must carry out actions that are likely to prevent ill effects of economic change, (2) above;
- In order to achieve 1) and 2) and because of 3), 4) and 5) we shall need randomised controlled trials;
- Because of 6), 7) and 8) a large number of subjects will need to be studied over a period of at least 2 - 3 years;
- Because of 3), 4) and 5) many factors should be assessed in each subject. We shall show that these should include economic, psychological, sociological and pathological factors;
- All measurements made should be assessed for imprecision (random error) and for bias (correctable error) so that the limits of the observations are established and false conclusions may be avoided.

We may note that studies which demonstrate associations can at most give us ideas for further test before they will answer the questions posed at the head of this paper. They will not show that the ideas are correct or incorrect. It should also be noted that we are calling for tests of interventions designed to help people who might otherwise be harmed by economic change. No such studies have been reported.

We shall need to put forward hypotheses of cause and effect in the system economic change, health and well-being. This we shall now consider.

General Concept of
Social Changes, Stress and Disease

Figure 1 shows the Stress Lab's/WHO Centre's concept schematically. It is the system in which individuals or groups of people (box 4) seek to satisfy their needs and wishes.

For example let us suppose that a person has all his real needs and all that he wishes and is therefore in a state of equilibrium. Let this state be suddenly threatened by severe change in natural resources (box 1), e.g. an earthquake, or change in social arrangements (box 2), e.g. he is told that he will lose his job at the end of the week. If this threatens him physically or if he thinks if threatens him both ways, physically and psychosocially, (as could be in both our examples), physical and/or psychosocial stressor (box 3) will come into action. The stress response (box 5) will depend on his current physical and psychological abilities and his appreciation of their capability to handle the situation (his current psychobiological programme - box 4).

Thus if he has experience of earthquakes and knows them to be of little consequence <u>there will be little or no stress</u> response. If he thinks being out of work will be a disgrace or will bring hardship to himself or to his family, his stress response will be great.

There are many types of stress response. Most are specific to the particular kind of stressor. Two types of response are caused by so many different types of stressor - psychosocial or physicosocial - that we call them "General Stress" responses. Both these responses consist of a psychological, social, and physical component. Both have fairly well defined and separate brain-body pathways. Both are very ancient responses existing, as far as we can tell, in many animals as well as man. Both have useful functions and both probably carry risk if they occur under the wrong circumstances.

We call these general stress responses "Cannon" and "Selye" stress. The first consists of the psycho-social-physical triad of Anxiety, Fear, Anger, Arousal; Physical Activity; and Activity of the Adrenal Medullary-Sympathetic system. "Selye" stress consists of the triad of Depression; Withdrawal; and Activity of the Adreno-Cortical system.

We speculate that the useful functions of "Cannon" Stress are to prepare the animal for coping with a situation by some form of short term physical activity. The useful function of "Selye" Stress is probably to enable the organism to withdraw from an apparently hopeless situation, perhaps till the situation changes, or perhaps, to rethink and learn a new way of dealing with it.

Our ideas on the conditions under which these responses may be harmful are also speculative and depend upon two kinds of consideration. The first is that both responses cause widespread psychological behavioural and physiological changes that under some circumstances are regarded as risk factors (or precursors) (box 6) for a wide variety of diseases (box 7), e.g. precursors such as anxiety, depression; risk taking behaviour: dangerous driving, overuse of alcohol, cigarettes or food; raised bloodpressure, diminished efficiency of the heart; diminished myocardial uptake of Oxygen, decreased glucose tolerance, etc.

The second reason for concern is that the general stress responses seem to be designed for problems that are common for animals and were common for humans until 100 years ago but are no longer appropriate to the latter. Both responses are excellent for problems that can be solved in a few minutes by extra physical effort or in a few hours by completely giving in to the situation. Few of our problems today can be solved in a matter of minutes or by physical effort or by giving up. Yet the stressors that elicit responses for these purposes and their accompanying "percursors" of disease, occur and recur for some people many times a day.

With this in mind we may state the General Theory of Social Change, Stress and Disease as: Psychological, Social, Physical or mixed stressors arise when human beings seek, or perceive the need, to satisfy needs and wishes. If the real needs are nor satisfied or needs and wishes are perceived as unsatisfied, stress responses occur. General Stress responses can, under present social conditions, often be inappropriate and disease can result from secondary changes caused by the general stress responses. The Stressor, Stress Response, precursors, disease, can be exacerbated, changed, or reduced by interacting variables (box 8) of a psychological, social, or physiological nature acting on Society (box 2), the individual (box 4), the psycho-physicosocial stressors (box 3), stress responses (box 5), precursors (box 6) or disease (box 7).

Key Hypotheses in the General Concept

By the key hypotheses I mean those which if tested and not disproved are likely to give us a much greater understanding of our problem and therefore a much greater facility for tackling it. Similarly a key hypothesis if shown to be false, should enable us to modify our approach and research considerably.

In the case of social change, stress and disease (Fig. 1) these are about social stressors (box 3) and stress responses (box 5).

Thus, although a very large number of social situations (box 2) - any - may produce stressors, we hypothesize that the psychosocial stressors themselves (box 3) are few in type and namely threaten
- personal, family or community survival
- sense of love or belonging
- sense of status or self-esteem
- sense of self-expression or creativity
- sense of being in control of one's situation.

These can be operationally defined and assessed fairly easily. Secondly we hypothesize that ill effects are most likely to arise when the stress response is inappropriate to the situation, i.e. the problem cannot be solved in a short time and a stress response continues; or the problem elicits "Cannon" Stress but is not soluble by a short, sharp, exertion; or it elicits "Selye" Stress and cannot be solved by 'giving up' completely for a few hours. It will also cause ill effects even if the response is appropriate to the situation, if the individual has already an impaired structure or function in certain tissues or organs, e.g. impaired coronary circulation.

Key Hypotheses in the System of Economic Change, Stress and Disease

I think what we know about economic instability or change and health fits in with the general theory and these two hypotheses. The deliberations here and elsewhere fit in with our general theory that there is something about economic change, which is always likely to be a threat to somebody, this has been shown to be associated with disease at a later date. Further general stress responses, precursors of disease and minor disease itself, have been shown to be more common in subjects threatened with loss of work than in similar subjects not so threatened and greater in those of the former group who are not protected by interacting variables such as kin and community support, early solution of the problem etc.

The two key hypotheses from the general theory are relevant to

Economic Change and Health. They can be framed here as:
- <u>Hypothesis of Psychosocial Stressor</u> - "The pathogenic stressors in the 'Economic Change - Health' system are for instance a threat to - sense of survival, love or belonging, self-esteem, status, self-expression or self-control of the situation".
- <u>Hypothesis of Mechanism</u> - "The pathogenic mechanisms are inappropriate 'Selye' or 'Cannon' Stress responses".

If we are able to show that the first hypothesis or psychosocial stressors are true, it would be possible simply by assessing the change in an individual through 7 types of psychosocial stressors, to know whether he/she is exposed to a potentially dangerous or healthy situation. We have good practical methods for doing this.

Similarly, if the second hypothesis of mechanism is correct, we should have a "compass" by which we would know if interventions were improving the situation or making it worse for the individual. We would be able to do so in a matter of hours before anything serious happened rather than waiting for months or years for precursors of disease to occur. It would be necessary to assess 'Cannon' or 'Selye' Stress. We have ways of doing so in psychological, social and physiological terms.

Suggestion for the Strategy and Tactics of Future Research on Economic Change and Health

The probability that economic change carries a risk for health and well-being through psychosocial stressors, remains likely but unproven. There is some evidence that economic change fits with the general theory of social change, stress, and disease through 'Selye' or 'Cannon' Stress mechanisms. It is not possible yet to give evaluated advice to those who want answers to the questions appearing at the beginning of this paper.

Further research should be directed to show whether harm can arise from economic change and how it can be minimised.

This can best be done by evaluating interventions designed to keep away ill health and lack of well-being from those who are about to be subjected to economic change of various kinds. This can also be done simultaneously, for little more than the same cost, by testing key hypotheses.

At the same time data on the quantitative relationships of the elements (factors) thought to be of importance in the social change-stress-health system will be collected and stored.

"Bread, Butter and Jam"

This strategy of research is known as "bread", "butter" and "jam".

The purpose of the evaluation, which is the bread part of the sandwich, is to show to people concerned the effects of health/social action: what kind of benefits will be produced, how much and for whom; what kind of harm will be produced, how much and for whom; and what will the cost be. It will be an evaluation which will allow action to be improved by learning from mistakes. It should be carried out with the cooperation and participation of all, or representatives of all kinds of people concerned, e.g. workers, worker's families, management, medical department, trade union representatives, community.

It will require a study design for prospective randomised, controlled intervention.

The purpose of testing key hypotheses, which is the butter part of the sandwich, is to get a better understanding of the way the social change, stress, disease system works. Through this better understanding intervention will be better understood and success or failure of intervention or risk from social change may be detectable and therefore correctable at a very early stage - a matter of hours rather than months or years.

The purpose of data collection on quantitative relations between factors thought to be of importance is so that eventually, when enough data from different studies are collected, we may approach the highly speculative task of making a simulation model. This is to overcome the problems of research findings being outmoded, by the march of social change, before they have been established.

This would be very expensive to approach on its own. It is very unlikely to succeed. By combining it with the other two approaches we get necessary data for nothing. In addition we will have retrospective data with which to test our model. If our key hypotheses testing has been sucessful we shall also have a deeper understanding of what makes the

the whole thing tick and this can go into our model. It can be built
out of retrospective data but will need testing on prospective data.
If it works it will be the "jam".

The need to learn from mistakes in trying to improve the lot of many
of those who are about to be exposed to severe economic change, arises
every day. Surely it would be possible through WHO to find a dozen
places in which this situation will occur _and_ in which people are
willing _and_ able to evaluate intervention for safety, efficacy and
cost in studies lasting between 1 to 3 years.

It would improve our understanding if these interventions, which might
all be different, were done in a coordinated way and in each case the
same key hypotheses were tested and the quantitative data on relations
were collected and later pooled to attempt "Simulation" of the society,
stress, health system.

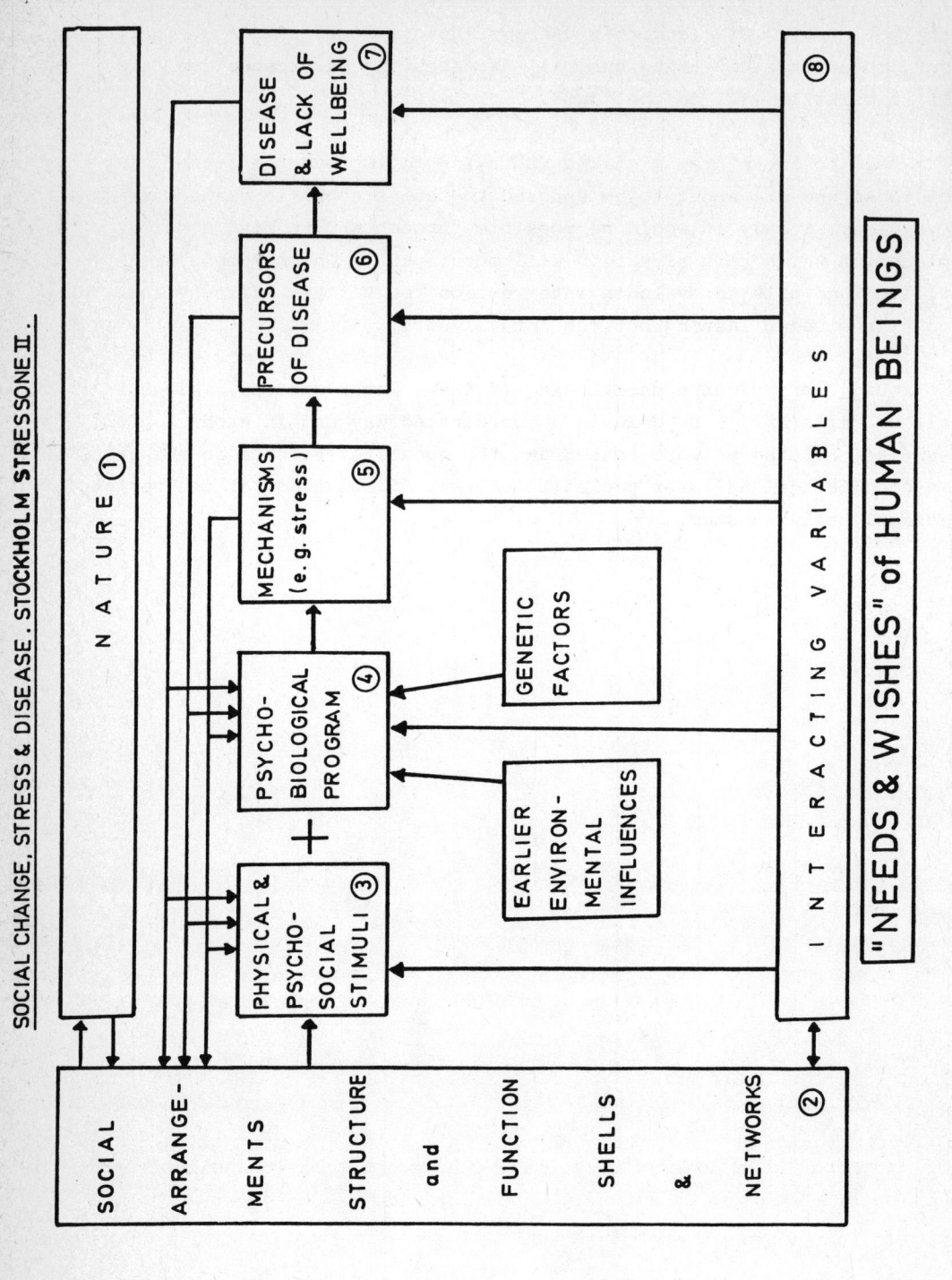

SOCIAL CHANGE, STRESS & DISEASE. STOCKHOLM STRESSONE II.

NATURE ①

| ② SOCIAL ARRANGEMENTS STRUCTURE and FUNCTION SHELLS & NETWORKS |

③ PHYSICAL & PSYCHO-SOCIAL STIMULI

④ PSYCHO-BIOLOGICAL PROGRAM

GENETIC FACTORS

EARLIER ENVIRONMENTAL INFLUENCES

⑤ MECHANISMS (e.g. stress)

⑥ PRECURSORS OF DISEASE

⑦ DISEASE & LACK OF WELLBEING

⑧ INTERACTING VARIABLES

"NEEDS & WISHES" of HUMAN BEINGS

KAGAN '76

RECESSION & HEALTH - A RESEARCH STRATEGY

Stephen J. Watkins

Department of Epidemiology and Social Research
University Hospital of South Manchester
Manchester, Great Britain

The work of Harvey Brenner (1) has shown that there is a statistical association between levels of unemployment in the community and indicators of ill health in the same community. The assumption is usually made that this association is causal in that either unemployment itself or the fear of unemployment or both are damaging to health. Although I personally believe that this is at least part of the explanation of the association, it must be said that this is far from proved and there are other explanations of the finding.

It is a basic principle of epidemiology that if A causes B and A causes C then an association will be observed between B and C. Since unemployment is an indicator of recession, it would therefore be expected to correlate with any phenomenon caused by recession, whether or not it was itself an intermediary in the causation. The fact that it correlates better than other indices of recession might merely mean that it is a better indicator of recession than those other indicators.

The question therefore must be asked "How can recession cause ill health?" The following mechanisms need to be considered.

1. <u>Unemployment:</u> The obvious hypothesis that unemployment or the stress caused by the fear of unemployment directly damages health and therefore accounts for the association may well be correct. I think it probably is partially true, although I think other factors may contribute. We must beware of the assumption that if we demonstrate in case/control of longitudinal studies that unemployment damages health therefore it accounts for the whole of the association. The association may be a complex of different effects, including unemployment and the fear of it but also including some of the other mechanisms which I will now postulate.

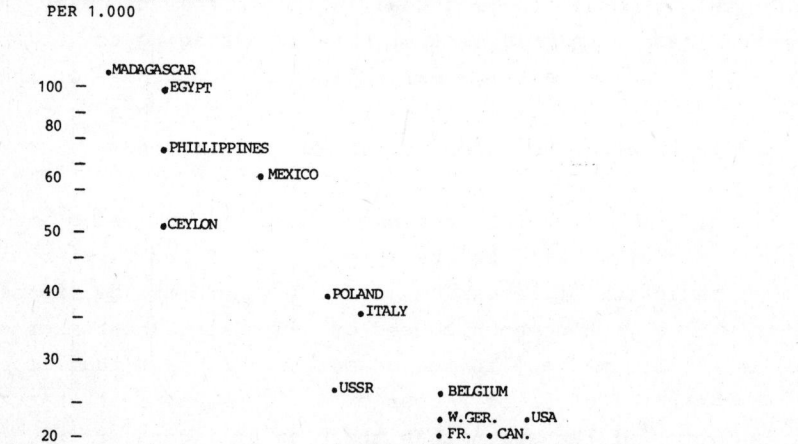

2. __Economic Failure:__ We know that economic success is in some way associated with improved health. This is evident from time trends in which countries have become healthier as they have become richer. Brenner's work itself demonstrates this general trend and it was necessary to detrend the data in order to look at the effects of recession.

The association is also evident from international comparisons.

INFANT DEATH RATES 1966 AND GROSS NATIONAL PRODUCTS/HEAD IN 18 COUNTRIES

INFANT DEATH RATE PER 1.000

```
100 -  • MADAGASCAR
        • EGYPT
 80 -
        • PHILLIPPINES
 60 -          • MEXICO
 50 -  • CEYLON
 40 -         • POLAND
                • ITALY
 30 -
           • USSR    • BELGIUM
                   • W.GER.  • USA
 20 -              • FR.  • CAN.
          • JAPAN  • UK.
                     • AUSTRALIA
 15 -           • NETHERLANDS
                  • SWEDEN
```

    100   200   500   1000   2000   GROSS NATIONAL PRODUCT $ US PER HEAD

I could obviously present other similar data for other years or other health indices but I will not insult you by presenting material with which you will all be very familiar. Suffice it to say that these international relationships of health with economic success are so well established that a recent Norwegian study of ischaemic heart disease in relation to economic conditions in childhood by county has used infant mortality rate as its __economic__ indicator (2).

The same relationship of economic success to health is evident from social class comparison within countries. This is extremely thoroughly documented in relation to the United Kingdom, together with some data from other countries in the British Government publication "Inequalities in Health", commonly known as the Black Report (3).

The following figures are sex/social class specific death rates per 1.000 for the age range 15 to 64 in England and Wales in 1971:

Social class	male	female
1	3.89	2.15
2	5.54	2.85
3N	5.80	2.76
3M	6.08	3.41
4	7.96	4.27
5	9.88	5.31

This social class gradient is observed for almost every cause of death and can also be seen in indices of morbidity, although the figures are then sometimes confused by the tendency for higher social classes to make more use of the Health Service relative to their level of morbidity, thereby artificially elevating morbidity indices which are based on health service use.

So from time trends, international comparisons and social class comparisons we can draw the clear conclusion that economic advance has been associated with improved health. It would therefore be expected that the economic failure of recession would produce ill health by a reversal of that mechanism.

It isn't clear what the mechanism is. Few of us will believe that dishwashers make people healthy. Reasonable hypotheses might include higher social spending, better nutrition, better housing, greater opportunities for leisure and life satisfaction, better working conditions, etc. Some hunches can be generated by looking at countries which lie above or below the regression line in international comparisons, and there emerges a vague suggestion that higher social spending and a more egalitarian income distribution improve health indices at a given level of national income.

But all that we can really say is that the association of health with economic success is there and is obviously relevant when we are considering the health effects of economic failure.

3. **Stress:** Brenner invokes stress as an intermediary in the causation of ill health by unemployment and the fear of it. It may also be an intermediary in some of the other mechanisms which I am suggesting. However quite apart from unemployment or the fear of it or the stress of life changes or changed personal lives, the general level of stress in society is bound to increase in recession. It becomes more difficult to maintain public services, to collect donations for charity, to conclude wage deals, or to make profits. So the managers of all kinds of organisations, whether public services, companies, trade unions or voluntary organisations face a more difficult or less satisfying job. Workers are less sure that they will be able to maintain their standard of living. Housewives in the West face higher prices, perhaps out of proportion to increases in the household budget, whilst housewives in the socialist countries face instead longer queues for scarcer products. Those who live on state benefits become acutely aware of political debate about whether their meagre income is or is not an unacceptable drain on the economy. One may not be unemployed or have any fear of unemployment and yet recession will still cause stress.

4. **Working Conditions:** Shearman and Jenkins (4) quote an old Haitian proverb "If work were good for you the rich would have found a way of keeping it all to themselves".
It is not surprising therefore that Brenner's work has drawn criticism from those whose ideology finds it hard to accept that removal from the alienating environment of work can be bad for you.
Thus Eyer (5) has argued that if different time lags are used it can be claimed that the association of ill health with recession is actually an association with the delayed effects of the preceding boom.
I am a member of the National Executive of a trade union, the Association of Scientific, Technical and Managerial Staffs, which attaches great importance to health and safety at work and to shorter working hours. I certainly believe that work can be damaging to health.
But I am also aware, since my union is the sixth largest union in the British Trades Union Congress with members in a wide range of British industries, of the problems being faced in the midst of recession by those who sell their labour.

Eyer has missed the point that it is in recession that the labour market becomes more adverse to those who sell their labour. It is in recession that the capacity of workers to resist exploitation is diminished. Health and safety at work becomes deemphasised in the mere struggle for survival (6). Working conditions become less important than the protection of jobs. Workers who are faced with the prospect of redundancy and with the knowledge that it will be very hard to win a pay increase equal to the rate of inflation are less likely to worry about industrial democracy or job enrichment or job satisfaction. Indeed standards of safety, relaxed working methods, hard won working conditions are likely to come under attack from employers keen to reduce the unit cost of labour. Overwork will often result from reduced manning levels.

This buyer's market in labour, with the deteriorating working conditions that accompany it is more likely to damage health than the conditions of boom, where more workers may be exposed to the hazards of work, but in conditions where they are much more able to defend themselves against them.

5. <u>Deteriorating Social Services:</u> We meet in West Germany the week after a political crisis that centered on disagreements in the coalition Govt. about the extent and nature of cuts in public expenditure. In Britain we have a crisis in which local councils elected on a commitment to increase spending are being brutally prevented from doing so by a Government which has elevated the reduction of public spending to an article of faith pursued with semi religious zeal. Throughout the Western world we see the political idea that the social services upon which the basic infrastructure of a civilised society rests must be reduced. This outdated idea, based on an outdated concept of what is "productive" is now dominant in the thinking of most Western governments except that of France.

These cuts in spending damage health in a number of ways. Direct reductions in health services and personal social services are the most obvious. In Britain we have seen reduced spending on fire prevention and on accident prevention and quite serious reductions in the levels of road maintenance. Last winter I personnally had occasion to provide medical assistance at the scene of a road traffic accident caused by reductions in the road gritting programme.

6. <u>Changed Personal Lives:</u> Our personal lives, our marital relationships, our relationships with our children, our friendships, our social networks are important to our health. We know that laboratory animals develop less atheroma when they are cuddled than when they are not. We know the importance of social networks in psychological illness for example the follow up of the Granville train disaster demonstrated that those with strong social networks were less likely to develop psychiatric reactions after the disaster (7). Social networks have also been shown to reduce the incidence of complications of childbirth (8). The death rate is lower in those who are married than in those who are single. The following are British figures for 1970-71:

SMR	male	female
all	100	100
married	94	92
single	128	118
widowed	158	122
divorced	138	103

The nine year follow-up of an American community has shown reduced mortality in those with most social support (10).

Changes in these relationships occur in recession. People delay marriage, they delay childbearing. The stress of recession causes marital disharmony.

The recent work by Brown (9) has demonstrated the importance of an intimate marital relationship in preventing depression in women and there are now suggestions that this may be true for men as well and so we can appreciate the significance of reports of increased demands in the United Kingdom on marriage counselling services, quite apart from the direct human tragedy and health effects of increase in those attending battered wives refuges.

These indentifiable effects may well be only the tip of an iceberg of more subtle changes.

Each of these features of recession will show a correlation in a community over time with unemployment insofar as unemployment is an indicator of recession. Hence a research strategy aimed at uncovering the reason for an association between levels of unemployment and indicators of ill health must investigate all of these.

The association which Brenner has described and put an equation to may be a complex of different effects - the direct health effects of unemployment in the unemployed, the fear of unemployment and the effect of deteriorating working conditions in those still in employment, frustration in the achievement oriented managerial and professional groups, deteriorating social services for those who need them, and deteriorating personal relationships in us all.

INVESTIGATING THE FACTORS OTHER THAN UNEMPLOYMENT

1. <u>Economic Failure:</u> The main difficulty we face in looking at this factor is that we do not know what it is about economic success that is associated with health, and so we really don't know what should be the independent variable in our case/control or longitudinal studies.

    There is a suggestion from international data that more egalitarian income distributions may be associated with better health for a given level of GDP. We could look at the effects of recession on income distribution. If we could calculate income specific mortality rates we could standardise our health indices for the effect of the changed income levels.

    It may be that it is not simply income that is important but life style. It may be that at any level of income life-style is healthiest in those who have always been at that income level, less healthy in those who have planned for an increase and have had their expectations frustrated, and least healthy in those who have suffered a severe income drop. Certainly if I were forced to live on £30/week I would do so less efficiently than those who now live at that income level. The poor have always known better than the rich how to handle their money. We must look at the effect that recession has on life styles and the effects that the changed life styles have on health. It is not however just the life styles of the unemployed that we need to investigate but also the life styles of those whose circumstances have changed more subtly.

    Recession may have meant different things in different countries. We might like to compare the health effects of recession in countries which have different experiences, for example those which have cut public spending sharply and those which have cut it more gently, those whose nutritional habits have changed and those who have not, etc.

2. <u>Stress:</u> I think we should try and document the levels of stress in different groups in society. It would be interesting to compare cholesterol levels and blood pressure now with those before the recession, where we have baseline measurements to look back to.

3. <u>Working Conditions:</u> The problem we will face in investigating the working conditions hypothesis is that those industries in which the market in labour will have become most adverse to those who sell their labour will be the same industries as those in which fear of unemployment is the greatest. It will be difficult to disentangle the two effects. It may be possible however to identify cohorts of workers who feel relatively little fear of unemployment but who still face pressures on working conditions. An example might be those who work in profitable sectors of a loss making company, or those who work in companies which have announced rationalisation plans and who know that their plant is not amongst those scheluded for closure.

There may be groups of workers such as computer programmers or skilled secretaries whose skills are still in short supply even in recession and for whom the labour market therefore is less adverse than for other workers and yet who still fear redundancy because of the upheaval it would cause. On the other hand such workers may fear redundancy less because they know they can get another job, whilst the generally changed attitudes to employer/employee relations may counteract the objective situation of their particular section of the labour market, so you can really argue this either way.

. <u>Deteriorating Social Services:</u> We should look at the health of those who are dependent on state benefits. We should also document the deteriorations that have taken place in public services and try and assess their health implications.

. <u>Changed Personal Lives:</u> We should document the changes in personal lives which take place in recession.

INVESTIGATING EMPLOYMENT

The first question we must ask when we turn our attention to unemployment per se must be whether unemployment itself is damaging to health or whether the correlations which have been demonstrated are entirely indirect. The next question must be "What is it about unemployment that damages health?"

1. <u>Does Unemployment Damage Health?:</u> Evidence that unemployment is not only the indicator of recession, but also one of the intermediaries in the causal chain that produced the association must derive from studies of the health of unemployed individuals.

    The work most commonly quoted in this respect is that of Kasl & Cobb (11). However it must be borne in mind that in their study the majority of those studied found work again very quickly. Their study therefore looks at the health effects of life change rather than of unemployment. Indeed that is exactly what its purpose was and it is only in a colder economic climate that we have tried to use its findings to support a case which the study was never designed to test and for which it is therefore, not surprisingly, inappropriate in design.

    Their study did look at the health of the long term unemployed and found it to be poor. However the long term unemployed in their study were those who had failed to obtain new employment in a buoyant labour market, and on looking back at the health of those same people before the closure of the plant they found that their health was poor then. In other words it was their ill health which prevented them finding work again rather than their unemployment which damaged their health. Any study which supports to demonstrate adverse health effects of chronic unemployment must cope with this problem.

    One way to do this is to measure health before unemployment as well as during it and compare those who had similar health status at the beginning of the experience but differ in whether or for how long they suffered unemployment. This approach has been followed in the study of unemployed school leavers carried out by the Applied Psychology Unit at Sheffield (12).

    This study measured a mental health score of a group of school leavers, some of whom subsequently did not find jobs. Those who did not find jobs had worse scores than those who did when the score was taken again, even though their sources had been the same on the first occasion before the experience of unemployment.

Another way would be to repeat Kasl & Cobb's study in a group of workers who are unlikely to find reemployment because of the depressed state of the local labour market.

The criteria for an ideal study would be as follows:
(1) There would be the complete closure of a factory, thereby removing the question of selection for redundancy.
(2) There would be a control factory in which there were no redundancies at all, thereby removing the question of selection out of the unhealthy in the control factory.
(3) The two factories would otherwise be comparable.
(4) We should have sufficient warning of these events to take measurements of health in both factories before the closure.
(5) We should have sufficient cooperation from both the study workforce and the control group to enable measurements of health to take place regularly for at least 3 years.
(6) In order to eliminate the effect of selecting out the healthy back into jobs the comparison would need to be between the entire study sample and the entire control sample. If the study were not to lack precision as a result of this it would be necessary that it should be carried out in an area where the labour market was very depressed so that very few of those made unemployed would find alternative work. Greater precision should probably be obtained by confining the study to older workers who are least likely to find alternative employment.
(7) Ideally we should have measures of health in both workforces before the closure was announced. This is impracticable unless they can be obtained from previous occupational health service records.
(8) Ideally the fear of unemployment should have been the same in both workforces before the closure announcement, and the factory which is the control should then be free of any such fear. This is probably impracticable. The only situation I can think of where it might be met would be one of two comparable plants where a reduced market necessitates the closure of one but where the other will then have a secure future, and nobody knows until the closure announcement which one is to close.
(9) The two factories should be in the same town to equalise other effects.

In any society which had any pretence to humanity it would be impossible for these criteria to be met because they require that the fears and hopes of human beings should be treated in a brutal and uncaring way. It would of course be unethical to create these conditions - indeed it is necessary for anybody with a commitment to health to argue against their creation. Rather than carry out this study I would prefer that we could make it impossible. That is of course true of any study of human suffering.

Since we do live in an uncaring society in which the hopes and fears of human beings are treated brutally, it is possible that circumstances might arise which will approximate to the above. I don't think we should underestimate the difficulties - the criteria I have suggested are very difficult to meet or even approximate to. Unless they are at least approximately met a study of this kind would add little to the mass of suggestive data which we already have. I set out about twelve months ago to plan such a study in Liverpool and nothing coming remotely close to the ideal has arisen. I think we must look throughout the whole of Europe for that circumstance which comes closest to the criteria and mount the study there.

Another possible situation which would offer scope for study would be one in which selection for redundancy amongst the workforce or a subgroup of it had been random. This is not on the whole the way that selection takes place but there may be occasions in which this method would be used and I think we could perhaps make known to trade unions that we would like to be informed of any situation in which random selection for redundancy has taken place. If this did happen then it would remove all the difficulties about comparability of controls. If it happened in a very depressed area where prospects of reemployment were slight then we would have a study which came very close indeed to our criteria.

The details of measurement of health and other aspects of methodology of such a study are very similar to those discussed in other papers. Indeed, since Gill Westcott(13) and I anticipated the spirit of cooperation which this conference is designed to encourage by planning our studies together, I suspect that I will have very little to add in the way of methodology to the points she will make in her paper. I would also at this stage like to acknowledge her contribution to the strategy I have described in my paper.

Although I have presented the idea of designing a study to dispel the lingering doubts that exist on the question "Does unemployment cause ill health?" I would not wish to underestimate the strength of the evidence that we already have. Indeed when I say that any further study must be very close to perfect I am implying that there is very little to be gained from further imperfect studies and the reason that I say that is that we already have quite enough data to have established a working hypothesis.

The studies presented at this conference, the studies cited by the participants to this conference, the studies cited especially in the literature review which preceded the paper by Len Fagin (14) and the studies cited in the bibliography by Newell (15) all add up to a situation in which I think it would be perverse to believe other than that unemployment damages health, even though I think there is scope to test the hypothesis further. We must beware of falling into the trap of believing that there is such a thing as a scientific fact, and we must beware of the trap of allowing policy makers to believe that the process of eliminating remaining doubts is an excuse for ignoring that which can be reasonably inferred from existing knowledge.

In science and politics alike it is unreasonable to await certainty. Therefore I think it is reasonable to turn to the second of the two questions I asked when opening this section.

2. How Does Unemployment Damage Health?:

Unemployment is a number of different things.

1. Stress: The fear of unemployment is itself stressful and those who now are unemployed may have suffered that stress for a considerable length of time and may now be suffering the after-effects. In addition stress will be suffered as a result of the unemployment itself and the fear of the future, the stress of seeking jobs, the worries about finance etc. The sources of stress are well documented in the review by Spruit (17) presented at this Conference.

2. Life changes: We know that life changes cause ill health from the data we already have on job changes, bereavement and retirement. Unemployment will likewise be a life change and will cause ill health until the individual becomes adjusted to his new state. However unlike bereavement or a new job the individual is not supposed to adjust to his joblessness.

3. Social networks: I have already mentioned the importance of social networks to health. Work is an important source of social interaction.

4. Poverty: To be without work is also to be without the money that work brings.

5. Lack of status: A person's job is a source of social identity.

6. Lack of purpose to life: I am not aware of any scientific evidence of the importance to health of having a purpose to life, but I think there is a great deal of anecdotal and experiential evidence of that.

If we are to decide the contribution which each of these factors makes we to need to look at the health experiences of groups of people whose experience of unemployment is different and of groups who share some but not all of the experiences of the unemployed.
One approach would be to take a large group of unemployed people and look at the different health experiences of different subgroups. This is the approach which Gill Westcott is taking in her Scunthorpe study. She will be able to look at the effect of finding other meaningful life activity, or of having a spouse who is still employed, or of having past experience of unemployment, or of being young or old, or of having a particularly strong or weak work ethic, or of having strong social networks away from work.

The other approach is to design a number of studies which isolate particular aspects by the way they draw their controls.
For example to look at the effect of money we could look at the health of workers laid off on guaranteed incomes who suffer many of the other aspects of unemployment but not to the same extent the financial aspect, and we could compare the health of the unemployed with the health of low paid workers.

We could also look at the differences in the health of unemployed people in countries which have differing levels of unemployment benefit.

The Sheffield study which I have already cited (12) has shown us that the effects of unemployment on the mental health of school-leavers were worse in those with a higher score on a measure of commitment to the work ethic and this finding needs to be followed up. Fröhlich (18) has shown the same in his paper to this Conference.

It would be nice to be able to isolate the social effects from the financial effects and I would like to suggest a study which might do that. If we could define a group of families who had suffered a loss of family income as a result of the unemployment of the male spouse and an equal number of families who had suffered the same loss of family income due to the unemployment of the female spouse, and if the two groups of families were otherwise well matched then we could compare the health of the employed and unemployed spouses. The two groups would automatically be matched for loss of income. They would automatically be matched for any other factor which affects the two spouses equally. We would need to include an equal number of "male unemployment" and "female unemployment" families in order to ensure that the two groups were matched for sex. Insofar as the stress of unemployment falls equally upon each partner the proposed two groups would be matched for stress, although this would not be so to the extent that the unemployed person feels more stress than their spouse, hence the importance of matching the two groups of families as closely as possible. The only aggregate difference between the two groups therefore would be that one group suffered the financial and social effects of unemployment, whereas the other group suffered equal financial effects but only suffered the social effects indirectly through empathy with the spouse. The main difficulties with this proposed study would be that the study group would be untypical of unemployed people, and that we do not really understand the extent to which empathy between spouses would subject the control group to experiences which we are supposing to be isolated to the study group.

Another interesting group to study are a group of managers in a large company which has told them that it has no long term job for them but that it will not make them redundant until they have, with its help, found other work. It would be interesting to see to what extent this more humane and caring approach mitigates the stress of having the label "no longer wanted here" attached and being forced to change jobs. Since there will allways be declining industries it is important for us to know best to redeploy staff. It will be interesting to compare the effects of this gentler method with the sharp shock approach which Kasl & Cobb studied.

THE PURPOSE OF A RESEARCH STRATEGY

Some will believe that the purpose of a research strategy need merely be the advancement of scientific knowledge. I think however that we should have some end in mind for the findings we seek to make.

Some will believe that the purpose of further study is to add to the evidence that unemployment is bad for you in order to bring pressure to bear on politicians. I am sure that all of us in this room would wish to see the entire conference rendered meaningless by the sudden abolition of unemployment.

The abolition of unemployment is feasible. There is always useful work to do and the "socially useful work" approach to unemployment would be to employ people on doing it. Programmes of public works, expansion of caring activities and education, and the allocation of money to public services to spend on goods which can be made in the industrial sector, such as public transport equipment, kidney machines, or aids for the disabled (19) (20) could be expanded to that level at which they absorbed the unemployed. Alternatively, or in combination with the other approach, we could follow the "work sharing" approach to unemployment in sharing out the available work and giving everybody more leisure instead of forcing an unhealthy excess of leisure on some, but an unhealthy excess of work on others.

Whenever these commonsense approaches to unemployment are advocated the reply is to ask how will they be funded.

It must be understood that no resources are saved by having a person unemployed instead of working.

It must also be understood that no resources are saved by having 4 people work for 40 hours a week and a fifth not work at all rather than have all five work for 32 hours.

Certain calculations in the United Kingdom have suggested that the cost of keeping somebody unemployed is equal to the national average wage (16) in which case the eradiction of unemployment should cost nothing. But even if there is a cost it is only the cost of providing to those people who would otherwise have been unemployed their full share of the nation's standard of living. If that cost has to be met out of taxation, i.e. out of the standard of living of the rest of the community, then it is no more than simple justice. To argue that this can't be afforded is to argue that a random section of the population should be selected to suffer the full burden of economic crisis so that the standard of living of everybody else may be marginally higher than it would otherwise be, and that in order to do this we will forego the goods and services which the unemployed could have produced and the leisure which work sharing could have given us. This argument is either immoral or insane or both.

Some may argue that there is here a further purpose for a research strategy, in that it might help to demonstrate that a policy of the kind I have set out would improve health. This might, after all, not be the case if the only reason for the association of unemployment with indices of ill health was the simple fall in GDP per capita, and therefore to demonstrate that more than just that is involved might strengthen our case.

That is certainly true, but I think it must be said that we do not need more research to tell us that unemployment is bad for people and we do not need more research to tell us that a policy which eradicated it would be a good thing.

Future generations will see unemployment as a wasteful and unnecessary cruelty imposed upon people by unimaginative Governments who believe that the solving of economic equations is more important than understanding the human realities which their indices imperfectly express.

Nonetheless if the Governments of the world so fail in their moral duty as to allow the continued existence for a few more years of the conditions which will make possible this research strategy then I believe there is a purpose in pursuing the strategy, even though I personally would prefer it to be rendered impossible.

One such purpose is to supply Governments with further evidence, which they ought not to need, of the case for a rational approach to work sharing and socially useful work.

The other purpose is more fundamental. We need to be able to answer the question "Why does economic success promote health?" and thence to answer the question "What pattern of economic activity is optimal for health?"

The purpose of an economic system is to enhance the well being of its members. At present our economic systems attach overwhelming priority to those aspects of well being which may broadly be termed "Wealth" and take inadequate account of those aspects of well being which may broadly be termed "Health".

This is so whether we are talking about planned economies or market economies and it need not be so in either. A planned economy could aim to optimise a combination of indices representing different aspects of well being whilst in a market economy the market decisions could be based upon the optimisation of well being rather than wealth so that decisions which emphasised life satisfaction or leisure or health or friendship at the expense of money were more likely to be made both by individuals and by communities.

If public health is to become central to economics in this way then we need to be able to answer the question "What pattern of economic activity would be optimal for health, and if we depart from that pattern in order to move closer to the optimum for some other aspect of well being what health price do we pay?"

We are not even remotely close to being able to answer that question. Studying the health effects of recession and hence unravelling the reason that economic failure causes ill health may be the first step in moving towards the answer to that question.

(1) BRENNER, M.H.: Mortality and the national economy II: Principal factors affecting post-war British mortality trends. In this volume (1981)

(2) FORSDAHL: Are poor living conditions in childhood and adolescence an important risk factor for arteriosclerotic heart disease? British Journal of Preventive and Social Medicine 31, 91-95 (1977)

(3) DHSS: Inequalities in health. Report of a research working group. London: Dept. of Health and Social Security (1980)

(4) JENKINS, C., SHERMAN, B.: The collapse of work. London: Eyre Methuen (1979)

(5) EYER, J.: Does unemployment cause the death rate peak in each business cycle? A multifactor model of death rate changes. International Journal of Health Services 7, 4, 625-662 (1977)

(6) HEALTH AND SAFETY EXECUTIVE: Accidents in the construction industry. London: HMSO (1980)

(7) BOMAN: Behavioural observations on the Granville train disaster and the significance of stress for psychiatry. Social Science and Medicine 13A, 463-471 (1979)

(8) NUCKOLLS, KB., CASSELL, J., KAPLAN, B.H.: Psychosocial assets, life crisis and the prognosis of pregnancy. American Journal of Epidemiology 95, 431-441 (1972)

(9) BROWN, G.W., HARRIS, T.: Social origins of depression - a study of psychiatric disorder in women. London: Tavistock (1978)

(10) BERKMAN, L.F., SYME, S.L.: Social networks, host resistance and mortality - a nine year follow up study of Alameda Country residents. American Journal of Epidemiology 109, 186-203 (1979)

(11) KASL, S., COBB, S., GORE, S.: Changes in reported illness and illness behaviour related to termination of employment. International Journal of Epidemiology 1, 2, 111-118 (1972)

(12) STAFFORD, JACKSON, BANKS: Employment, work involvement and mental health in less qualified young people. Journal of Occupational Psychology 53, 291-304 (1980)

(13) WESTCOTT, G.: Proposed research on the effects of unemployment on health in Scunthorpe. In this volume (1981)

(14) FAGIN, L.: Unemployment: A psychiatric problem as well? In this volume (1981)

(15) NEWELL, S.: A bibliography with abstracts on the psychological impact of unemployment on the individual and the family. Cardiff: Welsh National School of Medicine (1981)

(16) WHITING, E.: Unemployment costs. Financial Times, Nov 24, 1980 (letter)

(17) SPRUIT, I.P.: Unemployment, the unemployed, and health. An analysis of the Dutch situation. In this volume (1981)

(18) FRÖHLICH, D.: Economic deprivation, work organisation and health. Conceptual ideas and some empirical findings. In this volume (1981)

(19) LUCAS AEROSPACE SHOP STEWARDS' COMBINE ALTERNATIVE CORPORATE PLAN.

(20) MEDICAL PRACTITIONERS' UNION: Stop knocking the public services. In: Medical Manpower and Career Structure. London: Association of Scientific, Technical and Managerial Staffs (1979)

THE EFFECTS OF UNEMPLOYMENT ON HEALTH AND PUBLIC AWARENESS OF THIS IN THE FEDERAL REPUBLIC OF GERMANY

Klaus-Dieter Thomann

Frankfurt, Federal Republic of Germany

Health matters are in the main politico-economical and sociopolitical matters. Decisions in economic policy always indirectly affect health. Everyone employed in the field of social medicine knows this from experience. Economic policy is itself dependent on questions of ownership and social power structures.

In a country with a capitalist business structure like the Federal Republic of Germany, capital is invested where expectation of profit can be realized. Rationalisation is carried out to be able to produce at lower costs. A change in the location of companies and the search for a location are subject to the same law. In Frankfurt/Main, approximately 2000 workers and employees are at present out of work due to a factory having shut down. There is no new employment in view for them. Whether jobs are created or rationalized out of existence is subject to a mechanism which the individual dependently employed man or woman can only indirectly influence. The unemployment prevailing in western countries is characteristic of "market economy".

The government, political parties, employers' associations, trade-unions and the employed can alter the level of unemployment by bringing socio-political and politico-economical influence to bear in one way or another. The worst effects of unemployment can thus be alleviated by socio-political measures. The problem cannot be mastered in the existing economic system.

To be able to exercise any influence on the effects of unemployment on society and on health, these effects must first be known. Only a consolidated examination of the effects of unemployment and adequate acquaintance of the public with these effects can be a basis for purposeful measures in health policy or politico-economical corrections in course. Only then can one recognize and foresee what consequences the policy of reductions in social expenditure conducted at present in several western countries has.

In assessing the effects of unemployment on health, a few observations on the history of our country are necessary:

1. The problem of high unemployment is relatively new to the Federal Republic. For approximately two decades, unemployment was ignored on account of its low level. It was generally maintained that "Who wants to work will find work".

2. Social security for short-term unemployment was comparatively better than in the economic crisis at the end of the twenties and beginning of the thirties. The effects on society and on health were consequently reduced.

3. Medicine in the German Federal Republic is therapy-orientated and not prophylaxis-orientated which, in turn, is linked with the structure of our health service. The next point is inseparable from this:

4. Social medicine is underdeveloped in our country. Although problems are perceived by the medical profession, no systematic stock-taking of the social effects on health has ever taken place (since 1945). There is no "socio-medical awareness" in the medical profession. Consequently, no notice has been taken of the effects of unemployment on health. Medical sociology initiated at universities has not been able to bring about any general change in the attitude of the medical profession.

A factor which also must not remain unnoticed in the bad appearance and social prestige of the unemployed. Since unemployment is often not seen as a politico-economical problem, there is a tendency to impute the blame to the individual. The unemployed person is quick to feel himself a failure. He is dissatisfied with himself and the people around him are dissatisfied with him. A lot of people are still of the opinion that a great majority of unemployed are dodgers and loafers who are not seriously interested in a job. The media do not effectively oppose this prejudice. Newspapers are continually playing up individual examples to demonstrate that the unemployed is himself to blame for his fate. In 1977, the news magazine "Der Spiegel" published a title-story from which it was to be understood that the equation of out of work with work-shy was correct. Even in government circles, prejudice is stirred up against the unemployed. A former Minister of Economics for Hesse referred to the unemployed as "fools, simpletons and flops".

Discussion on unemployment is at present characterised by alleged abuse of the "social system". If the consequences of unemployment are discussed, it is mainly the financial outlay caused by unemployment-benefit that is mentioned. Only just recently, the Minister of Economics, Lambsdorf, made proposals for reducing unemployment-benefit.

Any discussion held only worsens the public image of the unemployed still further. According to a survey carried out by the Allensbach Public Opinion Research Institute, 59% of the citizens of the German Federal Republic are convinced that "among those at present unemployed, there is a considerable number who simply do not want to work". The general negative representation of opinion additionally leads to psychological destabilization of the unemployed.

The deprecatory attitude of the public in turn has an effect on the public authorities, on the parties and also on the medical profession. To get to know better the attitude of the different institutions and the effects of unemployment on doctors' patients, various surveys were carried out.

To get some insight into recorded effects of unemployment on health, in October 1977, H. Mausbach and I wrote to approximately 30 practising doctors and doctors teaching in universities, requesting them to tell us of their experience of and their opinion on the effects of unemployment on health. More than a half of those we wrote to honoured us with a reply. With one exception, those consulted acknowledged the importance of this problem, however, they considered that their patients were too few in number to allow any objective and quantifiable declaration. Many of these doctors wanted to see the present research deficit made good by extensive and relevant investigations. The managing director of the Department for Internal Medicine at the Medical College, Hanover, Prof. Hartmann considered "such investigations to be imperative". The head of the Sigmund Freud Institute in Frankfurt/Main, Cl. de Boor, wrote that he is convinced "that, for many of the unemployed, the psychological stress situation induced by unemployment can lead to a multitude of disorders in psychological and physical stability". As a consequence, the Sigmund Freud Institute organized a work conference in October 1979 under Cl. de Boor's leadership on the psychological effects of unemployment on health. With a great number of examples, the speakers corroborated the thesis that unemployment is a highly important pathogenic factor.

That individual observations are not enough and that the social environment (town/country, social contacts, other activities, etc.) plays a role not to be underestimated, is stressed in a letter received from the chairman of the Association of University Teachers and Assistant Lecturers of General Medicine, Prof. Häussler, who has been practising for 32 years in the vicinity of Esslingen. He informed us that he has not been able to detect any remarkable impairment to health caused by unemployment and surmises:

"The reason for this is possibly that the unemployed resident here mostly have - as is pertinant to the Swabian way of life - their own house and can occupy themselves at home when unemployed. The reason can also be that, in a community of this kind (6000 inhabitants), the whole climate of social life is very much better consequently here, for example, isolation does not occur especially on account of the numerous social contacts in clubs."

The only point of view which categorically dismissed any connection between illness and unemployment came from Dr. Jan Pohl, president of the German Society for Psychosocial Medicine, who does not wish to acknowledge social factors in the pathogenesis and progress of a disease in the sense of a dogmatically interpreted psychosomatic conception. In his letter, he maintained, among other things, that there is no indication whatever of there being negative effects of unemployment on health. Psychosomatic disturbances always have serious causes pertaining to life-history and cannot be produced by unemployment.

From 1977 to 1981, the number of unemployed scarcely dropped below a million. To what extent are the medical profession and the various institutions aware of unemployment and its effects at the present moment?

To obtain a random sample, in the summer of 1981, letters were sent to 50 doctors of general medicine and to 10 psychiatrists in Saarbrücken, an area with a permanent unemployment rate of approximately 9%. In addition to this, the consultation was extended to 10 assistant lecturers in general medicine in different parts of the German Federal Republic. Those written to were asked "whether or not, in their area, they had made observations demonstrating an increase in damages to health as the probable or provable consequence of unemployment". To simplify matters, a questionnaire containing questions on the psychological and physical effects of unemployment was enclosed.

Only 6 of the doctors approached by letter sent a reply. The low return quota of approximately 10% of the questionnaires sent out shows that interest in this problem is not great. Discrimination against the unemployed and the thesis of "unemployment having been brought upon oneself" could have repressed the problem both in the patients and in the doctors.

What relevant statements could be drawn from the replies? Only one doctor of general medicine observed psychological effects of unemployment and mentioned: "exacerbation of psychoses, nonspecific neurotic symptoms such as: cases of a tendency to somatization, depressive syndromes, alcoholism". The same doctor detected somatic effects - cases of liver damage and the activation of stomach ulcers were mentioned. Disorders in the psychological sphere often lingered even after unemployment had ended Three further doctors, who had not observed any psychological or physical effects in unemployed patients, nevertheless recognized "social effects" such as a "loss of the sense of their own value particularly in the older generation" or a "lack of training particularly in women". One of the doctors replying reflected on whether the prevailing predisposition to alcohol in unemployed is not primary and loss of job secondary.

In his unemployed patients totalling approximately 100, a further doctor observed positive effects of unemployment on health. He recorded: "With one or two exceptions, joyful relief from the stress of work, plenty of opportunity to make lucrative earnings on the side and cultivation of hobbies". This doctor also considered further epidemiological investigations to be superfluous. A total of three doctors of general medicine favoured further epidemiological investigations, two rejected them and one did not comment on this question.

Of the ten university teachers approached by letter, four replied. None of them had observed physical effects of unemployment and only two had seen psychological effects. "Signs of disorders of the autonomic nervous system, sleeplessness, depressive syndromes, unsociableness, inferiority complexes" and "depressive psychosis and addiction to drink" were mentioned. In the opinion of the professors, the biggest problem lay in "loneliness" and in the "reduction of a person willing to work "to the level of a "useless being". The editor of a standard work for general medicine, Haehn, observed neither effects of unemployment on health nor social effects and consequently also rejected further investigations as superfluous.

Although the result of the survey is not representative, the fact that the questionnaire was sent out during holiday time playing a role in this, it remains to be put down on record that, even in a region with high structural permanent unemployment,

1. only a small section of the doctors show interest in the problem and
2. the majority of the practitioners in their own practices have not realized the possible connection between unemployment and ill-health.
3. Several of the replies gave indications of unemployment having an effect detrimental to health.

The lack of awareness of the problem in the section of the medical profession consulted is no isolated occurrence. Already in 1977, I had asked the Federal Ministry for Youth, Family Affairs and Health to comment on the problem of unemployment. At the time, I received the reply that no representative results of investigations were available.

In July 1978, the German Society for Social Psychiatry and a further two therapeutist organizations sent a petition to the Federal Minister of Labour on behalf of 8,000 members. The petition drew attention to the increasing mental stress as the result of unemployment. In particular: an increase in the number of addicts, attempted suicides, depressive symptom and intensification of existing psychological stress due to removal from the process of work were mentioned. The organizations sharply and severely objected to the problem being psychologized. Instead, they pleaded "for a new orientation in economic and social policy .... which would make man, his needs and his right to work the centre of attention". The petition met with lengthy response in the daily press. The reaction of the Ministry was restrained and noncommittal. The reply expressed the hope that the number of unemployed would soon drop. A new orientation in economic policy was not considered.

To get some impression of the extent to which the various parties, the government and the politico-economical and sociopolitical organizations were aware of unemployment and its effects, I questioned the following institutions in the summer of 1981:

the Christian Democratic Union (CDU)
the Christian Social Union (CSU)
the German Communist Party (DKP)
the Free Democratic Party (FDP)
the Grüne Aktion Zukunft (ecologist party) (GAZ)
the German Social Democratic Party (SDP)

the Federal Ministry for Youth, Family Affairs and Health
the Federal Ministry of Labour
the Committee for Youth, Family Affairs and Health of
the German Bundestag (Lower House of Parliament)
the Federal Health Authorities
the Federal Medical Society
the Federal Headquarters for Health Education
the German Federation of Trade Unions (DGB)
the Federal Association of Employers' Associations and the Employers' Association Saarland
the Federal Association of General Practitioners and Doctors of General Medicine
the List of Democratic Doctors in the Medical Society Hesse

In their reply, the CDU indicated that they knew "about the connection between health and unemployment" "however, they could not go into this in detail". In a documentary report of this party prepared on February 21, 1980, they again refer to the connection and recommend the agencies of the National Health Insurance Scheme to carry out appropriate investigations The party was not going to strive for any fundamentally new orientation in economic policy.

The CSU could not make any concrete statements about the problem under discussion.

The DKP's reply on the one hand sketches the social impairment and the impairment to health and, at the same time, produces politico-economical and politico-occupational alternatives. Reference is made to the party's health policy proposals in which substantial influence on the mental health of the population is apportioned to unemployment. International investigations were carried out to substantiate that unemployment is "a health problem of the first order". The DKP stresses that "the most important politico-economical and sociopolitical objective from the point of view of the working population .... is effective measures to combat unemployment, particularly unemployment among the young". They make a string of concrete suggestions such as better protection against termination of employment, a law against mass layoffs, reduction in working time, etc.

The FDP could not make any statements.

The GAZ could not make any general or specific statements.

Through the Bremen Minister of Health, Senator Brückner, the SPD reported that the party could not "treat" the question of impairment to health "exhaustively" "since, to my knowledge, there are no exact data and research available on the connections between unemployment and illness". The general aim of the Social Democratic Party's social and health policy is to create jobs and eventually to alleviate factors of disease caused by unemployment.

So much for the parties.

The following institutions declared that <u>they knew nothing about the connection between unemployment and ill-health</u> or that <u>they were not competent to reply</u>:

the Bundestag Committee for Youth, Family Affairs and Health
the Employers' Association, Saarland
the German Federation of Trade Unions, Saar region
the Association of panel-doctors, North Württemberg
Professional Association of General Practitioners and Doctors of General Medicine
the Federal Headquarters for Health Education

The Federal Association of German Employers' Associations pointed out that they had no data on the connection between unemployment and ill-health and continued "on the other hand, it would be very difficult to prove empirically disturbances in health to be the result of unemployment".

The Federal Medical Society passed the inquiry on to experts. The undersecretary of the Federal Ministry for Youth, Family Affairs and Health referred to the WHO conference held in November 1980 in Copenhagen and declared that "further studies on this complex of problems would undoubtedly be beneficial and necessary".

A demand for further epidemiological investigations was raised by the List of Democratic Doctors in the Medical Society Hesse. They referred to cases of impairment to health which are both known and assumed to be caused by persistent unemployment. Politico-economical decisions which would bring about a reduction in unemployment - e.g. a reduction in the weekly working hours and control of rationalization plans both by those affected and by their unions - is most important. The medical society pronounced themselves in favour of informing the public about the economic causes and the psychosocial effects and effects on health of unemployment, in order to reduce prejudices in the population against the unemployed and to facilitate their integration.

If the last reply is not taken into account, the same state of affairs as that seen in the case of doctors with their own practices becomes evident with almost all of the institutions approached:

<u>Apart from a very few exceptions, unemployment is still not recognized in the German Federal Republic to be a health problem</u>.

The reasons for this can be guessed: the genesis of a social disease has not just one cause. Impairment to health which is caused, fostered or made worse by unemployment cannot be detected at a glance. To be able to recognize the pathogenic effect of the loss of one's job, a certain social receptiveness is required. The social case-history must be carefully put together. Prevailing social discrimination against the unemployed hinders this receptiveness. Consequently, due to a lack of receptiveness, the detrimental effects of unemployment can be ignored by public awareness.

In the medical sector, there is a link between the unawareness of the problem and the non-recognition of the symptoms. It is an old medical fact derived from experience that symptoms which are not known cannot be recorded and incorporated in a clinical picture. Hence, lack of knowledge about the connections hinder ill health being observed. Within the administrative bodies and institutions, a lack of knowledge leads to the mental and physical disorders in unemployed patients being belittled.

<u>What conclusions are to be drawn</u>?

1. The present results of <u>international research</u>, which show an intrinsic connection between unemployment and ill-health, must be made known to the public.

2. <u>Large-scale sociomedical studies</u> on the relationship between unemployment and health are urgently required in the German Federal Republic. Already in the preparatory stage, these studies should be used as an opportunity to inform the population about the problem. By this means, prejudices

against the unemployed could be abolished and the social aspect of health could gain in importance.

Besides a large-scale epidemiological study, the following additional studies should be considered:

3. <u>Individual case studies</u> of unemployed persons who had fallen ill would, in view of widespread mistrust of social medicine, more likely find acceptance with the medical profession than mere theoretical studies.

4. In a relatively small project, appropriate medical practices could be selected in which systematic inquiries into the state of health of unemployed patients could be made.

5. <u>Analysis of health insurance scheme sick lists</u>: In the health-insurance data, both illnesses accompanied by the diagnoses and whether or not the persons in question are unable to work or are unemployed are recorded. In an evaluation of a random sample of sick lists from the Allgemeine Ortskrankenkasse (German form of compulsory health insurance) carried out by way of trial, gastro-intestinal diseases and cardiovascular diseases, for example, were found overproportionately frequently in unemployed patients.

6. The employment offices carry out a large number of medical examinations of unemployed persons. The existing data could be analyzed retrospectively. At the same time, it would be of value to carry out new studies in a way that would yield a definite conclusion on the connection between unemployment and ill-health.

If studies carried out in the future produce results proving the detrimental effect of unemployment on health, the public should be informed of this intensively and in good time. In this way, the scientists involved could operate prophylactically and initiate an economic policy which is more markedly orientated towards full employment.

STUDY ON THE INFLUENCE OF ECONOMIC DEVELOPMENT ON HEALTH
Report on the WHO Planning Meeting*
Copenhagen, 11-13 November 1980

1. Introduction

There is universal agreement in Europe and North America that improved standards of living have contributed to the long-term decline in mortality rates through improved nutrition, education and medical facilities. Somewhat more controversial is the thesis that people exposed for long periods to socioeconomic instability, especially the unemployed, are likely to die earlier. This thesis suggests that there is a need to reassess health policies which, according to the strategy of WHO and its Member States, should secure health for all by the year 2000, i.e. a level of health that will permit to lead socially and economically productive lives.

Stimulated by the pioneering work undertaken by Professor M. Harvey Brenner of the Johns Hopkins University, Baltimore, Maryland, taking into account the great interest shown by Member States in the implications of the present economic climate and following a recommendation by the European Advisory Committee for Medical Research, the Regional Office for Europe held this Meeting to plan the above-mentioned Study, which will be carried out by a number of institutes at their own or their countries' expense.

The Meeting was attended by 15 temporary advisers from 11 countries and 5 staff members of the Regional Office for Europe. Mr. K. Barnard was elected Chairman of the Meeting and Professor M.H. Brenner and Dr. D. Schwefel rapporteurs. Dr. Zöllner served as Secretary.

1.1 Scope and purpose

Dr. J. Asvall, Director, Programme Management, welcomed the participants

---

*) unedited by WHO. The issue of this document does not constitute formal publication. It should not be reviewed, abstracted or quoted without the agreement of the World Health Organization. Authors alone are responsible for views expressed in signed articles.

on behalf of Dr. Leo A. Kaprio, Director of the WHO Regional Office for Europe. He commented that the Planning Meeting would discuss an issue so far neglected by WHO. There was universal agreement in Europe and North America that improved standards of living had contributed to the long-term decline in mortality rates through improved nutrition, education and medical facilities. Somewhat more controversial was the thesis that people exposed for long periods to socioeconomic instability, especially the unemployed, were likely to die earlier. This thesis suggested that there was a need to reassess health policies which, according to the strategy of WHO and its Member States, should secure health for all by the year 2000, i.e. a level of health that will permit people to lead socially and economically productive lives. Being sufficiently precise and idealistic at the same time, this strategy had been recognized as being vital for Europe and not only for developing countries. In highly industrialized countries the health impacts of socioeconomic development and technological advances had to be assessed as well.

In order to achieve health for all by the year 2000, priority was placed on primary health care, which was seen as being no longer the prerogative of medical services only.

The Regional Office for Europe of the World Health Organization had asked all Member States to meet this challenge. The resulting Regional Strategy for Attaining Health for All by the Year 2000, which was adopted at the thirtieth session of the Regional Committee, drew attention to a new perspective in health, which emphasizes:
(1) promotion of lifestyles whicn are conducive to health;
(2) reduction of health risks and conditions which are preventable;
(3) reorientation and extension of health care systems towards primary health care;
(4) strengthening of relevant programmes in support of the other three strategies.

The participants of the Meeting drew attention to the following points: lifestyle should be interpreted to mean not only individual behaviour, but social networks and community actions as well; analysis of the relationships between lifestyle and health was required; there should be a shift towards humane and logically consistent models of health care; and the health professionals should participate in its implementation.

The Regional Committee had insisted to include in the second strategy the following paragraph:

> "To reduce poverty: at country level, poverty can be reduced by such measures as social security, subsidized housing or housing allowances, land reform, fiscal readjustments to benefit low income groups and general socioeconomic development. A genuine policy of peace, détente and disarmament could and should release additional resources for such measures as reaffirmed in resolution WHA33.24."

This addition reflected an increase in social and economic problems in European countries. Economic instability, increasing social insecurity and long-lasting unemployment in several countries of the Region - especially as they affect younger people and the quality and equality of opportunities for women - could have a vital impact on health. Countermeasures were needed both inside and outside the health care sector and required both technocratic and solidarity among people.

The Regional Office was therefore seeking scientific evidence and expert advice on the influence of economic development on health.

1.2 General understanding

Research studies demonstrating the effects of socioeconomic development on health could

- strengthen the bargaining power of health authorities in relation to other sectors of the economy;
- promote intersectoral collaboration and encourage activities by other sectors aimed at attaining health for all by the year 2000; and
- increase the effectiveness of health care activities.

This would be the case particularly:

- if research is able to trace the cause-effect linkages of the chain or tree of factors that related economy and health;
- if reliable forecasting of the relevant trends can be carried out;
- if research concentrates on the population groups suffering most from economic change, recession and unemployment, i.e. presumably teenage school-leavers and younger women; and
- if, at the same time, it can be proved that better health reinforces social and economic development.

Studies should therefore concentrate on shedding light on the social and economic benefits and costs of socioeconomic development and especially on its impact on wellbeing, morbidity and mortality rates.

2. Thesis: economic instability increases mortality; long-term economic growth decreases mortality

2.1 Indicators

2.1.1 Health indicators

The overall mortality rate (either age-adjusted or age-specific), as well as the corresponding mortality rate by cause (suicide, homicide, accidents, cardiovascular diseases, malignancies etc.), are taken as the principal indicators of a population's health. Thus, the mortality rate is being used as an indicator in two ways. First, it actually measures the number of deaths per unit of population and, by derivation, the population's longevity. Second, the mortality rate, especially by cause, is assumed to reflect changing patterns of morbidity. In this way, the mortality rates due to suicide, homicide and hypertension, for example, are used to reflect respectively the incidence of depression, violence, and high blood pressure.

2.1.2 Economic indicators

(a) Long-term economic growth. This is measured by the long-term (i.e. at least 20-years) exponential trend in real income per capita. The benefits inherent in long-term economic growth are both direct and indirect. Directly, especially in populations in which infectious diseases are significant sources of morbidity and mortality, the trend is an indicator of the availability of nutrition, climate control, and sanitary engineering. Indirectly, the trend reflects better education (especially with respect to health); also, it is an indirect indicator of the extent to which structural unemployment is likely to be damaging. With long-term economic growth, the shift from older to newer industries and occupations would ideally result from the attractions of the higher income and job status offered by the newer industries, or, at the very least, from the push by the older industries which are losing markets and therefore income. During long-term economic growth, economic loss to workers is minimized.

Finally, two important indirect benefits of economic growth are continous investment into identifying causes of morbidity and mortality, and continuous investment into effective health technologies.

Consistent findings of an inverse relationship between socioeconomic status and mortality rates, at least in France, the UK and USA, are evidence for the overwhelming significance of socioeconomic factors to health. Of equal importance are the findings of comparative studies that the level of gross national product per capita is the single most important predictor of prevalence of diseases, and frequently of incidence as well.

(b) <u>Rate of unemployment</u>. Economic instability is partly indicated by the rate of unemployment. Unemployment as an indicator also refers to the incidence of economic loss in the population. Thus, in general, the unemployment rate is assumed to assess or at least indicate losses of employment and income. Where the unemployment rate does not properly measure the extent of loss of employment and income, other measures, such as the employment rate and relative income of specific population groups, may be more appropriate.

Two types of unemployment are to be distinguished. Cyclical unemployment is often less serious, since it occurs in industries in which the work force has become adapted to such changes. Cyclical unemployment is, however, also an indicator of cyclical losses of income and employment to the owners of small and medium-sized enterprises. An alternative indicator of cyclical changes in the economic situation of the self-employed, therefore, would be the rate of bankruptcy.

The second major type is "technological" of "structural" unemployment. It occurs as a result of (i) innovations which are introduced to reduce the need for labour or (ii) the decline of specific industries due to technological change or international competition. Structural unemployment is therefore also an indicator of economic losses to the self-employed and of income losses to workers.

(c) <u>Rapid economic growth</u>. Economic instability results also from rapid economic growth. While rapid economic growth is rarely harmful to the population which gains income and job status, it constitutes a period of economic and social "reintegration" for the population experiencing economic losses. Several major sources of stress are involved in the reintegration process, in addition to the original economic loss. These stresses may involve migration and loss of community networks, substantially lower economic and social standing, work in unfamiliar occupations and/or industries, and finally, striving to regain one's previous economic and social standing. The last of these situations involves "overwork", i.e. working beyond one's usual capacity; it is associated with driving oneself hard, time pressure and overexertion and hence cardiovascular risk, sometimes referred to as "type A" behaviour.

(d) Disaggregated indicators. There is a need to disaggregate the above-mentioned indicators by groups of population. It has, e.g., been maintained that economic instability is considerably greater among populations of lower socioeconomic status. This might in turn contribute to their higher mortality rate by way of stress and its implications for lifestyle in terms of heavy use of alcohol and tabacco, for example.

2.2   Linkages between economy and health

2.2.1   Models

Throughout the three-day Meeting the participants, when speaking of "the model", referred to that by Professor M.H. Brenner in the Lancet (Lancet, 2: 568-573(1979)). This particular presentation of the argument linking economic change and health as presented by Professor Brenner is basically theoretical and elaborates previous models in those earlier articles and books by Professor Brenner that are referred to in the Lancet paper. During the first part of the Meeting, however, Professor Brenner offered additional elaborations on the general model of the impact of the economy on health. The model now includes also intervening risk factors, such as those measured by per capita consumption of alcohol and tobacco, average weekly hours worked in manufacturing industries, and production of synthetic organic chemicals.

It is argued that factors both directly and indirectly associated with long-term economic growth, as well as economic instability and uncertainty, have important effects on morbidity (not included due to data limitations) and mortality. These effects can be measured at least on a population basis.

For each subpopulation, i.e. different age, sex, occupational or industrial groups, somewhat different submodels are relevant. Further, for each major cause of morbidity or mortality, a somewhat different sub-model of the general model will apply. Finally, it is assumed that in different countries or regions of different countries, subject to different economic and social policies and cultural influences, once again other different submodels will be appropriate. The latter points to the need for differentiating countries with liberal economies from countries with highly developed universal welfare systems and countries with planned economic systems (where unemployment is minimal but there are important structural changes in employment patterns associated with economic growth).

3. Antithesis: some critical remarks

On the macro level the relationship between socioeconomic development and health is analysed by Professor Brenner as follows: indicators such as the unemployment rate and the growth of GNP are linked statistically with mortality rates, sometimes using general rates, sometimes age-specific and sex-specific rates. The results are then interpreted as indicating a link between socioeconomic conditions during a particular period and subsequent health. This reasoning entails, however, considerable problems regarding models, indicators, computational techniques and interpretation of results, including the danger of "ecological fallacy".

3.1 Indicators

The main indicators are:

(a) mortality rates for selected conditions such as cardiovascular diseases, suicide, etc., and for specific demographic segments of the population according to age and sex;
(b) growth rate of GNP, exponential growth rate of per capita income and unemployment rates.

3.1.1 Health indicators

In view of the longstanding controversy as to definition, objectivity, reliability, validity, comparability and utility of mortality statistics, the participants of the Meeting made only very few additional critical remarks. The analysis of time series of mortality rates might be biased because of changing patterns of (i) diseases and causes of death, (ii) care, (iii) classification and reporting practices and (iv) control on the reliability of data. Mortality, morbidity, impairment (as diagnosed by professionals), disability, handicap and wellbeing (as diagnosed individually or socially) are quite distinct and often incomparable dimensions of health. In any case, mortality is quite removed from what is generally understood as health.

3.1.2 Economic indicators

In spite of an ample reservoir of indicators for socioeconomic development such as migration, divorce, mobility, and so forth, only few indicators have been used in the model. One of these, economic growth rate, reflects all major developments including changes in technologies, production processes, composition of goods and services, patterns of money and credit markets, international trade patterns and so on. This indicator can therefore be interpreted as a general trend factor which partly explains the variance of other trend variables. At the same time it has frequently been shown that the socioeconomic meaning of this indicator differs for different population groups.

Shortcomings of this indicator are illustrated indirectly by the intrinsic biases of the unemployment indicator.

3.1.2.1. Problems in defining unemployment in the narrow economic sense

The first problem is the variation in the definition of the active labour force or the employable population. In different countries and at different times, various definitions have been used, especially regarding the labour-force participation of
- women,
- the self-employed,
- the chronically disabled,
- the unemployable,
- school leavers,
- the hidden unemployed.

The second problem is the variation in the registration of the unemployed; there are large differences according to institutional settings and security schemes.

The third problem is that employment normally refers only to the labour market, leaving aside all people working in the subsistence sector of economy, namely housewives, family workers, some labourers in agriculture, etc. Here one often finds overwork without formal employment status being necessary.

The fourth problem arises when different types of unemployment are to be considered: cyclical, frictional, seasonal, structural unemployment on the one hand and short-term versus long-term unemployment on the other.

The fifth problem relates to the question of whether the <u>incidence or the prevalence of unemployment</u> is to be reported.

The sixth problem - which applies to all social and economic indicators - stems from the consequences of World War II: many European countries were so severely affected that time series going back to the forties or further are difficult to interpret.

3.1.2.2 The social meaning of unemployment

In Professor Brenner's model, the term "unemployment" is used not only as an indicator of unemployment but, in a much broader sense, as an indicator of (i) economic instability and (ii) the preconditions and consequences of instability at different levels of society. In this respect the unemployment variable has been interpreted in different and sometimes conflicting ways to pertain to:

(a) <u>economic problems</u>
- cost of technological or economic change
- loss of income
- low fiscal control over the black labour market
- lack of interaction between employer and the market
- absenteeism and disability;

(b) <u>labour market problems</u>
- rapid labour turnover
- expulsion from work
- loss of job in the "white economy"
- increase in the black labour market
- misuse of security laws by employers
- disrupted work conditions
- job insecurity for all;

(c) <u>social problems</u>
- inadequate participation of women in the labour market
- social problems for whole families and their dependants
- limited or excessive mobility
- increase of work within the family
- lack of attractiveness of lower status jobs
- loss of social status;

(d) <u>mental health problems</u>
- job displacement of people
- lack of adaptational abilities
- stress for the unemployed
- loss of communication with people
- loss of identity
- dissatisfaction
- loss of meaning of the world
- social stigmatization.

These aspects of the socioeconomic and emotional meaning of unemployment were used by the participants of the Meeting to demonstrate the vague and sometimes contradictory meaning of unemployment.

This confusing picture is complicated by the fact that unemployment has different socioeconomic and psychical consequences according to
- age (e.g. young school leavers, the older employees)
- sex (e.g. unemployment has different consequences for women as compared to men)
- family structure (e.g. unemployed with or without family)
- social class (e.g. blue collar versus white collar workers)
- region (e.g. with high versus low rates of unemployment)
- personality type (e.g. A versus B)
- phases of the business cycle (e.g. depression versus boom)
- family wealth (e.g. availability versus inavailability of income from sources other than employment)
- social security system (depending on extent and coverage).

This chameleon-like multidimensionality and heterogeneity of the unemployment indicator is even more problematic if one takes into account that
- effects spread from the unemployed individual to his social group;
- unemployment is used to point sometimes to individual consequences

and sometimes to general characteristics of society;
- anticipation or fear of unemployment could have the same consequences as real unemployment;
- there seems sometimes to be coexistence of unemployment and overwork;
- the same situation may be interpreted differently by different people;
- there could be positive and negative effects of unemployment at the same time;
- the level of aggregation used to interpret consequences of unemployment is chosen in an arbitrary manner;
- all these problems change over time in intensity and relevance.

The definition, objectivity, reliability, validity, comparability and utility of the unemployment variable are blurred by so many factors that one can have doubts regarding the statistical interrelation of this indicator with the similarly blurred indicator of mortality. This points to the need to exercise extreme caution in interpreting results.

3.2 Linkages between economy and health

3.2.1 Models

It is by no means a single and unique model which is used to explain the empirical relation between economic instability as indicated by the unemployment rate, etc., on the one hand, and mortality rates on the other. Reconstructing Brenner's model, one of the participants, Dr. Wlodarczyk, identified a series of different submodels. These submodels relate health with
- the economy via long-term economic growth, unemployment, short-term rapid economic growth and government expenditure on welfare with economic (in)stability and (in)security;
- the economic instability and insecurity via migration, urbanization and cumulative influences of various stressful events, and more generally disruption of basic social patterns involving family and community as indicated e.g. by divorces;
- long-term economic growth via rising real per capita incomes;
- recession via loss of income and social status, dangerous life habits, breakdown of families and social structures and individual depression, to name but a few.

These _ad hoc_ submodels do not share a consistent set of characteristics; sometimes they appear consistent with the empirical data and sometimes widely divergent. Some of the submodels seem to contradict common sense; this is especially the case when rates of unemployment are related to the infant death rate or the mortality of people aged 85 and over, or when unemployment rates are linked with mortality, without specifying whether those who die are the unemployed or not. From a sociological point of view those linkages are not illogical, but point to the need to consider explicitly accelerator effects of labour force changes on the economically, physically or mentally more sensitive groups of the population, e.g. infants or the elderly.

3.2.2   Implicit hypothesis

It is assumed that economic instability can act in two ways to increase the risk of mortality. First, it involves economic loss and reduces socioeconomic status, thus negating or minimizing the gains to longevity and health that long-term economic growth would ordinarily have brought about. In this sense, economic instability is to be understood as a source of disruption or elimination of the beneficial physical aspects of economic growth.

Second, and of equal if not even greater importance, economic instability is assumed to be a major source of psychosocial stress in society, since it involves both loss and the striving to recover the economic and social loss, as well as disruption of the social support networks during both the periods of loss and recovery. In this regard, there is assumed to be a "network" or "spread" effect in which the stress on losers of employment and/or income also affects their families and those who are dependent on them for economic, social or emotional position or support. Thus, the elderly and very young whose situation is dependent economically or emotionally on middle-aged family members will in turn suffer first as a consequence of economic loss to the middle-aged. The network, or spread, effect therefore creates an ecological set of relations in which the family or other social network must be taken as the "unit" of analysis, in terms of microstudies to be conducted in this field.

The network effect has been discussed in terms of the "multiplier" principle of stress, by which the stress of one individual increases that of a related individual. This principle is to be distinguished from that of the "accelerator" principle, according to which a single stress, such as unemployment, increases the probability of occurrence of secondary and tertiary stresses in the same individual (e.g. migration, adaptation to new position, adaptation to lower socioeconomic status). The model does not have a clear hypothesis on which population groups will suffer excess mortality.

Substantial research literature supporting the psychosocial stress effects of economic instability include (1) clinical depression aspects of loss and reparation, (2) impact of cumulative stresses or "life changes" on morbidity, (3) impact of social change on cardiovascular illness, (4) significance of "Type A" pressured behaviour as a risk in coronary disease, and (5) epidemiological studies on unemployment.

Interpreting the relationship between economic development and health leads to an almost unlimited set of micro-assumptions, such as
- the lower the socioeconomic class of a person, the higher the possibility of her/his being unemployed;
- the higher the skills of a person, the higher the probability that she/he will migrate when unemployed;
- the higher the amount of overwork, the higher the risk of unemployment;
- the stronger the work pressure, the greater the risk of heart disease;
- the higher the risk of unemployment, the higher the risk of heart disease;
- the greater the dependency of people, the more people will be affected by the unemployment of relatives;
- the higher the unemployment, the lower the incidence of accidents;
- the greater the changes of life, the more difficult the adaptation process;
- the more pronounced the loss of status, the more severe the mental and social problems.

Hypotheses such as these are by no means linked to the macro model of Professor Brenner, but are nevertheless used by readers for interpretation. They point to interesting areas of research.

3.2.3 Intervening variables

Several major health risk factors are understood to intervene in the causal chain linking economic growth and instability to morbidity and mortality. One of the principal beneficial intervening factors derived from economic growth is the reduction in average working hours per week in manufacturing industries. This factor presumably acts to minimize exposure to occupational hazards and fatigue. It also provides for greater leisure and recreation, including socio-emotional interchange, exercise, and recuperation from the psychological or physical fatigue of work.

Two intervening factors which presumably have acted to minimize the health benefits of long-term economic growth are the production of carcinogens (especially synthetic organic chemicals) and the per capita consumption of calories leading to conditions of overweight.

Two "lifestyle" factors which are believed to be intervening factors deriving from long-term economic growth as well as economic instability are the per capita consumption of alcoholic beverages and tobacco products.

Other possible intervening variables on the national level have been mentioned, e.g.
- production of chemicals
- distribution of risk factors
- occupational structure
- investment in social security
- social welfare in terms of housing, education, nutrition, etc.
- international and internal migration
- socioeconomic attributes of regions
- changing balance between professional qualifications.

The inclusion of intervening variables would underline the fact that mortality is not influenced by unemployment only and that unemployment has many effects apart from early death. The relevance of intervening lifestyle indicators for, as well as the changing impact of health services on, a reduction of disease-specific mortality has recently been shown by Professor Brenner.

3.2.4 Time lags

It is clear that excess mortality lags behind unemployment. There is no theoretically or epidemiologically based model presented to account for the different lags included in the equations for different ages, sexes and diseases. Instead, the best statistical fit is used to determine the distributed lag structure, resulting in implausibilities when checked against the common medical wisdom. It is true that many cancers have lag time of 20 years before reaching a clinical phase, while again other diseases have shorter lags. In many cases, such as suicides and homicides, lags are not known at all. The model would have more power if it could differentiate between diseases and population groups involved.

The question regarding lags between economic variables and mortality points again to micro questions and to the urgency of theoretical underpinning, e.g., using the concept of stable populations. The difficulty is that a tested comprehensive theoretical model is not available. The model therefore is a compromise between fragments of different theories belonging to several disciplines, the ingenuity and imagination of the researcher and the availability of data.

3.3 Techniques

There are different techniques available to analyse statistically the relationship between changing economic and mortality rates. The choice of technique depends on
- the degree of *a priori* knowledge
- the degree of sophistication of the model
- the degree of interaction between variables
- the amount of data available
- the number of variables to be considered
- the relevance of the multicollinearity problem, etc.

There seems to be no definite consensus as to which technique can be used in this case to avoid spurious and artificial results, i.e. especially
- different methods of regression (e.g. ordinary least squares vs. Almon-lag estimation)
- spectral analysis
- other modern methods of time series analysis (e.g. Box-Jenkins techniques).

3.4 Explanation and prediction

The model indicates associations, not cause-effect relationships: economic development has something to do with death.

Up to now the predictive power of the model has not been assessed. The model only shows closeness or fit to actual data.

It was argued that prediction based on data not used in the estimation procedure could be regarded as a further and stricter test of the model. It is important to test this, since the usefulness of the model for policy purposes, e.g. health planning measures, depends on its predictive power.

While it appears correct that a real test of the model - especially with respect to possible specification errors - is provided by prediction based on an independent set of data, one should keep in mind that, due to the stochastic nature of the estimated relationship, a poor predictive performance for smaller sets of observations cannot be taken to "falsify" the model. With respect to the policy significance of the model, it should also be pointed out that there is the question of how far ahead one can predict. This needs to be tested on existing data.

4. The relevance of criticism of the Brenner Model

4.1 The overall theoretical structure and the predictive model

While the Meeting took as its basic point of departure the predictive model presented in the earlier cited Lancet article, Professor Brenner presented a more detailed predictive model for the United States, 1950-1976. Also discussed were the elements, or basic building blocks, of an overall theory of the relation between national economic changes and health.

Since the conference initially focused on the Lancet article's predictive model, there was a tendency to regard that model as representing the theoretical superstructure. A resulting problem was that the variable "unemployment rate" tended to be understood as a principal concept - which it is not - rather than as one of several indicators of the rates of recessional and structural economic loss in a population. As an indicator, the unemployment rate can be interpreted in either a unidimensional or multidimensional manner depending on its role in the design of specific research problems.

The theoretical superstructure itself involves two factors which are conceptualized as responsible for changes in a population's mortality rate: (1) growth and development of three main types of resource; namely wealth, knowledge and social organization (including social integration); and (2) the proportional allocation of resources within each of the three main types. Thus, societal wealth can be allocated (or distributed) proportionately among, for example, nutritional, defence, health care, or educational needs. Knowledge investments can be allocated to the production of wealth via increased productivity of technology, or to the testing, evaluation and modification of technology so as to increase its beneficial impact on a population's health. For social organization, an important allocation problem is in the distribution of occupational skills and management authority among the labour force.

The problem of allocation (or distribution) of societal resources has a theoretically optimum, or "balanced", solution, for any society at any particular period in its development. Thus, "imbalance" in allocation of resources results in insufficient investment in the resolution of certain societal problems, and relative overinvestment in other problem areas. Comparative underinvestment in specific areas leads to a higher rate of societal errors of adaptation in those areas. For a society experiencing high rates of technological growth, it is especially important that investments in knowledge leading to higher productivity do not run too far ahead of investments in knowledge which are necessary to the testing and modification of technology so as to make it consistent with human adaptational requirements.

In general, the higher the quantity, and level of development, of resources available to a society (wealth, knowledge, social organization) and the closer the optimum (or "balance") are proportional resource allocations at any given time, the greater is its adaptive capacity (and therefore the greater the longevity, the higher the health levels, and the lower the mortality rate at all ages, of its population).

The effects of resource growth and development, and the rational allocation of resources, are to increase the capacity of a society to fulfil its adaptive requirements. The adaptive requirements of a population include the following: nutrition, climate control, maintenance of biological immune systems, parasite control, physical security, maintenance of physical capacity (versus exhaustion), and social integration.

Social integration involves the needs, or drives, of social animals for relations based on principles of socioemotional expression and bonding, reciprocal exchange systems and altruism, and social stratification. Social integration can be damaged relatively quickly by a decline in, or disruption of, the flow of resources. The general mechanisms are hypothesized to be as follows. A decline in resources for a general population is reflected, for specific subpopulations, in losses of resources, decline in the rate of remuneration (inconsistent with norms of distributive justice), insecurity and anxiety over future losses, chronic economic unpredictability (uncertainty), and loss (or change) of employment. These primary effects on subpopulations experiencing loss can be conceptually summarized as decline in, or threat of loss, of: (1) material resources; (2) social esteem - the social value of persons - and thus self-esteem; and (3) meaning and purpose of economic and social participation.

Secondary effects of the decline in societal resources (for the subpopulations affected) involve damage to societal networks: the basic systems of exchange of goods and services, substantive communications, and socioemotional expression. These secondary effects can be conceptualized as the multiplier effects of stress, since they represent the mechanism whereby one individual's stress leads to a greater probability of stress among other individuals within the subject's social exchange network. The multiplier is to be analytically distinguished from the other major type of "spread" effects of stress, namely the accelerator effects in which the incidence of a single major stress to an individual's social position initiates and exacerbates further stresses within the same individual's life course.

Secondary effects of the decline in societal resources on the process of social integration include the following three elements:

(1) Decline in sharing of resources - the instrumental dimension.
(2) Increase in socioemotional distance, or decline in supportive emotional interchange. This tends to occur as a result of the communication of psychological distress, or the disruption of communication, associated with: depression and withdrawal, aggression

and hostility (related to frustration), anxiety, and tension.
(3) Increase in spatial distance associated with migration from areas of relatively poor economic opportunity to those of greater opportunity. In the more extreme cases of this "push-pull" phenomenon of migration, symptoms of anomie or social "uprooting" may occur.

4.2 The accelerator principle: intervening variables

The extent to which there are important factors which intervene between economic loss and morbidity or mortality is frequently attributable to the "process of acceleration" of stress. The most general principle here is that the greater the decline in resources, resulting from economic loss, the greater is the difficulty in adapting to any and all subsequent problems and stresses, since resources are the instruments of adaptation. Thus, for example, if income is lost, future solutions to adaptive problems which require material wealth will be compromised.

The trauma of loss should be understood as having effects separate from those of living, subsequently, at a lower socioeconomic standard, i.e., with fewer resources. Loss, however, initiates the lower socioeconomic standard. The initial decline in resources will vary in its subsequent impact in at least two different subpopulations. In the first subpopulation, the initial economic injury is extremely damaging, and probably results in loss of job or major investment (as in bankruptcy by self-employed). Such a great loss is frequently followed by movement into another occupation or industry which may involve a second important loss in job status and income - especially for those at middle age or older. This second loss, then, results from the need to adapt to a new economic and social position. Finally, after securing a new position, problems of relative deprivation and status inconsistency often develop.

The second subpopulation which experiences economic loss is considerably larger than that for whom the loss results rapidly in job termination or destruction of a firm. In the second subpopulation, the economic loss is substantial but the economic organization is still viable in the short and medium term. Since, however, the organization still appears to have the potential for economic survival, the staff may endure a prolonged period of chronic anxiety, tension and overwork in order to prevent the threat of total loss from becoming a reality.

The tendency to chronic overwork in such an organization is also partly due to the decline in resources that results from the original economic loss. The decline in resources leads to the situation that investment funds and credit necessary to maintain current staff and provide for the future are lacking. Thus, even in the short run, the organization in this condition will be understaffed and underfunded, so that the remaining staff must work harder and longer hours in order to maintain a minimal level of overall performance. Under such more difficult working conditions, the organization's standard of performance may deteriorate, causing conflict among staff, which further contributes to the ultimate destruction of the organization.

Two additional pathways of the acceleration principle are: (1) economic loss, leading to a decline in social support, thereby increases the subsequent probability of morbidity; and (2) economic loss, leading to stress-related illness via intervening variables, thereby increases the subsequent probability of a second loss (e.g., of employment or of the inability to secure new employment).

4.3 Choice of indicators

The choice of indicators to test the general theoretical argument will vary depending on the country, subpopulation, and time span under study. The selection process should take into account the criteria listed below.
(1) There should be more than trivial variation in an independent variable, or else it will empirically explain very little, even though it would otherwise appear to be highly relevant to the overall theory.
(2) The choice of indicators, pertinent to theoretical considerations, should be relevant to the empirical conditions specific to the time span, culture, nation, subpopulations, and diagnostic classifications of morbidity and mortality under study.
(3) The choice of independent variable indicators will be limited by degrees of freedom; i.e., sample size (of time units) and the number of issues considered crucial for prediction and statistical control.
(4) The choice of indicators will be limited by issues of multicollinearity. This factor requires that a minimum number of independent variables expressing somewhat overlapping health risks can be tolerated in the predictive equation. Ideally, independent variables should be entirely uncorrelated with one another.
(5) As pointed out in the Meeting, the choice of indicators and varia-

bles will be limited by issues of validity and reliability.
(6) A sufficient number of indicators should be present in the predictive model so that the effects of all-important factors influencing the dependent variable have been estimated and controlled. This prevents over- and under-estimation of coefficients and standard errors.
(7) The choice of indicators should also conform to the requirements of a well-integrated model, ideally reflecting a logical structure of the theoretical propositions.

In the model used to explain the major trends in US mortality during 1950-1976, for example, the following indicators are used: exponential trend in real per capita income (indicating the long-term trend in wealth and consumption); average weekly hours worked in manufacturing industries (indicating structural and cyclic changes in weekly hours of physically taxing work); the unemployment and bankruptcy rates (indicators of cyclic and structural economic loss); per capita consumption of alcohol and tobacco, and the production of synthetic organic chemicals (indicators of major health risks associated with "adaptive error").

4.4 Choice of time-series techniques

There are two principal methods for the quantitative analysis of relations among variables over time, namely spectral analysis including autoregressive moving average techniques (ARMA and ARIMA) and time-series regression analysis. The time-series regression techniques have been more widely used in econometrics, demography, and the social sciences because of their flexibility. The spectral techniques are constrained because they: require a comparatively lengthy period of study (i.e., numbers of observations); make little allowance for extended multivariate analysis, and are basically designed for univariate and bivariate work; do not allow for estimates of changes in the strength of relations or for new variables to enter the causal system; and do not easily allow for estimation of distributed lags. Nevertheless, in principle, there is no reason why these two types of time-series analysis should bring the researcher to different conclusions.

Pooled time-series regression techniques are also appropriate for use in this problem and maximize the use of a relatively small time sample. However, the pooled technique requires that the relation between critical independent variables and the dependent variable be similar across subpopulation groups. This criterion is usually not met in the research in this area.

Another commonly used regression procedure for time-change analysis estimates relations among variables that are in change form(e.g., the percentage in per capita income and in the mortality rate during 1960-1970). This technique is an excellent supplement to the time-series regression procedure and should produce results consistent with it provided that the same time span is involved in each of the two analyses.

4.5 Estimation of time lags

The problem of proper estimation of the lag period between the incidence of major economic stress and different measures of health status, including mortality, is indeed complicated by the absence of a comprehensive theory of the impact of stress on ill health. Essentially lacking is full knowledge of the pathobiological mechanisms whereby social stress alters organismic susceptibility to physical and mental disorder and death. At the same time, we are not entirely without such theory, and there is now a substantial amount of cumulative empirical data available.

First of all, there must necessarily be some time lag between the response of the human organism to stress and the development of illness and, finally, to mortality. Moreover, one would expect that disorders of function not based on the development of chronic disease, namely suicide, homicide or accidents, would occur relatively rapidly (perhaps within several months) of the proximal impact of major economic stress. Chronic diseases, however, associated, for example, with cardiovascular or immune system disorders, would be expected to develop over a period of years if there were a causal connection to previous economic stress. Empirical evidence, in addition (especially the tradition of research begun by Holmes and Rahe), indicates that many of the severe responses to cumulative stress can be measured over a period of two years, though the effects of such stress can be seen over at least the following decade.

Also, several principles that can be used in the lag analysis include: (1) more vulnerable populations to illness or mortality (e.g. the aged, previously ill, infants) should respond more rapidly to economic stress with elevated mortality rates; (2) populations which are more highly exposed to economic stress are at greater risk of a rapid morbidity and mortality response; (3) the mortality of populations initially in marginal economic circumstances (such as lower socioeconomic groups in industrialized countries, and national populations at lower GNP levels), or in less socially integrated societies, should increase more rapidly in relation to economic stress than that of other populations.

The technique utilized in the _Lancet_ article allows one to ascertain, first, whether over the entire period of a decade, economic loss, as measured by the unemployment rate, is associated with elevated mortality rates (via the polynomial distributed lag procedure). In a second phase of the analysis, one examines whether within each five-year period following increased unemployment there is also increased mortality. Finally, in a third phase, it is possible to ascertain which of each of the five years following increased unemployment are the important contributors to mortality. This technique then permits one to identify the single most important predictive lag of economic loss for subsequent mortality. This lag will usually represent the optimum "fit", namely the most efficient predictor having the lowest standard error. It is this "optimum" lag of the economic stress variable that can be selected for predictive regression equations where the analysis has serious degrees-of-freedom constraints and a choice among several indicators must be made.

4.6 Issue of prediction

It is clearly important to show the ability of the research model to predict (to future events), if only for the purpose of estimating its usefulness as a planning instrument. However, the predictive ability of a specific research model, which was constructed with the purpose of explaining variations in a phenomenon which covers a specific historical period, may only extend a short period beyond the original span examined. This limitation on predictive ability of a specific research model, as distinguished from the overall theoretical formulation, will depend upon: (1) changes in the strength of the relations; and (2) the emergence of a new independent variable as an important additional cause of temporal variation in the dependent variable.

5. Research needs

5.1 General remarks

Criticisms, the problems encountered and the implicit hypotheses formulated point to the actual research needs at different levels of analysis; countries and regions at the macro-level, population and social groups at the intermediate level and the individual at the micro-level.

The following outlines in telegraphic style different aspects to be considered:
(1) Purposes of the study: basic research, applied research, action research, policy guidance, managerial decision aid.
(2) Specific topics: socioeconomic development and health, unemployment and health, economic business cycles and health, costs and benefits of unemployment, health implications of the shift of the sectoral balance towards the communication sector.
(3) Areas of application: geographic, sectorial, groups at risk, etc.
(4) Explanation: association, cause-effect, etc.
(5) Methodology: econometrics, sociology, psychology, anthropology, epidemiology, clinical trials.
(6) Problems of definition and measurement: see earlier discussion; mortality, morbidity, measures of wellbeing.
(7) Data required: general statistics, specially collected data.
(8) Instruments: questionnaires, in-depth interviews, expert meetings.
(9) Constraints of data collection: confidentiality.
(10) Resources: time, money, manpower.
(11) Quality control and assurance.
(12) Research economics: small studies vs. large studies.
(13) Possibility for international cooperation, coordination and comparability.

Priorities have to be formulated in view of this large set of research aspects, the need to open the "black box"; need to concentrate on the complicated network linking the variables, in order to build up knowledge in a stepwise fashion.

Participants of the Meeting mentioned especially the following requirements for the national studies and the overall international study:
- concentration on relevant groups at risk such as young school leavers and the older employees, in order to guarantee the political significance of research;
- focus also on action research, where scientific and ethical crite-

ria are balanced and people participate not only to ensure the relevance of questionnaires and other instruments of research;
- good quality control or research, especially when complex research designs such as non-concurrent prospective study design are used and where confounding factors may intervene. Also avoidance of including easily measurable but irrelevant variables;
- shift of study focus from testing associations towards indentifying cause-effect relationships;
- inclusion of politically relevant variables, even if they may be difficult to measure;
- development of conceptual frameworks for linking the studies.

In line with the important work of Professor Brenner, some of the studies should also focus on the replication and improvement of macro-models. This would involve a closer look at the unemployment variable and its apparent incomparability between socialist and other countries. Other studies should concentrate on other levels of analysis, even if this would imply the need to control a larger number of variables.

The Meeting concluded that studies carried out at different levels of analysis and in different countries would give a better understanding of the situation within 3-5 years.

5.2 Studies on the macro-level

At the macro-level of analysis, Professor Brenner's approach[a] would be adapted, replicated and tested in order to estimate and predict by multiple regression the magnitudes of (a) a relation between steady economic growth and a decrease in overall mortality, and (b) a relation between short-term economic instability/unemployment and increased mortality.

5.3 Studies at intermediate levels

Studies at intermediate levels of analysis may include regional disaggregations of the macro-model, community studies on intervention programmes and studies on selected industries and population groups.

---

[a] Brenner, M:H: Lancet,2:568-573 (1979).

5.3.1 Disaggregated macro-level

Regions within national economies can have quite distinctive patterns of growth, stability and economic and social wellbeing. Disaggregation of the macro-model into regions has several potential advantages over the aggregate model:

(a) the construction of meaningful conceptual models for the complicated path between health and development;
(b) close look at diverse patterns of growth and composition of prospering and declining industries;
(c) use of meaningful indicators for economic development and economic instability;
(d) the application of specific instruments for collecting data - e.g. questionnaires, estimates based on expert consensus.

These studies would be aimed at testing key hypotheses and underlying mechanisms. Starting with a path model - the most unsophisticated type of simulation model - disaggregated macro-studies could ultimately lead to explanatory predictive models.

5.3.2 Community studies

Community studies would focus on the spread effects of different interventions to reduce the negative socioeconomic consequences of economic instability and/or unemployment or on different reactions of people towards unemployment and/or economic instability. They would seek to fill the existing gaps in knowledge about the links between the economy and health, health levels being expressed in terms of morbidity, risk and lack of satisfaction and wellbeing.

Using a conceptual model of relevant features of the community, a baseline assessment should be made both before and after an important social and economic event such as the closure of a major firm, with consequent mass unemployment, or the initiation of intervention programmes.

This baseline assessment should concentrate on:
- demographic aspects including migration
- social aspects including changing structure of families and social classes, and social security,
- labour aspects, including factors of work absenteeism,
- psychosocial aspects including life styles and reactions to stress,

- economic aspects including changes in production and consumption patterns, costs of intervention and/or change,
- health aspects in terms of consultations and other utilization indicators and in terms of "subjective" and "objective" indicators of health.

For such investigations a control group study design is needed. This study could be prospective or, in the interest of research economy and of reflecting the current situation, noncurrent prospective/retrospective. It should be mentioned that for implementing the latter design specific instruments for retrospective data collection have to be developed and tested. Community studies should not be a monolithic undertaking; sometimes the need will arise to study specific hypotheses by using subsamples of the population. Sometimes — depending on the sociopolitical context of the study - local authorities will have to be more intensively involved than usual. Sometimes the study would benefit by action research, by involving the affected people.

5.4 <u>Studies on social groups</u>

The major advantage of studies concentrating on the effects of socioeconomic conditions on the health status is their specificity and concreteness. The first step is identification of relevant groups to be studied in depth, e.g.
- age groups;
- groups with specific risk;
- groups living in specific social environments;
- groups with high self-scoring with regard to social problems;
- groups with a certain similarity of characteristics such as symptoms, risk factors, school leaving;
- highly educated groups without specific tasks demanded in the labour market;
- the self-employed;
- groups which need special attention to reduce the negative consequences of instability and/or unemployment;
- groups which are more easily harmed by instability and/or unemployment;
- groups under heavy stress at work and/or home.

The identification of the groups to be studied could depart from a simple cross-tabulation of social and/or demographic variables with data on or estimations of, the pattern of diseases, risk or wellbeing. This cross-tabulation should be complemented by other methods of empirical research, as e.g. group discussions with social workers using Delphi panels.

The study design to be chosen in this area of research will most probably be the cohort study design with control groups. The study may be prospective and/or retrospective concentrating on the life history of members of the group. Another possibility which has to be discussed in much more detail is to try to add relevant socioeconomic data to ongoing cohort studies.

5.5 Studies at the micro-level

There is no clear-cut boundary between studies on groups and micro-studies. Micro-studies focus on the individual and endeavour to approach cause-effect relationships very closely. Typical questions for micro-studies include:
- To what extent is the time lag between social event and ill-health related to differences between individuals and how are the links between social event and ill-health to be taken into account on the psychosocial, psychological and physiological level?
- How intensive is the relationship between dissatisfaction and illness?
- What are the particular stresses of unemployment for different individuals?
- To what extent does reduction of risk factors decrease ill-health?

Numerous other questions to be studied at this level of analysis have already been mentioned in this report.

The cohort study design seems most suitable. But due to various institutional and political settings in the different research areas a universally applicable study design cannot be proposed. To be sure, case studies at the "hypermicro-level" should be designed carefully, making extensive use of biographical methods for the preparation of meaningful prospective experimental designs.

5.6 Linkages between levels of analysis

At present there seems to be a sharp methodological gap between study designs at the macro- and micro-levels; there also seems to be a wide acceptance of a research philosophy favouring an individualistic research approach oriented towards duplicating the research philosophy of the natural sciences. There should, therefore, be methodological guidelines on how to link studies on the level of society and studies on the level of the individual.

6. The next step in the study

6.1 Ongoing studies and options

The participants gave an outline of some ongoing or definitely planned studies which are endeavouring to shed light on some aspects which, in the framework of macro-models, remain concealed in that large, unknown black box that lies between socioeconomic development and health or mortality.
- One study aims at tracing the chain of events between physical stresses, psychosocial stresses, behavioural reactions and risk of disease.
- Another analyses social, psychological and physiological aspects of the unemployed vis à vis a control group.
- A third interprets the relationship between business cycles and mortality in terms of stress and overwork.
- A fourth attempts to identify dissatisfaction as a risk factor of disease.
- A fifth seeks to identify the psychological and social wellbeing of unemployed as compared to employed people.
- A sixth investigates the organizational conditions for increasing the effectiveness of health care services.
- A seventh includes in a microcensus among others, questions on wellbeing, health conditions and different types of unemployment.
- An eighth has detected a positive correlation of only 0.3 between life change and illness, and
- the last study has encountered difficulties in obtaining information on mortality and economic conditions, analogous to that used for the USA by Professor Brenner.

All studies show that the blackbox between mortality and health and economic conditions must be opened, in order to strengthen the effectiveness, advocacy and bargaining power of services, authorities and people endeavouring to improve the health for all.

Participants expressed interest in carrying out one or the other aspect of the following research, or assisting in its planning:
- replication and improvement of the Brenner model;
- test of the predictive power of this model;
- disaggregation of the model into regional and/or sectoral levels within countries, taking into account several intervening variables;
- supplementary studies related to ongoing epidemiological cohort studies, especially in the fields of mental health and of cardiovascular diseases;
- studies on the wellbeing of selected social groups, e.g. the elderly and unemployed;
- comparative studies following up the "fit" unemployed and those certified as "disabled", and their families;
- studies on the relationship between stress and cardiovascular diseases for individuals of different social and emotional make-up.

It should be pointed out that many potential contributors to the Study on the Influence of Economic Development on Health were not present at this Meeting. Efforts should be made to ensure participation by other research institutes and by sponsors in this area of research.

6.2 Research coordination

The WHO Regional Office for Europe should act as an intermediary between research groups. The role of EURO would be especially welcomed with regard to the following aspects:
- collection of research protocols from individual research groups;
- assurance of confidential review of the quality of research proposals, perhaps by means of contacting relevant institutions;
- circulation of reviewed research proposals and draft papers to participants and other relevant researchers;
- support in terms of bibliographic surveys and reading lists;
- establishment of contacts between relevant research institutions;
- assurance of a certain degree of comparability of (collaborative) studies;
- reinforcement for national authorities to be interested in studies

based on a survey of what relevant social groups exist in the countries to be studied;
- demonstration of vital interest in this area by financing coordination meetings.

It was agreed that the Regional Office could implement this role best by helping to coordinate the Study through a few key institutes able and willing to provide central facilities for information processing, methodology and reporting, and should endeavour to secure the collaboration of OECD (which has already provided economic data for the macro-level study), ILO, the Commission of the European Communities and the Council of Europe.

6.3 Follow-up meeting

The Institute for Medical Informatics and Health Services Research of the GSF Research Centre (MEDIS) of the Federal Republic of Germany offered to hold a follow-up meeting in Munich from 9 to 11 September 1981, in order to help WHO and national experts to continue the discussion on research in the area. A detailed call for papers would be sent to all the participants of this Planning Meeting and additional experts.

The participants of the Meeting welcomed this announcement and expressed their hope that other institutes would follow this initiative and thus contribute toward better understanding of the vital links between socio-economic development and health for all.

LIST OF PARTICIPANTS/AUTHORS

Ludwig BAPST, lic.oec.
Interdisciplinary Research Centre for Public Health
Rorschacher Str. 103c
CH-9007 St. Gallen
SWITZERLAND

Keith BARNARD, M.A., D.S.A.
Deputy Director
Nuffield Centre for Health Services Studies
The University of Leeds
71-75 Clarendon Road
Leeds LS2 9PL
UNITED KINGDOM

Dr. Heinrich BAUER
Diabetes-Klinik
D-3118 Bad Bevensen
F.R.G.

Dipl.Psych. Niels BECKMANN
Arbeitsgemeinschaft für Angewandte Psychologie
Am Weiher 17
D-2000 Hamburg 19
F.R.G.

Patrice BERGER
GIS Economie De La Santé
162, avenue Lacassagne
F-69424 Lyon Cedex
FRANCE

Dr. Christopher A. BIRT
Stockport Health Authority
Bramhall Moor Lane, Hazel Grove
Stockport SK7 5AB
UNITED KINGDOM

Prof. M. Harvey BRENNER, Ph.D.
Division of Operations Research
Dept. of Health Services Administration
The Johns Hopkins University
615 North Wolfe Street
Baltimore, Maryland 21205
U.S.A.

Christian BRINKMANN
Institut für Arbeitsmarkt- und Berufsforschung
der Bundesanstalt für Arbeit
Postfach
D-8500 Nürnberg 1
F.R.G.

Ralph A. CATALANO, Ph.D.
Professor, Program in Social Ecology
Associate Director, Public Policy
Public Policy Research Organization
University of California, Irvine
Irvine, California 92717
U.S.A.

Malcolm COLLEDGE*
School of Behavioural Science
Northumberland Annexe
Newcastle Polytechnic
Northumberland Road
Newcastle-upon-Tyne NE1 8ST
UNITED KINGDOM

Charles D. DOOLEY, Ph.D.
Professor, Program in Social Ecology
Public Policy Research Organization
University of California, Irvine
Irvine, California 92717
U.S.A.

Prof. Dr. Wilhelm van EIMEREN
Direktor
Medis-Institut der GSF
Ingolstädter Landstr. 1
D-8042 Neuherberg
Post Oberschleissheim
F.R.G.

Dr. Leonard FAGIN
Consultant Psychiatrist
Claybury Hospital
Woodford Bridge, Woodford Green
Essex IG8 8BY
UNITED KINGDOM

Dieter FRÖHLICH
Institut zur Erforschung sozialer Chancen
(Berufsforschungsinstitut)
Kuenstr. 1 b
D-5000 Köln 60
F.R.G.

Klaus-Dieter HAHN
Arbeitsgemeinschaft für Angewandte Psychologie
Am Weiher 17
D-2000 Hamburg 19
F.R.G.

Dr. Jürgen JOHN
Medis-Institut der GSF
Ingolstädter Landstr. 1
D-8042 Neuherberg
Post Oberschleissheim
F.R.G.

Prof. Dr. Aubrey R. KAGAN
Laboratory for Clinical Stress Research
Fack
S-104 01 Stockholm 60
SWEDEN

Stanislav V. KASL, Ph.D.
Professor of Epidemiology
School of Medicine
Dept. of Epidemiology and Public Health
Yale University
P.O. Box 3333
60 College Street
New Haven, Connecticut 06510
U.S.A.

Michael KINGHAM*
Faculty of Community and Social Studies
Newcastle Polytechnic
Northumberland Building
Northumberland Road
Newcastle upon Tyne NE1 8ST
UNITED KINGDOM

Marten LAGERGREN
Nordic School of Public Health
Medicinargatan
Göteborg
SWEDEN

Dr. Andrés LOPEZ-BLASCO
Instituto Alfonso el Magnanimo
Plaza Alfonso el Magnanimo 1
Valencia 3
SPAIN

Klaus PREISER*
Wellinghoferstr. 77
D-4600 Dortmund 30
F.R.G.

Dr. Heikki SALOVAARA
Järnvägsgatan 41
S-29300 Olofström
SWEDEN

Priv.-Doz. Dr. Detlef SCHWEFEL
Medis-Institut der GSF
Ingolstädter Landstr. 1
D-8042 Neuherberg
Post Oberschleissheim
F.R.G.

Jes SØGAARD, cand.rer.soc., research associate
Institut for samfundsmedicin
Odense University
J.B. Winsløwsvej 17
DK-5000 Odense C
DENMARK

drs. Inge P. SPRUIT
Rijksuniversiteit te Leiden
Instituut voor Sociale Geneeskunde
Wassenaarseweg 62
Postbus 9605
NL-2300 RC Leiden
NETHERLANDS

Dr. med. Klaus-Dieter THOMANN
Praunheimer Weg 84
D-6000 Frankfurt/M. 50
F.R.G.

drs. H. VERKLEY
Rijksuniversiteit te Leiden
Instituut voor Sociale Geneeskunde
Wassenaarseweg
Postbus 9605
NL-2300 RC Leiden
NETHERLANDS

Dr. Stephen J. WATKINS
Senior Registrar in Community Medicine
South Manchester Health Authority
Mauldeth House, Mauldeth Road West
Manchester M21 2RL
UNITED KINGDOM

Gill WESTCOTT
Nuffield Centre for Health Services Studies
The University of Leeds
71-75 Clarendon Road
Leeds LS2 9PL
UNITED KINGDOM

Dr. Jay M. WINTER
University Lecturer in History
and Fellow of Pembroke College
Pembroke College
Cambridge CB2 1RF
UNITED KINGDOM

Dr. Włodzimierz Cezary WŁODARCZYK
Institute of Occupational Medicine
8, Teresy Street
P.O. Box 199
90-950 Lodz
POLAND

Dr. Herbert ZÖLLNER
Regional Office for Europe
World Health Organization
8, Sherfigsvej
DK-2100 Copenhagen
DENMARK

---

*M. Colledge, M. Kingham and K. Preiser
were not able to participate in the Symposium
but submitted papers.

ACKNOWLEDGEMENTS

Our thanks are due to the below mentioned publishers and journals for their permission to reprint the following papers:

1. BECKMANN, N., HAHN, K.-D.: Unemployment and life-style changes. Revised German version in: *Mitteilungen aus der Arbeitsmarkt- und Berufsforschung*, 15, 1, pp. 69-77 (1982). Kohlhammer Verlag

2. CATALANO, R., DOOLEY, D.: The health effects of economic instability: A test of the economic stress hypothesis. *Journal of Health and Social Behavior* (in Press)

3. COLLEDGE, M., KINGHAM, M.: Involuntary unemployment and health status: A regional case study utilising sociological and micro-epidemiological perspectives. Extended version published in *Medicine in Society*, Vol. 8, No. 2 (1982)

4. KASL, S.V.: Strategies of research on economic instability and health. *Psychological Medicine*, Vol. 12, No. 3 (1982). Cambridge: Cambridge University Press

5. WINTER, J.M.: Unemployment, nutrition and infant mortality in Britain, 1920-1950. In: J.M. Winter (Ed.): The working class in modern British history (forthcoming). Cambridge: Cambridge University Press